A Companion to Life Course Studies

Since the end of the Second World War, society has been characterised by rapid and extensive political, economic, scientific and technological change. Opportunities for education, employment, human relations and good health have all been greatly affected by those changes, as have all aspects of life. Consequently, each post-war generation has been like no other before or since.

Britain, uniquely, has five large-scale life course studies that began at intervals throughout that period. They have shown how lives are shaped by individual characteristics, their past and current experiences and opportunities, and so reflect their times. This book describes those fundamental changes that affected life chances differently in each generation, and how governments struggled to accommodate the changes with new policies for improving and managing the nation's capital in terms of education, family policy, health, human rights and economics.

A Companion to Life Course Studies provides a resource for the interpretation of the findings and design differences in the five studies, and the stimulus for new comparisons of the life course between these differing generations that would contribute to policy and to understanding.

Michael Wadsworth directed the first birth cohort study until 2006, reconfiguring it as a study of physical and mental change with age, adding a study of the following generation, and the collection of DNA, and writing a history of its findings during the first thirty-six years in their historical and social context in *The Imprint of Time*.

John Bynner directed the Centre for Longitudinal Studies and the 1958 and 1970 cohort studies within a comparative life course study framework until 2003. He also directed the Wider Benefits of Learning Research Centre and the National Research and Development Centre for Adult Literacy and Numeracy.

Routledge Advances in Sociology

1. Virtual Globalization
Virtual spaces/tourist spaces
Edited by David Holmes

2. The Criminal Spectre in Law, Literature and Aesthetics
Peter Hutchings

3. Immigrants and National Identity in Europe
Anna Triandafyllidou

4. Constructing Risk and Safety in Technological Practice
Edited by Jane Summerton and Boel Berner

5. Europeanisation, National Identities and Migration
Changes in boundary constructions between Western and Eastern Europe
Willfried Spohn and Anna Triandafyllidou

6. Language, Identity and Conflict
A comparative study of language in ethnic conflict in Europe and Eurasia
Diarmait Mac Giolla Chríost

7. Immigrant Life in the U.S.
Multi-disciplinary perspectives
Edited by Donna R. Gabaccia and Colin Wayne Leach

8. Rave Culture and Religion
Edited by Graham St. John

9. Creation and Returns of Social Capital
A new research program
Edited by Henk Flap and Beate Völker

10. Self-Care
Embodiment, personal autonomy and the shaping of health consciousness
Christopher Ziguras

11. Mechanisms of Cooperation
Werner Raub and Jeroen Weesie

12. After the Bell
Educational success, public policy and family background
Edited by Dalton Conley and Karen Albright

13. Youth Crime and Youth Culture in the Inner City
Bill Sanders

14. Emotions and Social Movements
Edited by Helena Flam and Debra King

15. Globalization, Uncertainty and Youth in Society
Edited by Hans-Peter Blossfeld, Erik Klijzing, Melinda Mills and Karin Kurz

16. Love, Heterosexuality and Society
Paul Johnson

17. Agricultural Governance
Globalization and the new politics of regulation
Edited by Vaughan Higgins and Geoffrey Lawrence

18. Challenging Hegemonic Masculinity
Richard Howson

19. Social Isolation in Modern Society
Roelof Hortulanus, Anja Machielse and Ludwien Meeuwesen

20. Weber and the Persistence of Religion
Social theory, capitalism and the sublime
Joseph W. H. Lough

21. Globalization, Uncertainty and Late Careers in Society
Edited by Hans-Peter Blossfeld, Sandra Buchholz and Dirk Hofäcker

22. Bourdieu's Politics
Problems and possibilities
Jeremy F. Lane

23. Media Bias in Reporting Social Research?
The case of reviewing ethnic inequalities in education
Martyn Hammersley

24. A General Theory of Emotions and Social Life
Warren D. TenHouten

25. Sociology, Religion and Grace
Arpad Szakolczai

26. Youth Cultures
Scenes, subcultures and tribes
Edited by Paul Hodkinson and Wolfgang Deicke

27. The Obituary as Collective Memory
Bridget Fowler

28. Tocqueville's Virus
Utopia and dystopia in Western social and political thought
Mark Featherstone

29. Jewish Eating and Identity Through the Ages
David Kraemer

30. The Institutionalization of Social Welfare
A study of medicalizing management
Mikael Holmqvist

31. The Role of Religion in Modern Societies
Edited by Detlef Pollack and Daniel V. A. Olson

32. Sex Research and Sex Therapy
A sociological analysis of Masters and Johnson
Ross Morrow

33. A Crisis of Waste?
Understanding the rubbish society
Martin O'Brien

34. Globalization and Transformations of Local Socioeconomic Practices
Edited by Ulrike Schuerkens

35. The Culture of Welfare Markets
The international recasting of pension and care systems
Ingo Bode

36. Cohabitation, Family and Society
Tiziana Nazio

37. Latin America and Contemporary Modernity
A sociological interpretation
José Maurízio Domingues

38. Exploring the Networked Worlds of Popular Music
Milieu cultures
Peter Webb

39. The Cultural Significance of the Child Star
Jane O'Connor

40. European Integration as an Elite Process
The failure of a dream?
Max Haller

41. Queer Political Performance and Protest
Benjamin Shepard

42. Cosmopolitan Spaces
Europe, globalization, theory
Chris Rumford

43. Contexts of Social Capital
Social networks in communities, markets and organizations
Edited by Ray-May Hsung, Nan Lin, and Ronald Breiger

44. Feminism, Domesticity and Popular Culture
Edited by Stacy Gillis and Joanne Hollows

45. Changing Relationships
Edited by Malcolm Brynin and John Ermisch

46. Formal and Informal Work
The hidden work regime in Europe
Edited by Birgit Pfau-Effinger, Lluis Flaquer, and Per H. Jensen

47. Interpreting Human Rights
Social science perspectives
Edited by Rhiannon Morgan and Bryan S. Turner

48. Club Cultures
Boundaries, identities and otherness
Silvia Rief

49. Eastern European Immigrant Families
Mihaela Robila

50. People and Societies
Rom Harré and designing the social sciences
Luk van Langenhove

51. Social Theory in Contemporary Asia
Ann Brooks

52. Foundations of Critical Media and Information Studies
Christian Fuchs

53. A Companion to Life Course Studies
The social and historical context of the British birth cohort studies
Edited by Michael Wadsworth and John Bynner

A Companion to Life Course Studies

The social and historical context of the British birth cohort studies

Edited by Michael Wadsworth and John Bynner

Routledge
Taylor & Francis Group
LONDON AND NEW YORK

First published 2011
by Routledge
2 Park Square, Milton Park, Abingdon, Oxon, OX14 4RN

Simultaneously published in the USA and Canada
by Routledge
711 Third Avenue, New York, NY 10017

Routledge is an imprint of the Taylor & Francis Group, an informa business

British Library Cataloguing in Publication Data
A catalogue record for this book is available from the British Library

Library of Congress Cataloging in Publication Data
A companion to life course studies: the social and historical context of the British birth cohort studies / edited by Michael Wadsworth and John Bynner.
p. cm.
1. Cohort analysis. 2. Social capital (Sociology)–Great Britain–Case studies. 3. Families–Great Britain. 4. Great Britain–Economic policy. 5. Great Britain–Social policy. 6. Social change. I. Wadsworth, Michael E. J. (Michael Edwin John) II. Bynner, J. M.
HB849.47.C66 2011
304.6 1–dc22
2010039200

ISBN13: 978–0–415–49540–0 (hbk)
ISBN13: 978–0–203–87858–3 (ebk)

Typeset in Times New Roman by Prepress Projects Ltd, UK
Printed and bound in Great Britain by CPI Antony Rowe, Chippenham, Wiltshire

Contents

Figures

Tables

Contributors

David Ashton is Emeritus Professor at the University of Leicester and Honorary Professor at the University of Cardiff. He founded the Centre for Labour Market Studies at the University of Leicester in 1990. He has published extensively in the areas of labour market analysis, comparative vocational education and training systems, training, skills and high performance working.

John Bynner is Emeritus Professor of Social Sciences in Education at the Institute of Education and editor of the *International Journal for Longitudinal and Life Course Studies*. He directed the Bedford Group for Life Course and Statistical Studies, the Centre for Longitudinal Studies, the Wider Benefits of Learning Research Centre and the National Research and Development Centre for Adult Literacy and Numeracy. His publications include *Tracking Adult Literacy and Numeracy Skills* (2009) (co-edited with Steve Reder).

Lynda Clarke is Head of the Department of Population Studies at the London School of Hygiene and Tropical Medicine. Previously she undertook social research at the Thomas Coram Research Institute and the Office for National Statistics, and was Director of Family Demography at the Family Policy Studies Centre. Current work includes collaboration in international studies of fathers in South Africa, and the impact of imprisonment on men and their families in the United States and Britain.

Gary McCulloch is Brian Simon Professor of History of Education at the Institute of Education, University of London. He is a former president of the History of Education Society (UK) and a former editor of the journal *History of Education*. His recent publications include *The Struggle for the History of Education* (2011) and *Cyril Norwood and the Ideal of Secondary Education* (2007).

Lindsay Paterson is Professor of Educational Policy at Edinburgh University. His current research interests are in the twentieth-century history of Scottish education, social mobility and the relationship between education and civic values.

Hugh Pemberton is Senior Lecturer in Modern British History at the University of Bristol. His research focuses on British economic and social policy since 1945. He is the author of *Policy Learning and British Governance in the 1960s* (2004), co-editor (with Lawrence Black) of *An Affluent Society? Britain's*

'Golden Age' Revisited (2004) and co-editor (with Pat Thane and Noel Whiteside) of *Britain's Pensions Crisis: History and Policy* (2006).

Ceridwen Roberts is a Senior Research Fellow in the Department of Social Policy and Social Work at the University of Oxford. Formerly Director of the Family Policy Studies Centre she also held research and research management posts in the UK Government Department of Employment and in academia as an industrial sociologist, and she was the UK expert on the European Commission's Observatory on the Social Situation, Demography and Family.

Ken Roberts is Professor of Sociology at the University of Liverpool, and a founder member of the Executive Committee of the Leisure Studies Association. His first book on leisure was *Leisure* (1970), and his most recent is *Leisure in Contemporary Society* (2006, 2nd edition). He has been President of the International Sociological Association Research Committee on Leisure, Chair of the World Leisure Organization's Research Commission, and Senior Fellow of the American Leisure Academy and the World Leisure Academy.

Michael Wadsworth is Emeritus Professor in the Department of Epidemiology and Public Health at University College London Medical School and Honorary Senior Scientist at the MRC Unit for Life Long Health and Ageing. He directed the first British national birth cohort study for more than twenty years. His publications include *The Imprint of Time: Childhood, History and Adult Life* (1991) and *Changing Britain, Changing Lives* (2003) (co-edited with Elsa Ferri and John Bynner).

Preface

The idea for this collection came from our experience of working on the British birth cohort studies over many years. These five large-scale longitudinal surveys continue to make unique contributions to the social, behavioural and health sciences, and to understanding how the changing social and economic context impacts on the aspirations, opportunities, education, income, lifestyles and health of the populations they study. The first of these studies began in 1946, less than a year after the end of the Second World War, and the most recent began fifty-four years later in 2000, and so they cover a period of extensive and rapid change in British society. The historical context of these studies has, however, received relatively little attention in the interpretation of their findings. We believe that it has become increasingly apparent, as the years of data collection accumulate, and as comparisons between the studies became ever more relevant, that an historical perspective is needed.

In an earlier collection co-edited with Elsa Ferri in 2003 (*Changing Britain, Changing Lives: Three Generations at the Turn of the Century*) we showed the range of information and the span of the life course covered by the three longest-running British birth cohort studies, and gave examples of the value of comparing findings from them. In this present collection our purpose is to show the extent of change in British society since it affected all five studies during the sixty-five years since the first study began. That extensive change required each of the five studies to be responsive to the rapidly developing research and policy questions that dominate the period, and to the new methods of measurement and data collection that developed during that time in the social, behavioural and health sciences.

The chapters in this volume have been written to illustrate the extent and pace of change in the socio-political and economic context in Britain. They describe and interpret changing policies and their implementation, as governments endeavoured over the period to increase equality of opportunity and access to health and welfare services and to define and implement human rights whilst accommodating to the pressures from national and global economic change and scientific and technological innovations.

This book is intended to be of value to readers of research from the birth cohort studies, to those planning new work using these resources, and to readers with a general interest in the history of the period. We hope that the book will be a valuable source of reference, and will stimulate new cross-cohort comparisons that will show how the changing social and economic context of life and of opportunity impacted on the life course of each cohort and contributed to the differences between the generations that the cohorts represent.

We were encouraged to assemble this collection not only by our experience with the cohort studies, but also by colleagues with whom we developed the independent think tank Longview (http://www.longviewuk.com) and its associated online journal (*Longitudinal and Life Course Studies* – http://www.journal.longviewuk.com – which is now the journal of the *Society for Longitudinal and Life Course Studies).* Longview contributed materially by funding an initial meeting of authors.

We are grateful in particular to our colleagues who contributed to this collection by writing chapters, as well as to colleagues at Longview and elsewhere for their critical comments and encouragement.

Michael Wadsworth and John Bynner

1 Introduction

Michael Wadsworth and John Bynner

Introduction

The sixty-five years from the end of the Second World War until 2010 was a period of extensive and continuous change in Britain. It began in a time of national austerity, poor standards of living, food rationing and costly health care, which was much less effective than today. Opportunities were limited for educational attainment and social mobility. The workforce was largely male and the majority was employed in manual work, living in rented accommodation and in families with mostly one earner and two married parents. Historical documentation of the changing times may be seen in *The Audit of War* (Barnett 1986) and *Austerity Britain 1945–1951* (Kynaston 2007). Subsequently radical changes occurred in Beckevery aspect of British life including the nation's demography, as discussed in *Twentieth-Century British Social Trends* (Halsey and Webb 2000), and the health and welfare services, described in *Empire, Welfare State, Europe* (Lloyd 1994). The development of modern institutions and their relation to contemporary identity formation are the subject of *Modernity and Self Identity* (Giddens 1991). Halpern (2005) describes changing social networks and ties in his *Social Capital.*

Even during the war the coalition government had been greatly concerned with the question of how to bring change that would effectively be investment in the nation's human capital. The Beveridge Report published in 1942 expressed the challenge in terms of the pressing need to deal with the five giant evils of physical want, disease, ignorance, squalor and idleness, or in today's less biblical terms poverty, ill health, poor educational opportunity, substandard housing and unemployment. All of these topics were addressed by the 1945 post-war Labour government's extensive welfare state programme. That programme, together with the new developments in science and technology that set the pace as key drivers of the economy in the post-war world, brought a great swathe of change in, for example:

- the nature of work and skill acquisition in response to de-industrialisation and to computing technology, which made new demands on education from the earliest ages;

- the growth of the economy, adjustment to globalisation, and de-regulation as well as change in international affiliations from the Commonwealth to the European Union, and increasing competition from Asia;
- growing affluence for ever larger numbers of people during the 1950s and 1960s accompanied by a widening gap between rich and poor, and social exclusion concentrated in disadvantaged neighbourhoods and communities;
- increasingly effective health care, reliable control of fertility and improvements in the standards of living, which brought radical change in the age structure of the population and reduction in infant mortality, and changed the timing of parenthood and the nature of family life;
- the nature of communications through the development of television, the internet, and wireless and telephone systems, changing the nature of entertainment and giving unprecedented access to information;
- the expansion of public and personal means of travel, widening outlooks and expectations, the possibilities for migration, the risk of infectious disease transmission, and the range of food available.

By contrast there was greater stability in cultural and political orientations and interests. Although there were fluctuations, the core democratic values and norms remained largely impervious to the pressures of a changing world, and political extremism on continental lines consistently failed to take root.

Over the same post-war period British governments have had to manage the effects of these changes in terms of the consequent demands and expectations for greater equality of opportunity, income, wealth, education and health, for freedom of expression, and for reconsideration of the rights and responsibilities of governments, employers and citizens. Governments of every political persuasion were interventionist, and each was concerned about the continuing development and maintenance of human capital.

For individuals these political, scientific and technological changes profoundly affected ways of life in work, leisure and health expectations, and in perceptions of self, the family, community and society, and increased differences between the generations in family and working life, health and lifestyles. The structure of the life course was also transformed through the prolongation of the time spent in education, the postponement of marriage and partnership, and increasing longevity past retirement. Such fundamental changes promoted the development of ideas about the individual as a free and autonomous agent, no longer necessarily confined, as in the past, by class, gender, family and community, nor by traditional concerns for deference (Giddens 1991). The price to be paid was the growing complexity of the choices to be made in all domains of life and the increased prevalence of globalised risk (Beck *et al.* 1994) to which Anthony Giddens devoted his 1999 Reith lecture series 'Runaway World'. This aspect of change was driven by the twin pressures of technological transformation and globalisation, and the ever-rising demand for qualifications. The raising of educational levels and of opportunities for a wider perspective through travel and the internet brought new questions about the basis of contemporary identity and human rights and responsibilities.

This book is concerned with the nature of social and economic changes in the post-war period in Britain, and how they have been experienced in the lives of the population. This is encompassed by the data collected from respondents in the British birth cohort studies, which supply the means of investigating their effects. An introduction to the birth cohort studies follows with their main features summarised. We then turn to the aims of the book, which deal with the nature of national change over the years since the end of the Second World War. Chapter outlines follow in the key areas of politics and citizenship, family structure and policy, educational policy, economic policy, labour market, employment and skills, health and health care and the changing pattern of leisure.

Measuring social change

Britain has a long tradition of measuring societal change as an essential means of showing its course and extent, interpreting its causes, arguing the need for policy change and making decisions about how to accommodate and adapt to it. Starting in 1801 and taking its modern form in 1841 when details of all household members were recorded, the census has provided data about the current state of the nation. Governments have used registration data to produce population vital statistics on births, deaths, marriage and health, and have used the census and other forms of inquiry to collect what is now an extensive range of information on housing, the economy, industry and the workforce. In addition, governments have undertaken inquiries involving research and the collection of expert views on complex topics on which to base policy initiatives that affect the whole nation. For example, the Central Advisory Council for Education established by the 1944 Education Act undertook a series of enquiries including the Crowther Report (1959) on secondary education, the Newsom Report (1963) on those who left school at the earliest opportunity, the Robbins Report (1963) on higher education and the Plowden Report (1967) on primary education. These follow in the tradition of earlier major enquires such as those commissioned by the influential Inter Departmental Committee on Physical Deterioration (1904), and Royal Commissions on Children's Employment (1840), the Poor Laws and Relief of Distress (1909), the Distribution of the Industrial Population (1940), the Taxation of Incomes and Profits (1952), the Distribution of Wealth and Income (1979) and the Long-Term Care for the Elderly (1999).

There is an equally long British tradition of data collection by individuals and non-governmental groups concerned with measuring living conditions, work opportunities and health. This work has been used to inform political arguments and to provide evidence of the need for change, particularly for improvement in social and economic circumstances and in health. Amongst the most influential of these were the data collections and publications of Booth (1891, first published in 1889) and Rowntree (1901) on poverty and its causes, the Carnegie Trust report

Disinherited Youth (1943, first published in 1939) and, of more recent times, the work of charitable organisations including the Joseph Rowntree Charitable Trust, the Nuffield Foundation, the Leverhulme Trust, the Wolfson Foundation and the Sutton Trust.

During the years between the two World Wars it was clear from the national statistics that fertility had been falling in Britain since the middle of the nineteenth century. Anxieties were expressed about the social implications of that trend (Beveridge 1925; Charles 1934; Carr-Saunders 1936; Glass 1946), and about the slow rate of fall in infant mortality (Titmuss 1943). These reports prompted the setting up in 1944 of the Royal Commission on Population (1949). An academic group, the Population Investigation Committee (PIC), was a considerable source of impetus and support for the Royal Commission. It also raised money from the Nuffield Foundation in 1945, while the Commission was still sitting, to set up a national study that would throw more focused light on the problems of fertility and infant mortality.

The PIC study was designed to show the national distribution and availability of maternity services to different socio-economic groups, the use of those services and their effectiveness in educating mothers and reducing infant and maternal ill health and mortality, the cost to families of childbirth, and the need for domestic help during pregnancy and the early neonatal period. Its findings were of relevance to the planners of the National Health Service that was to start in 1948. The study collected data in 1946 and published its findings in 1947 and 1948 (Joint Committee 1947, 1948). Its principal investigators, James Douglas and David Glass, then decided to follow up a national sample of those births in order to explore their subsequent health, growth and survival in relation to their health and family circumstances and care at birth (Wadsworth 2010).

Although the initial survey was planned as a single study, with the focus on health at the time of birth, this was to become the first of a series of British national lifelong longitudinal birth cohort studies inaugurated during the sixty-five year period reviewed in this book. It was an important development in the national tradition of studies of societal circumstances and poverty and its effects because it introduced the dynamic element of developmental time or change with age into what had previously been a tradition of 'snapshot' cross-sectional studies, as discussed in *The Dynamics of Modern Society* (Leisering and Walker 1998) and *From Transmitted Deprivation to Social Exclusion* (Welshman 2007). By introducing developmental time the first study provided data that was uniquely useful for policy and also for research into the interaction between societal change and individual development and change with age. It made it possible to address questions about, for example, how many and what kind of people escape from the constraints of a childhood spent in poverty.

This method of enquiry, beginning with the birth of its subjects, and continuing the study of them throughout life, has been used in five large-scale studies (four of them national) that began at intervals during the sixty-five years since the end of the Second World War and the beginning of the welfare state. Because of their concern with questions appropriate for policy, as well as research into development and change with age, the five studies map onto the history of many of the major policy questions and the progress of the study of individual development and health during the post-war period.

The national birth cohort studies

The first national birth cohort study began in 1946 and this was followed by four others; as Table 1.1 shows they cover the post-war years.

The design of each study and the nature of the measures and instruments used in the data collections have been responsive to the changing nature of the research and policy questions throughout the period. Although initially limited by the available information technology, it became possible for the studies to increase sample size. Sample design also had to respond to the population's changing socio-economic and ethnic mix, and the demand for more detailed developmental, psychological and health measures. Scientific and methodological development and innovation required the use of the most up-to-date measurement methods and instrumentation, which had to be accommodated while maintaining continuity with the earlier data collections and the earlier studies.

The first study initially collected data about all the births in a single week (16,695) and then selected for follow-up a sample (5,362) from those studied, which was stratified to ensure sufficient representation from the smallest social group (at that time those in non-manual employment), and which covered England, Wales and Scotland.

The next two studies, starting in 1958 and 1970, increased sample sizes (17,634 and 17,287 respectively) and included all the births in a single week; although Northern Ireland was included in the birth survey in 1970 the babies were not followed up.

The fourth study concentrated its sample into one geographic area in order to improve the chances of getting more detailed information about local services as well as the cohort members, and for ease of access to educational and medical records. All births from a period of twenty-one months in 1991/2 were selected to construct a sample for the study of sufficient size (14,541) to address questions about sub-groups and to study interactions with key outcomes and gene–environment interaction.

The fifth birth cohort study beginning in 2000 returned to a UK-wide sample in order to achieve national representativeness and a large sample (18,818), and used a 'clustered' sample design based on all births in 400 electoral wards. To ensure sufficient representation of sub-population groups of special policy interests there was also 'oversampling' of wards with high levels of census-recorded levels of deprivation and black and ethnic minority status residents. This time births in Northern Ireland were included in follow-up data collections, and samples from there and from Wales and Scotland were doubled to strengthen the scope for country-based analysis.

Each of the five studies has received government and research council support and all have been used extensively for both policy and scientific purposes. The

Table 1.1 Periods and ages of data collection up to 2011 in the five British large-scale birth cohort studies[a] (see Appendix 1 for more details of the studies)

Age at data collection	*1946 cohort (n = 5,362)*	*1958 cohort (n = 17,634)*	*1970 cohort (n = 17,287)*	*1991–2 cohort (n = 14,541)*	*2000–1 cohort (n = 18,818)*
Birth to 5 years	1946–51	1958–63	1970–5	1991/2–1996/7	2000/1–2005/6
6–16 years	1952–62	1964–74	1976–86	1997/8–2007/8	2006/7–2016/17
Early adulthood, 17–30 years	1963–76	1975–88	1987–2000	2008/9–2021/2	2017/18–2030/1
Middle adulthood, 31–50 years	1977–96	1989–2008	2001–20	2022/3–2041/2	2031/2–2050/1
Later middle adulthood, 51–64 years	1997–2010	2009–22	2021–34	2042/3–2055/6	2051/2–2064/5
Later life, 65+ years	2011–	2023–	2035–	2056/7	2065/6–

Notes

n sample size at the beginning of the study.

a 1946 cohort – MRC National Survey of Health and Development (NSHD); 1958 cohort – The National Child Development Study (NCDS); 1970 cohort – British Birth Cohort 1970 (BCS70); 1991–2 – Avon Longitudinal Study of Parents and Children (ALSPAC); 2000–1 – The Millennium Cohort Study.

early studies especially have been major sources of evidence for government and independent inquiries. The brief summaries given below outline the range of data collected and give key references. More detailed information about each study is given in Appendix 1, where the studies' websites are also listed.

The Medical Research Council (MRC) National Survey of Health and Development (the 1946 national birth cohort)

The 1946 study, established by James Douglas, began two years before the inauguration of the National Health Service as an investigation of maternity and infant health and care in pregnancy and at the time of birth, and the cost to families of the pregnancy and birth, as reported in *Maternity in Great Britain* (Joint Committee 1948). Data collections during infancy were concerned with the factors influencing health and growth, and findings from this stage are the subject of the study's second book *Children under Five* (Douglas and Blomfield 1958). In the school years the health measures were continued and measures of cognitive development were added, together with information from teachers and schools, in order to study the child's educational attainment and behaviour in relation to ability and home and parental characteristics. Findings were reported in two influential books, *The Home and the School* (Douglas 1964) and *All our Future* (Douglas *et al.* 1968). Data collections in early adulthood were concerned with employment, earnings and family formation in relation to characteristics and experiences of education and the circumstances of the family of origin, and also with reports of ill health. The findings of research during this period are described in *The Imprint of Time* (Wadsworth 1991); the *Roots of Delinquency* (Wadsworth 1979) deals with one aspect. From age thirty-six years the main concern has been to measure change with age of physical and mental health and function and to collect data on health-related habits, and a source of DNA. Collection of information about occupation, family and partnership, and social engagement has continued. The aim is to study lifetime influences on the processes and indicators of ageing, as described in *A Life Course Approach to Women's Health* (Kuh and Hardy 2002) and *A Life Course Approach to Chronic Disease Epidemiology* (Kuh and Ben Shlomo 2004). The study is increasingly used as a research resource.

The National Child Development Study (the 1958 national birth cohort)

Under the leadership of Neville Butler the second study collected information at birth on health and survival in very early life to provide data on the performance of the maternity services during the first ten years of the National Health Service. Comparable data protocols enabled comparison with findings from the 1946 study as well as supporting study of the reasons for poor birth outcomes and their persisting socio-economic gradient. *Perinatal Mortality* (Butler and Bonham 1963) and *Perinatal Problems* (Butler and Alberman 1969) report the findings. Mia Kellmer-Pringle was responsible for establishing the longitudinal nature of the study during the school years when cognitive and physical development were measured, and research was undertaken on health and development and on the impact of change in national educational policy, as reported in *From Birth to Seven* (Davie *et al.* 1972), *Children in Adversity* (Wedge and Essen 1982) and *Continuities in Childhood Disadvantage* (Essen and Wedge 1982). Reports of the later childhood surveys include *Growing up in Great Britain* (Fogelman 1983) and *Health and Class* (Power *et al.* 1991). Through the teenage years up to the age twenty-three survey, data collection was focused on educational achievement, vocational education and training, employment, family formation and parenting, health and lifestyle. Adulthood data collections have been concerned to cover within an overarching life course perspective stability and change in all the main domains of adult life – family, occupation, lifelong learning, health, income, intergenerational social mobility, family building and breakdown, temperament and behaviour, literacy and numeracy, and social and political attitudes and engagement. Major books reporting the findings are *Life at 33* (Ferri 1993) and *Risk and Resilience* (Schoon 2006). The dataset has been available since 1985 as a research resource for general scientific and policy use and includes a sub-sample survey on adult basic skills conducted in 1997 and a full biomedical screen of the cohort in 2004, including the collection of DNA.

The 1970 British National Birth Cohort Study

The third birth cohort study under the initial leadership of Neville Butler was intended from the outset to be a longitudinal study. Information was collected about pregnancy and birth shortly after the birth of the cohort members in order to study the relationship of the mother's social and biological characteristics with the child's neonatal care, health and survival, and compare findings with those from the earlier studies, as reported in *British Births 1970* (Chamberlain *et al.* 1975) and *British Births: Obstetric Care* (Chamberlain *et al.* 1978). During the school years information was collected from schools and teachers on school progress, attainment and behaviour and the curriculum experienced, and the children's health and family circumstances. Measurements of growth and biological function were also taken, including blood pressure at ages ten and sixteen years, assessment of personality, temperament and behaviour, cognitive development, diet and developmental indicators. A wide range of publications reported on health, development and educational outcomes including *The Social Life of Britain's Five-Year-Olds* (Osborn *et al.* 1984), *From Birth to Five* (Butler *et al.* 1986) and *The Effects of Early Education* (Osborn and Milbank 1987). Data collections during the adult years were designed within the same life course framework as the 1958 study. A wide range of data has been collected on individual development, partnership and family formation, occupational and earnings history and health, as reported in *Twenty Something in the 90s* (Bynner *et al.* 1997). In 2004 a comprehensive survey, including a literacy and numeracy assessment, was undertaken and described in a number of reports and books including *Illuminating Disadvantage*

(Parsons and Bynner 2002) and *Tracking Adult Literacy and Numeracy Skills* (Reder and Bynner 2009).

The Avon Longitudinal Study of Parents and Children

This study established by Jean Golding is the only one of the five to recruit the sample during pregnancy when information was collected on current health, together with a source of DNA from parents as well as children. As already described, this study also differs from the others in having an area-based sample, which made it possible to undertake detailed clinic-based assessment as well as easily collect local information, for example from general practitioner and hospital records. Information is also collected annually or more frequently on many aspects of health and development, and includes the measurement of growth and change with age of fitness, physical function (e.g. cardiovascular and respiratory function) and bone mineralisation, allergic response and experience of ill health and medication, as well as, in late childhood and the teens, indicators of diet and lifestyle, psychological development, mental health, and attitudes and behaviour. An overview is given by Golding and colleagues (2001) in *The Avon Longitudinal Study of Parents and Children*. Together with the equally detailed information on socio-economic and family environment, these measures have made it possible to study a wide range of outcomes that include, for example, cognitive, behavioural and emotional development, diet, maternal depression, behaviour difficulties, atopic problems, the development of cardiovascular risk and the role of obesity and genetic influences. This study also provides a research resource for many other studies.

The Millennium Cohort Study

This study established by a team led by Heather Joshi is concerned with children's development and health, and asked how the beginnings of social capital and capability were associated with household structures, parenting regimes, neighbourhood characteristics, and parental health and employment in twenty-first-century circumstances. Studies of the first nine months focused initially on the parents and were concerned with inequalities in health and development, and with the increased risk among teenage parents of poorer resources in human relationships and in financial and social capital. Findings are described in *Children of the 21st Century from Birth to 9 Months* (Dex and Joshi 2005). From age two years cognitive and behavioural assessment has been a major feature of data collection. *Children of the 21st Century, the First Five Years* shows the range of research conducted up to wave 3 of the survey when the children had reached age seven years (Hansen *et al.* 2009). Prominent studies include the impact of family circumstances and income on the early stage of the children's lives, parental choice in education and health, and risk factors for later health and well-being. This study was funded as a research resource and is widely used for science and policy purposes.

The strength of the birth cohort design

The great strengths of these *prospective* longitudinal surveys are their lifelong data, their samples' location in particular historical eras and their time-sequenced collection of data, with relatively short intervals between surveys, which reduce problems of recall. These features make it possible to study change in two dimensions at the same time, namely change in individual lives in terms of development and ageing, and in terms of historical time, which charts change in the social and physical environment, including the ever-accelerating course of technological change. Consequently the birth cohort studies have a number of advantages for scientific investigations of the factors that shape the human life course and its outcomes at different stages of life. They show the time ordering of events and experiences, and are therefore ideally placed to study *age effects*, such as processes of development and ageing. Knowing time ordering of sequences offers valuable means for elucidating causes of later outcomes in the physical and social spheres.

There are three further design advantages of the birth cohort study that stem from the location of each sample in its historical period. The first is that it provides the opportunity to study *cohort effects*, that is, the effects of circumstances and experiences that are unique to those born at a specified time. The second advantage is the opportunity to study *period effects*, that is, influences that vary across historical time. The third advantage is that the study samples are unselected for any characteristic except date of birth, and all except one have nationally representative populations.

Consequently, having five birth cohort studies covering a period of extensive social and economic change, the opportunity arises for quasi-experimental comparative studies that can ask, for example, whether the chances of escaping from the effects of a disadvantaged childhood improved. For example, in *Escape from Disadvantage* Pilling (1990) reports the follow-up at age twenty-seven of cohort members assessed at age seven by Essen and Wedge (1982) as having poor prospects in life, who at age thirteen were leading successful lives, finding that sustained teacher and parent aspirations for the children were key factors.

Because of their design the British birth cohort studies uniquely offer some particular kinds of research strengths that can show or confirm, for example:

- who escapes the effects of experience that is mostly adverse or risky in effect, such as poverty in childhood, smoking, long-term involuntary unemployment or prolonged stress, and what constitute the protective factors;
- trajectories of, for example, height growth, developmental indices, mathematical attainment, income, blood pressure and memory, and life histories of employment, family life and health that provide the opportunity to find out what promotes and what hinders favourable change over time;
- lengths of time and age periods of exposure to risk, for instance from prolonged exposure to stress;
- whether there are life course stages of particular vulnerability either to

damage or to acquisition of skills and competencies, and if so to show for how long such effects may impact the life course;
- how risk accumulates, for instance through adverse events, development, growth or experience, and to what extent that precipitates further adversity;
- whether hypothesised adversity, experienced at a vulnerable time in development, has a deleterious effect, and if so for how long during the life course, and how that effect is maintained.

These strengths make the birth cohort studies' data of unique value in addressing questions about processes of development and change with age, and for addressing a wide range of questions in the social and health sciences, including questions about the effects of policy programmes. Cohort comparison extends their scope for analysing social trends and their impact on life course processes, as shown, for example, in Joshi and Paci's (1998) study of sex differences in income, the work of Gregg *et al.* (1999) on family income, Blanden and Gibbens' (2006) study of the persistence of poverty, the study by Richards *et al.* (2009) of childhood mental health and later life chances, the work of Parsons and Bynner (2002) on basic skills and the risk of social exclusion, Schoon's (2006) study of risk and resilience, and Blanden *et al.*'s (2001) study of social mobility. There has also been a comparative study of a range of findings across the three earlier cohorts (Ferri *et al.* 2003). Further design enhancements have included extending data collection to the next generation of cohort members' children in the 1946, 1958 and 1970 studies. Sub-studies involving additional data collection for specialised topics using sub-samples (such as those showing symptoms of respiratory illness) have been an important feature of the 1958 study. Extending comparison to other countries, in the process of launching their own birth cohort studies, is attracting increasing interest, in which relatively new studies such as the Millennium Cohort Study are likely to play a prominent role.

The aim of this book

The aim of this book is to describe the significant aspects of the changing social, economic, policy and scientific and technological contexts during the period since the end of the Second World War. The intention is to inform those who use the findings of the British birth cohort studies for research and policy purposes, and to stimulate those who plan new research using the extensive life course data resource collected by these studies.

For researchers using the birth cohorts' data the book offers many examples of the changing context to stimulate new analysis, including quasi-experiments using data within cohorts and inter-cohort analysis. For example, knowing that members of the 1946 cohort lived their first ten years before the Clean Air Act was passed in 1956, and that later-born cohorts were consequently far less exposed to the health risks from atmospheric pollution from coal burning (associated with risk to growth in early life and to the optimum development of respiratory function), suggests a potentially valuable quasi-experiment. Another quasi-experiment that could compare the life course health of cohorts born at different times is possible in relation to the epidemics of poliomyelitis that occurred in the 1940s and 1950s in Britain before vaccines became widely used. Similarly, inter-cohort comparative studies may utilise the salient social differences over time that include the rise and the changing forms of youth culture, shifts in labour market and economic policy, changes in the education system and its effects in terms of the labour market returns to new qualifications, the increase in opportunities for higher education and the changing gender mix of those in higher education, the periods of raised risk of unemployment, the rise in parental separation and divorce, and the generation differences in social exclusion, community cohesion, social participation and social mobility.

The following chapter synopses show the wide spectrum of change in the context of life that occurred during the lives of the men and women studied in the five British birth cohort studies.

Lindsay Paterson's chapter on politics, citizenship and social capital identifies the post-war period as particularly concerned with social rights and increased educational opportunities. There were increasing demands for individual freedoms, decreasing deference and increased scepticism about structures of power. The perception of bureaucracy as destructive of freedom helped the Conservatives to office, but they brought also requirements for individual responsibility, extensive de-regulation, increased unemployment and de-nationalisation. Labour drew attention to the dangers of unregulated capitalism and to the fact that widespread poverty and gross inequalities were incompatible with shared citizenship. Over the period state power came to matter less as important aspects of sovereignty passed to the European Union, and to global and multinational companies and markets. Market-driven new management styles and performance monitoring added to the diminishing old relationships based on trust. Bastions of the old social order and ethics began to fail in a crisis of cultural values, and there were fears that the democratic community of equal citizens was being replaced by rampant individualism and aggressive ambition. There was a risk of polarisation as the diminishing working class lost its social institutions and declined in social participation. Nevertheless, despite a socially differentiated decline in social engagement, social trust, and trust and respect for the political system, there has been a significant increase in liberalism, for instance in relation to women's rights and in opposition to racism. Increased levels of education are associated with that trend.

Lynda Clarke and Ceridwen Roberts' chapter on family structure and family policy and practice shows the dramatic changes in family life in the post-war period until the present (in terms, for example, of falling fertility, an increasing proportion of births outside marriage, increased dissolution of marriages and the falling likelihood of childhood in a two parent family), and in factors that affect the family such as increasing gender equity, women's employment and recognition of rights of the child. In policy terms it is shown how in the early part of the period the implicit policy for families was mostly non-interventionist and concerned with family financial support. However, under pressure from the need for improved care for growing numbers of lone parent families, from the liberalisation of attitudes to sexual behaviour and from increasing gender equity at home and in the labour market, government policy became explicit, culminating in the Children's Act of 1989. That recognised the essential nature of parental responsibility, the rights of the child and local authorities' duty of care for children and families. Gradually policy evolved to embrace diversity in family arrangements, and recognised, in the Children Act of 2004 and the SureStart project, the long-term value of investment in children's health and welfare. A similar process of policy evolution is beginning to take place with regard to care for the elderly.

Gary McCulloch's chapter on education policy and practice shows a comparable evolution of policy in a changing society. An initial post-war rapid and extensive increase in the size of the school age population, followed by some decline, was a source of pressure that surged through the school system and into further and higher education. Pressure was also increasing to raise standards as the nation moved through the era of mechanisation and rapid technological development towards the knowledge-based economy. Increased government spending on education came to be seen as essential, but was accompanied by the requirement for accountability and measurement of change. At the same time education was also widely regarded as a marker of national progress towards equity of opportunity. Concepts and measures of individual capability were greatly disputed, and schools felt increasingly strong pressures for production of a capable future workforce, and from comparisons with educational achievements in other countries, as well as from those, especially parents, who were concerned with the fundamental changes in behaviour of young people at school and in society. Consequently pressures and demands on schools for initiatives of all kinds increased, new organisation of education and new methods of teaching constantly evolved, and pressure for accountability increased, as did the tendency for centralised management. Nevertheless, it is concluded that throughout the period education was increasingly seen by government as an essential social and economic investment.

The chapter by Hugh Pemberton on economic policy and practice is concerned with the equity of the transformation of the economy in the years since the end of the Second World War in terms of the redistribution of income and wealth, the general increase in consumption and affluence and the growing proportion of the population in employment. As in education, here too the state has played an increasingly interventionist role, and did so from immediately after the war ended and the period of post-war high and stable employment began. The welfare state may be seen both as a cause and as a function of that post-war economic growth, and that and the high employment of the time are argued to have increased public confidence. The notion of the welfare state also contributed to the development of new thinking about human capital. However, the monetarist policy of the 1980s, which included recognition of the importance of developing human capital, came at great social cost in terms of unemployment and a reduction in trust between the government and workers. The earlier reduction of inequality in incomes was reversed, and the burden of individual debt continued to increase. Studies of individuals' happiness showed no correlation with economic growth, but growth was correlated with a fall in trust between individuals. Insecurity was also generated by the decline of manufacturing industry and the rise of the service sector, although that change brought increased opportunity for women's employment and advancement in employment. However, significant pockets of high unemployment and relative poverty remain, despite increased public spending.

David Ashton and John Bynner's chapter on labour market, employment and skills shows the great change over the post-war period in the nature of the British labour market and its response to global change in markets and manufacturing and to scientific and technological development. In the immediate post-war period, characterised by growth and stability, the labour force was largely male, employment rates were high and routes to employment were well-defined. However, response to global market change and technological developments brought extensive restructuring. Manufacturing shrank, de-nationalisation occurred, higher education was expanded in line with the demands of the growing 'knowledge economy', replacements for apprenticeships were developed as skills requirements changed and governments increasingly 'market tested' new methods and developments. For the population the effect was an increase in unemployment, self-employment and job insecurity, and in the public sector in particular autonomy at work was reduced. However, more women were employed and developed careers. Nevertheless, despite government schemes to offer prospective labour market entrants opportunities for skill development, there was anxiety about the proportion of young people not in education, employment or training. Consequently there are substantial differences between the birth cohort studies in employment prospects, requirements for entry to the labour market and aspirations for occupation and preparation for work, as well as for family formation. Despite the extensive changes, the effects of the socio-economic circumstances of the family of origin can still be detected in educational attainment and employment.

Michael Wadsworth's chapter on health and health care shows the impact of vastly improved standards of living, and of extensive developments in science and technology, on increasing chances of survival, the number of years of disability-free life, reliable fertility control and efficacious curative and preventive care of mental and physical health, illness and disability. These improvements over the post-war years brought considerable cohort differences in health and development, while playing an essential role in changing the age structure of the population and postponing age at first birth. Nevertheless much greater risks of ill health, disability and premature death remain for adults and children who live in insecure, stressful and disadvantaged socio-economic circumstances. Current biologically plausible hypotheses about how adverse socio-economic circumstances and prolonged exposure to stress damage health and 'get under the skin' are all concerned with long-term effects across the life course and across generations, and increasingly include genetic effects. Public health is regarded as an indicator of social equity and a vital national investment in human capital that has the potential to help make Britain a fairer society. Its delivery is, however, complicated not only by the rapid development and cost of new treatments, especially in an ageing society, but also by adverse trends in predominant lifestyles and public scepticism about health-care messages at a time when important aspects of maintaining health are a matter of personal choice. It is further complicated by changing concepts of the boundaries between state and individual responsibility for health and of the civil and political rights of the individual.

The final chapter, by Ken Roberts, is concerned with leisure, stability and change. It is argued that socialisation into leisure-time lifestyles takes place up to and including early adulthood, and that since the end of the Second World War, as average time before first entry to the labour market continually increased, there have been three differing periods of such socialisation. First is the baby-boom period when adolescence coincided with the beginnings of teenage affluence, the loosening of conventional sexual morality, the beginning of pop and youth culture and rebellion against the establishment that was played out in individual behaviour and in the arts. The second period began in the early 1970s as holiday entitlement increased, car ownership rose, membership of trades unions and working men's clubs fell, satellite television broadcasting began and consumption of alcohol and recreational drugs increased. The third period, beginning in the early 1990s, is characterised by popular access to the internet and new methods of communication, a much increased range of commercial television compared with public service broadcasting, increased spending on alcohol, drugs and gambling and, despite a reduced concern for politics, an increasing interest in such single-issue campaigns as environmental protection. It seems likely that these cohort differences in leisure time will continue to emphasise differences between generations, and will help to transform expectations of the post-retirement years.

Conclusions

The period of concern, from the end of the Second World War until the end of the first decade of the twenty-first century, has been a time of unprecedented change in the nature of life and of society as science and technology innovations affected all aspects of life. In Britain it was a period of increasing government intervention to contend with change through development of new economic strategies and new policies for families and children, education, the labour market, health and even leisure time. In Britain and elsewhere it was also a time during which demands for evidence increased, from policy thinkers and policy makers, from practitioners in economics, education and health, and from the growing research community in the social and health sciences. The five large-scale birth cohort studies in Britain were set up and continued in response to that range of demands. The studies continue and in doing so provide a unique kind of data and new ideas for understanding the life course. They also extend the long-established national tradition of data collection for monitoring change and understanding its effects. The book provides the historical context of experience at different times that the cohort studies reflect.

References

Barnett, C. (1986) *The audit of war: the illusion and reality of Britain as a great nation*, London: Macmillan.

Beck, U., Giddens, A. and Lash, S. (1994) *Reflexive modernization: politics, traditions and aesthetics in the modern social order*, Cambridge: Polity Press.

Beveridge, W. (1925) 'The fall of fertility among European races', *Economica*, 13: 10–27.

Beveridge, W. (1942) *Social insurance and allied services (the Beveridge Report)*, Cmnd. 6404, London: His Majesty's Stationery Office.

Blanden, J. and Gibbens, S. (2006) *The persistence of poverty across generations: a view from two British cohorts*, Joseph Rowntree Foundation Report, Bristol: Policy Press.

Blanden, J., Goodman, A, Gregg, P. and Machin, S. (2001) 'Changes in intergenerational mobility in Britain', Centre for Economic Performance Discussion Paper 517, London: London School of Economics.

Booth, C. (1891) *Life and labour of the people*, London: Williams and Norgate.

Butler, N. R. and Bonham, D. G. (1963) *Perinatal mortality*, Edinburgh: Livingstone.

Butler, N. R. and Alberman, E. D. (1969) *Perinatal problems*, Edinburgh: Livingstone.

Butler, N. R., Golding, J. and Howlett, B. C. (1986) *From birth to five: a study of the health and behaviour of Britain's five-year-olds*, Oxford: Pergamon Press.

Bynner, J., Ferri, E. and Shepherd, P. (eds) (1997) *Twenty something in the 90s: getting on, getting by and getting nowhere*, Aldershot: Ashgate Press.

Carnegie Trust (1943) *Disinherited youth*, Edinburgh: T. & A. Constable.

Carr-Saunders, A. M. (1936) *World population: past growth and present trends*, Oxford: Oxford University Press.

Chamberlain, G. V. P., Chamberlain, G., Howlett, B. and Claireaux, A. (1975) *British births 1970*, London: Heinemann.

Chamberlain, G. V. P., Phillip, E., Howlett, B.C. and Masters, K. (1978) *British births, volume 2: obstetric care*, London: Heinemann.

Charles, E. (1934) *Twilight of parenthood: a biological study of the decline of population growth*, London: Watts.

Crowther Report (1959) *15 to 18*, Ministry of Education, London: HMSO.

Davie, R., Butler, N. R. and Goldstein, H. (1972) *From birth to seven: a report of the National Child Development Study*, London: Longman.

Dex, S. and Joshi, H. (eds) (2005) *Children of the 21st century: from birth to nine months*, Bristol: Policy Press.

Douglas, J. W. B. (1964) *The home and the school*, London: MacGibbon and Kee.

Douglas, J. W. B. and Blomfield, J.M. (1958) *Children under five*, London: Allen & Unwin.

Douglas, J. W. B., Ross, J. M. and Simpson, H. R. (1968) *All our future*, London: Peter Davies.

Essen, J. and Wedge, P. (1982) *Continuities in childhood disadvantage*, London: Heinemann Educational.

Ferri, E. (ed.) (1993) *Life at 33: the fifth follow-up of the National Child Development Study*, London: National Children's Bureau and Economic and Social Research Council.

Ferri, E., Bynner, J. and Wadsworth, M. (eds) (2003) *Changing Britain, changing lives: three generations at the turn of the century*, London: Institute of Education.

Fogelman, K. (ed.) (1983) *Growing up in Great Britain: papers from the National Child Development Study*, London: Macmillan.

Giddens, A. (1991) *Modernity and self identity: self and society in the late modern age*, Cambridge: Polity Press.

Glass, D. V. (1946) *The struggle for population*, Oxford: Oxford University Press.

Golding, J., Pembrey, M., Jones, R. and the ALSPAC team (2001) 'ALSPAC – the Avon longitudinal study of parents and children: 1. Study methodology', *Paediatric and Perinatal Epidemiology*, 15: 74–87.

Gregg, P., Harkness, S. and Machin, S. (1999) *Child development and family income*, York: Joseph Rowntree Foundation.

Halpern, D. (2005) *Social capital*, Cambridge: Polity Press.

Halsey, A. H. and Webb, J. (2000) *Twentieth-century British social trends*, London: Palgrave Macmillan.

Hansen, K., Joshi, H. and Dex, S. (eds) (2009) *Children of the 21st century: the first five years*, Bristol: Policy Press.

Joint Committee (1947) 'A survey of child-bearing in Great Britain: a preliminary report issued by the a Joint Committee of the Royal College of Obstetricians and Gynaecologists and the Population Investigation Committee', *Population Studies*, 1: 99–136.

Joint Committee (1948) *Maternity in Great Britain*, Oxford: Oxford University Press.

Joshi, H. and Paci, P. (1998) *Unequal pay for men and women: evidence from the British birth cohort studies*, London: MIT Press.

Kuh, D. and Hardy, R. J. (eds) (2002) *A life course approach to women's health*, Oxford: Oxford University Press.

Kuh, D. and Ben Shlomo, Y. (eds) (2004) *A life course approach to chronic disease epidemiology*, 2nd edn, Oxford: Oxford University Press.

Kynaston, D. (2007) *Austerity Britain 1945–1951*, London: Bloomsbury.

Leisering, L. and Walker, R. (1998) *The dynamics of modern society: poverty, policy and welfare*, Bristol: Policy Press.

Lloyd, T. O. (1994) *Empire, welfare state, Europe: English history 1906–1992*, Oxford: Oxford University Press.

Newsom Report (1963) *Half our future*, Ministry of Education, London: HMSO.

Osborn, A. F. and Milbank, J. F. (1987) *The effects of early education: a report from the Child Health and Education Study*, Oxford: Clarendon Press.

Osborn, A. F., Butler, N. R. and Morris, A. C. (1984) *The social life of Britain's five-year-olds*, London: Routledge.

Parsons, S. and Bynner, J. (2002) *Illuminating disadvantage*, London: National Research and Development Centre for Adult Literacy and Numeracy, Institute of Education.

Pilling, D. (1990) *Escape from disadvantage*, Brighton: Falmer Press.

Plowden Report (1967) *Children and their primary schools*, London: Her Majesty's Stationery Office.

Power, C., Manor, O. and Fox, J. (1991) *Health and class: the early years*, London: Chapman and Hall.

Reder, S. and Bynner, J. (2009) *Tracking adult literacy and numeracy skills*, New York: Routledge.

Richards, M., Abbott, R., Collis, G., Hackett, P., Hotopf, M., Kuh, D., Jones, P., Maughan, B. and Parsonage, M. (2009) 'Childhood mental health and life chances in post-war Britain'. Available at http://www.scmh.org.uk/pdfs/life-chances-report.pdf (last accessed 4 May 2010).

Robbins Report (1963) *Higher education*, Cmnd. 2154, London: HMSO.

Rowntree, B. S. (1901) *Poverty: a study of town life*, London: Macmillan.

Royal Commission on Population (1949) Cmnd. 7695, London: His Majesty's Stationery Office.

Schoon, I. (2006) *Risk and resilience: adaptations in changing times*, Cambridge: Cambridge University Press.

Titmuss, R. M. (1943) *Birth, poverty and wealth*, London: Hamish Hamilton.

Wadsworth, M. E. J. (1979) *Roots of delinquency: infancy adolescence and crime*, London: Martin Robertson.

Wadsworth, M. E. J. (1991) *The imprint of time: childhood, history, and adult life*, Oxford: Clarendon Press.

Wadsworth, M. E. J. (2010) 'The origins and innovatory nature of the 1946 British birth cohort study', *Longitudinal and Life Course Studies*, 1: 121–36.

Wedge, P. and Essen, J. (1982) *Children in adversity*, London: Pan Books.

Welshman, J. (2007) *From transmitted deprivation to social exclusion: policy, poverty and parenting*, Bristol: Policy Press.

2 Politics, citizenship and social capital

Lindsay Paterson

Introduction

The birth cohorts have rarely been used in discussions of politics, and only occasionally in analysis of citizenship. The studies are primarily about social experience, not opinions, and the researchers who have worked with them have tended to be interested mainly in the measurable facts of health, education, families and occupations. Though recent sweeps have asked about social attitudes and social participation, investigating these has not been at the core of their design, and the absence of prior measures at younger ages makes the understanding of change over time difficult.

Yet the politicians who had charge of the UK state during the period when all the cohorts grew up believed that what they did influenced these hard facts. The National Health Service, for example, was set up by these politicians, advised by influential currents of ideology, in order to improve the well-being of babies such as those included in the cohorts. The very existence of the first two cohort studies owed much to that same reforming impulse, the sense that research might be used to help improve society. The minimum we might say in defence of paying attention to politics here is that the state influences the context of the cohorts' experiences.

We can say more than that, however. Popular attitudes matter in a democracy, and so the changing beliefs of the cohort members, recorded once they had become adults, tell us something about how democracy changes. What can shape people in directions that eventually result in political change? What relationship was there, for example, between the growing availability and extent of education in British society and the shift to the political right that took place in the 1980s and 1990s? Cohort studies, when continued into adulthood, can help answer such questions.

They can also allow us to ask deeper questions about when people's values are laid down. Are they fixed from childhood, or are they amenable to influence, whether by changes in the dominant political mood or by deliberate intervention? If we interpret democracy as something more than merely electing politicians to state power, what about citizens' activism? Why do people take part in civic organisations? In a democracy, citizens' influences on government might have been shaped by government itself through policies to encourage the expression of their views. Longitudinal studies are well suited to analysing this kind of cyclical process.

These are then some of the reasons why politics and citizenship are relevant to the cohorts. This chapter starts with an outline of the main changes in electoral behaviour and political ideology in Britain during the six decades when the cohorts have been studied, paying particular attention to those features of political debate that are concerned with citizens' relationship to the state. (We deal in this discussion with Britain, not the UK as a whole, because, except in the Millennium Cohort Study of 2000, the cohort samples did not cover Northern Ireland.) The following section asks more explicitly about the models of citizenship that have prevailed during the same period: what ideas about authority and the legitimation of power have evolved in that time? The next section then asks what evidence there is on the patterns of citizens' democratic participation in the period, specifically what the birth cohorts themselves tell us about that. The final section suggests some further research questions relating to politics and citizenship that the cohort studies might enable us to investigate.

Politics

1945 to the early 1960s

Politics in the two decades after 1945 was largely about extending and consolidating the welfare state. The rudiments had been laid down already, mainly by the Liberal government that was first elected in 1906, although also in the gradual extension of state welfare even during the most difficult circumstances of the 1930s in response to advocacy by 'middle opinion' (Marwick 1964). Thus the basis was laid then for a full system of secondary schooling and for a proper system of public medicine. When Labour achieved its first ever majority in 1945, it was inheriting a legacy as well as pioneering something new. That ambiguity of political leadership was a defining feature of the welfare state as it developed.

The clear Labour victory of 1945 afforded the new government the legislative capacity to bring about fundamental reforms. But in truth the popular vote was quite evenly split between the two large parties, then and later: both continued to attract over 40 per cent until the 1970s (Butler and Kavanagh 1997; Butler and Butler 1985). The sense of legitimacy in 1945 and then for Conservative consolidation in the 1950s was based principally on the seats won, because that was the way in which the system operated. Legitimacy also came from the genuinely national character of the victories in each case, in the sense that minorities were not so overwhelmed as to be permanently alienated. In 1945, Labour won the majority of seats in each region of Britain. They did not do so in southern England in 1950 or 1951, and the Conservatives failed to achieve this in London, northern England, Scotland and Wales even in 1959, but only in Wales could the victory for the losing party be said to have been really emphatic. The sense of a common national destiny was strengthened also up to 1955 by the uniformity of regional change between elections in the share of the vote (Curtice and Steed 1982: 256).

Much the same might be said of the other great cleavage, social class (Heath *et al.* 1985: 30). The Conservatives always dominated the middle class and Labour the working class, but the very stability here was combined with the alternation in power to reconcile each large bloc to the direction of policy. It was not National Government of the kind that had dominated British elections in the 1930s, but the closeness, uniformity and predictability of the results in the first decade and a half of post-war elections did encourage a sense that ideology, after a brief resurgence around the 1945 election and lasting until about 1947, had permanently faded from its pre-war intensity at home and abroad.

So this delicate balance of popular advantage is better expressed in the sharing of ideology than in the mere statistics. The most visible element of that was Keynesianism in economic policy, the essence of which was, in the words of Skidelsky (1996: 48), 'a collection of ideas, policies, and institutions designed to maintain full employment'. Keynes himself was a patrician liberal, and his ideas were not immediately as dominant as they became. Thinkers on the free-market right – notably Hayek – continued to regard them as requiring such levels of state intervention as to risk the liberal freedoms that had been fought for during the war (Clarke 1996: 76). Some socialist thinkers, too, were at first suspicious of Keynes (Skidelsky 1996: 49), for instance Hugh Dalton who became Labour Chancellor of the Exchequer in 1945 (Pimlott 1985: 154–63).

But the memory of 1930s unemployment ensured that, for the time being, these doubts were confined to the political margins. Dalton became a Keynesian in practice, linking demand management – as Skidelsky notes – to redistribution. In the Conservative party the ideas associated with R. A. Butler shifted the mainstream thinking towards the centre (Timmins 1995: 164). There then emerged in the 1950s the phenomenon that the *Economist* magazine in 1954 called 'Butskellism' – the convergence of Labour and Conservative ideology as embodied in Butler and in the Labour leader from 1955 to 1963, Hugh Gaitskell.

The economic aspects of the debate are discussed fully elsewhere in this book. The justification of the social reforms was given in an influential lecture in 1950 by T. H. Marshall, professor of social policy at the London School of Economics and Political Science (Marshall and Bottomore 1992). There were three kinds of rights, he argued, and now was an opportunity to secure the third of them. The first kind were civil rights – freedom of speech, of conscience, of religion, of access to the law courts, of owning property – largely secured in countries such as Britain by the early nineteenth century. Second, there were political rights, especially the right to vote; for adult men this had been established in Britain in 1918, for women a decade later. But these two kinds of rights meant little in practice if there were gross inequalities of social rights, notably of education or of living conditions.

The main response to this kind of challenge was the report by another Liberal, Sir William Beveridge. He listed 'five giant evils' that had to be removed before social citizenship might be achieved: physical want, disease, ignorance, squalor and idleness (Lowe 2005). Economic policy was addressed to the first and last of these. Disease was the target of the new National Health Service inaugurated in 1948, its principle being that health care should be available to everyone free at the point of use. There was also an intention to prevent disease as well as to cure it, and so this also related to the fourth of the evils. But the main attack on squalid living conditions came through housing policy, over which the two large political parties competed to promise ever larger amounts of new building. Want was further addressed through state benefits. Ignorance was to be dealt with by a reorganised system of secondary schooling, in practice divided between academic and non-academic streams, but offering a systematically planned curriculum to everyone for the first time.

That the last of these reforms was in fact expressed (for England and Wales) in the 1944 Education Act of the Conservative minister, R. A. Butler, indicates how firm the political consensus was; Scotland, indeed, had reached much the same position a decade earlier. Lowe (2005: 98) notes that the reason that consensus could prevail was that the two parties could see state-provided welfare as serving two distinct, longer-term purposes – gradually bringing about a more equal society, for Labour, and securing the future of free markets, for the Conservatives. That these could co-exist was due to economic growth and to the favourable international conditions that allowed that to come about.

Binding this together, and helping to secure the sense of an over-riding national interest, was an attachment to Britishness that had probably never been stronger and has not, since then, reached that same peak. Britain, its citizens believed, had won the war. There had emerged a sense of common purpose based on common suffering that transcended all sorts of internal divisions – of region, religion, gender and even class: it was, in that sense, a 'people's war' (Calder 1969). We can also see now, however, looking back, that this united British identity owed more to older ideas of internal variety than to the centralised imposition that the term came to connote later. The old ruling class, as Crick (1991) has noted, were wise enough to understand that effective rule required the toleration of difference. Britain in the nineteenth century was one of the most decentralised polities in Europe, the role of the imperial centre being to manage external affairs while local elites were left to get on with the 'low politics' of social policy (Bulpitt 1983). This sense persisted into the post-war world, even though the end of actual overseas power was firmly in sight, most spectacularly in the fiasco of the Suez invasion of 1956, when it became clear that Britain was no longer able to lead the policing of the world order. These events led to the ending of the old ruling elites, with their judicious understanding of British diversity, but not quite yet.

1960s to the early 1990s

The consensus gradually decayed, most visibly in the shifting electoral patterns. General elections in the 1960s continued to place both large parties at over 40 per cent of the vote, but that changed from the 1970s. Other parties grew, notably the Liberals but also the nationalist parties in Scotland and Wales; this brought both the Labour and the Conservative shares below 40 per cent, which had not happened since 1929, and in no election since 1970 have both the large parties been over 40 per cent. Uniform regional swings between elections had long since stopped happening by the 1970s, resulting in what Curtice and Steed (1982: 258) describe as 'the North and urban areas moving cumulatively towards Labour and the South and rural areas cumulatively towards the Conservatives' (see also Crewe *et al.* 1995: 43–4). The changes were sometimes described as 'class dealignment', but both large parties lost support in all classes while the working class shrank and the middle class – through much upwards social mobility – became more diverse (Heath *et al.* 1985: 38–9; Andersen and Heath 2002; Evans *et al.* 1999; Goldthorpe 1999).

As in the earlier period, however, the significance of these changes lay in ideology as much as in the statistical patterns (Evans *et al.* 1999: 99). Labour was in government for eleven years between 1964 and 1979. In that time it introduced several significant measures of social liberalisation (to which we return), and also responded quite well to the increasing regional divergence of the economy as the old manufacturing base went into terminal decline and as some regions, notably London and the south-east of England, pulled away from the rest (Maclennan and Parr 1979). Labour was incapable of managing that collapse of the old economy, succumbing to a trade union militancy that was in part an attempt to resist the necessary restructuring, and thus losing any claim to national leadership. This decay of Labour's credibility, along with deeper unease about the character of the state and of state welfare, led to eighteen years of Conservative government thereafter. Keynesianism was dead in any case, partly because of the increasing exposure of the economy internationally, but partly also because of the critique from the right, substituting inflation for unemployment as the prime economic evil (Skidelsky 1996). In government, both parties recognised that society was becoming more demanding of individual freedoms, but the ideological rationale that was offered was sharply different, and – in Labour's case – was lost during the 1980s in a return for a while to a kind of socialist fundamentalism that the party had not accepted since the low days of the early 1930s. That contributed to the Conservatives' dominance by splitting Labour down the middle; the centrist segment that broke away in 1981 to form the Social Democratic Party merged in 1988 with the Liberals to form the Liberal Democrats.

The most powerful ideological critique over this whole period came from the right, now referred to as the 'new right', and was a development of Hayek's original doubts. Pierson (1991: 41–8) sums this up. There was a perception that bureaucracy interferes with the efficiency of the market. Bureaucracy was not even effective in delivering services: despite all the aspirations, poverty had not been eliminated, and inequality across most of the range of income and wealth had not fallen. State management was also morally repugnant, reducing the recipients of welfare benefits to dependency. So the welfare state destroys freedom. Despite the hubris of state personnel, no central planner can ever gather the data needed to plan effectively.

Part of the critique was an emphasis on the importance of citizens' taking charge of their own lives. The new right alleged that the professionals who staffed the welfare state had formed a powerful lobbying group with a vested interest in the persistence of the very social evils that its members sought to eradicate. The Conservative government of Margaret Thatcher elected in 1979 sought to reduce the scope of the state and to give individual citizens greater individual choice over, for example, housing, schooling and medical care. Reducing tax on personal incomes served the same end, because, even if that entailed an increase in taxes on goods and services, the management of household budgets was restored to the citizen. This government also hastened the growth of an economy based on services, and the decline of the old manufacturing industry. Because unemployment therefore grew rapidly, the overall share of gross domestic product taken by state expenditure barely fell (Dilnot and Emmerson 2000: 332); electoral considerations, if nothing else, precluded any wholesale ending of benefits to poor people, and poverty, benefits and social inequality grew rapidly (Gallie 2000; Atkinson 2000; Webb 2000). Much of the cost was financed by the discovery of oil in the North Sea (Harvie 1994: 286–308). The harmful effects were felt particularly in the old manufacturing districts as the regional policies of the 1960s were abandoned, and so the growing social inequalities were expressed partly as widening spatial polarisation (Dorling and Rees 2003; Martin 1993).

The shift in social values to which the new right was responding has been well summed up by Hirst (1995: 344): 'modern publics have become more demanding, better educated, and less deferential. Their attitude to public services has changed from one of gratitude to a consumer consciousness. They demand higher quality and also more diverse services of greater complexity.' Some writers have referred to these changes as being about growing individualisation, or a tendency to see social problems increasingly 'as personal inadequacies, guilt feelings, anxieties, conflicts and neuroses' (Beck 1992: 100; Giddens 1994): the responsibility for coping with risk then passes to the individual, no longer lying in the collective insurance that was afforded by the welfare state or, earlier, by numerous kinds of voluntary associations. There may be a difference here between individualism and individualisation, the former, in Mrs Thatcher's rhetoric, a return to Victorian ideas of self-help, the latter a new autonomy that might also decline into a new helplessness. Savage (2000: 117) even suggests that this may show, rather than individualisation, merely a new inclination for public issues (such as class) to be discussed in personal terms. Nevertheless, whether these distinctions are sustainable may also be doubted. When Beck writes that 'under the conditions of reflexive biography, "society" *must* be individually manipulated' (Beck 1992: 135, his emphasis), there does not appear to be any real conceptual divide from Mrs Thatcher's declaration in 1987 that 'there are individual men and women and there are families and no government can do anything except through people and people must look to themselves first' (see Young 1989: 490): the political ideology was in practice the means by which the new condition of existence (or of discussing existence) was made real.

This same mood led on the political left to 'new social movements', some of the most prominent of which have been organisations promoting women's rights, rights of gays and lesbians, concern for the environment, development in sub-Saharan Africa, human rights around the world and nuclear disarmament.

Campaigns against racism in Britain were ultimately a response to one of the effects of the end of empire, as migrants came to Britain from the ex-colonies in search of work. Lying behind the growth of these groups was an increasing scepticism of established politics and a sense of the unacceptability of the structures of power that had long dominated the British state. Nevertheless, several of the liberal responses came from the Labour governments of the 1960s and even the 1970s – liberalising laws on homosexuality, abortion, contraception and censorship, and legislating against invidious discrimination on grounds of race or sex. The leader in this respect was the most liberal Home Secretary of the century, Roy Jenkins, another slightly patrician liberal in the tradition of Keynes and Beveridge (though of lowlier origins).

Something of the same sentiment led to the long rise of nationalism in Scotland and Wales, starting with occasional by-election success for the nationalist parties in the 1960s and early 1970s, peaking for a while in the general elections of 1974, falling back after rather weak proposals for devolved assemblies received either no (Welsh) or lukewarm (Scottish) support in referenda in 1979, rising again when these countries repeatedly did not vote for the Conservative governments of the 1980s and 1990s, and then culminating finally in quite different referendum outcomes in 1997: a three-to-one majority in favour of a Scottish parliament, and a bare majority in favour of a Welsh national assembly. None of this signalled an end to Britishness (Paterson 2002), but it did indicate a reaction against the homogeneous understanding of it that dominated Mrs Thatcher's thought. For the first time in about two centuries, the British ruling elite had forgotten Crick's injunction about the wisdom of tolerance, but the new constitutional structures after 1997 may signal a return to that older tradition.

The challenge to the ruling conventions also came from above, after Britain joined the European Economic Community in 1973. This had been an aspiration of several governments in the 1950s and 1960s, but was postponed through a mixture of British prevarication and French obstruction, and the ambivalence remained, despite the endorsement of entry in a referendum of 1975 by a majority of two to one. Whatever the cultural doubts, however, or the doubts about erosion of sovereignty, the pragmatic realities of trade have always prevailed: realistically, as the old imperial markets vanished, the only option for the British economy was the growing European one, and so, as a percentage of all UK external trade in goods, the share taken by European Union countries rose from 27 per cent in the mid-1960s to 52 per cent in the mid-1990s (Tsoukalis 1997: 182).

1997 to the present

The final period is the return to power of Labour under Tony Blair, but chastened by two decades of new right dominance and by the sense that the left too had to respond to the social changes that had brought the Conservatives to power in 1979. Labour won clearly in 1997, the Conservatives having their lowest share in the twentieth century. Labour beat the Conservatives in all regions other than southern England outside London (Curtice and Steed 1997: 302). Class voting was, once again, submerged in the new ideological landscape (Evans *et al.* 1999; Goldthorpe 1999): the key change was the large-scale middle class support for Labour. The party maintained this new electoral coalition broadly intact in the 2001 and – more precariously – the 2005 elections.

The ideology was now described as 'new Labour', and for electoral reasons it portrayed itself, and was castigated by its leftist critics, as a continuation of Thatcherism. But that was inaccurate, and we may trace three elements of it that came to shape also the Conservatives' response (Paterson 2003). The first did have themes from the new right of the 1980s, but it also drew upon much older ideas from a reinterpretation of nineteenth-century liberalism, Mr Blair having said that social democracy was an aberration. The rhetorical emphasis on citizens' taking charge of their own lives seemed to encourage a modernised version of that social activism which had preceded the foundation of state-dominated systems of welfare.

The second element may be called developmentalism, characterised by Ronald Dore as quoted by Marquand (1988: 103): the intention is 'explicitly to promote the competitiveness of the nation seen as one actor in a cut-throat world economy'. Marquand himself – one of the centrist intellectuals who departed from Labour in the 1981 split – had long argued that the main failure of the twentieth-century UK state was its incapacity for developmental leadership.

The third theme may be described as new social democracy (Gamble and Wright 1999). This did have elements in common with the other two strands, but was different in its continuing insistence on the inadequacies of unregulated capitalism, on the role of the public sector and on the importance of redistributing power, wealth and opportunity (Smith 1994). This shifted the party towards the mainstream of European social democracy, in which the free market is seen as the only efficient way of organising production and exchange but in which the state is seen as the only just way of mitigating the social consequences of the market. There was therefore a return to the original belief that welfare and citizenship were intimately linked in the sense that widespread poverty and gross inequality were once more understood to be incompatible with shared citizenship; the evidence suggested that the policy change after 1997 was real, although also that it would take many decades to overcome the effects of the previous two decades (Hills and Stewart 2005).

Labour also promoted a new kind of Britishness. Although its most visible sign was the new devolved legislatures in Wales and Scotland (and Northern Ireland), there was also an important strand that saw it as a way of incorporating a variety of cultures into a common project without enforcing homogeneity. One of the most prominent advocates of that line was Gordon Brown, who became prime minister in 2007, and who argued in 2004 that 'the United Kingdom has always been a country of different nations and thus of plural identities', that 'Britain . . . was first to make a virtue of tolerance and liberty', part of which had been and might be again 'the mushrooming of local and national endeavour, of associations and clubs, a rich tradition of voluntary organisations, local democracy and civic life' (Brown 2004).

The state and citizenship

This half-century of political change accompanied profound changes in the nature of the British state, the character of its leadership and the practices of citizenship that underpinned it. One way of telling the story is as a gradual shift away from old elites to populism. Another is as a shift from old styles of professional leadership to a mechanistic control by markets or by the measurement of performance. A third way is of steady decline from a state ruled by a globally significant governing class, socialised in some of the leading educational institutions of the world, to a third-rate power led by mediocre talent in which political responsibility is shunned by the most able citizens. These and other stories are all true to some extent. What they have in common, however, is a sense that state politics came slowly but insistently to matter less, constrained by the leaking of sovereignty downwards to markets, civil society and (very recently) new centres of legislative power, and upwards to supranational agencies, especially in the European Union, and to global markets. Ruling groups were no longer accorded deference, and educational success was no longer a mark of unquestioned superiority.

A starting point for understanding what has happened is the account by Poggi (1978) of the changes that took place in the nature of the state between the nineteenth and twentieth centuries. He argued that the essential principle of the state as fully established by the nineteenth century was the rule of law, not only in the sense that we have noted earlier from T. H. Marshall, but also in that professional legal knowledge came to be the route into the ruling elites. Poggi argued that this slowly evolved into something quite different as the state came to assume responsibility for social development: generalist lawyers were replaced by specialist technocrats, qualified not across the whole field of government but only in particular branches of it. Poggi calls the resulting system by the middle of the twentieth century the technocratic state, but that is perhaps to pre-date it by a couple of decades, and there was a transitional period best described by a term adapted from Perkin (1989) as the professional state. What then matters in understanding the shared ideology of the ruling groups at the beginning of our period is their adherence to what Perkin calls 'the professional ideal'. The basis of this was recruitment according to measured merit: by the mid-twentieth century all the professions drew on the expanded system of secondary schools and the universities. The professional ideal also, Perkin says, rests on a principle of universality of provision, and thus is perfectly congruent with the principles of the welfare state. So the ideal was linked to the concept of the moral community of the nation of which the professionals were the leaders and guarantors.

The key institutions here were the universities, educating only around one in twenty of the age group in the 1950s, but drawing, through the academic parts of the new secondary system, on a wider social base in a more meritocratic manner than hitherto (Rubinstein 1986; Kelsall 1955: 134–45). The character of this leadership class was shaped by that education, a homogenising experience that would forge a common identity out of their rather diverse social origins. The key ideas remained those that had their origins in the late-nineteenth-century philosophical idealism of T. H. Green (Harris 1992). Bogdanor (2006) describes this as 'mandarin culture': through the university training of the welfare-state professionals, it embraced in a common mission the elites in Whitehall and those who were fighting the five giant evils in every local community, however remote from power. This was the social basis of what Middlemas (1979) calls 'corporate bias', the state's allying itself with influential institutions of civil society in order to bring about social reform.

The elite and somewhat meritocratic ruling culture then, in turn, helped to determine the nature of ordinary citizenship. Harris (1996) pointed out that much of the character of the British welfare state may be explained only if we understand that democratic ideas of citizenship continued to depend on the old pre-democratic notion that the right to vote was granted only to those who contributed, originally in the form of owning land, later by virtue of owning other property and then by paying rates or other taxes. The analogy of these legacies for the democratic welfare state was the contributory principle according to which large parts of it were financed by insurance, at least nominally. In this way, argues Harris, the whole social order continued to depend on a contract between ruled and rulers: benefits were conferred on people in return for that, not on the basis of their being simply citizens.

As the various challenges emerged to the foundational welfare state, this professional leadership became more thoroughly technocratic, hence amoral, and thus losing its ethical claims to legitimacy and opening itself to populist challenge and to the allegation that its leadership was not as effective as it claimed to be. That crisis underpinned the crisis of Labour in the 1970s. The party had become the exponent of technocratic management and yet, in government, was neither competent enough to sustain it nor coherent enough ideologically to give the state a new ethical basis. The most powerful assaults on the decaying moral order were those of the market and of the mechanistic interpretations of accountability that were introduced by the government of Mrs Thatcher. New styles of public management sought to hold professional staff to account by measuring their performance insistently (Dunleavy and Hood 1994; Farnham and Horton 1996). Only occasionally was this through actual markets, because the government shirked the controversy that would have resulted from any wholesale introduction of real markets into core public services; but the performance monitoring had the same effect of converting the old relationships of trust based on implicit hierarchy into something more mechanical and thus empty of trust. The professions that continued to be trusted were those that earned this through providing a visible service, such as doctors and teachers (as shown in regular surveys from the early 1980s; Ipsos Mori 2009).

The old sources of trust were undermined, too, by the changed character of education and by the decline of organised religion. By the 1990s, following the ending of the distinction between kinds of secondary school in the 1970s, over two-thirds of the age group was completing eleven years of full-time schooling (or its equivalent in a college); forty years earlier, the proportion had been under one-third (Smith 2000). Universities were, by the end of the century, teaching over one-third of young people, and so were no longer educating only a ruling elite. The controversies over standards of attainment that accompanied this expansion were therefore also debates about the cultural attributes of social leadership in a democracy: if large numbers were ostensibly reaching a level that only a small minority used to attain, then did that nominal level actually any longer equip them for power, and, if not, then how was the new, more accessible system of education to select those truly capable of governing?

The problem in this debate about the cultural meaning of educational standards has been to balance two definitions (Aldrich 2000; Wolf 2000). According to one, these refer to the attributes indicated by particular levels of performance in examinations. Here there is quite reliable evidence that matters deteriorated towards the end of the century (Tymms and Fitz-Gibbon 2001). Coe (1999) found that the standard of attainment of a student of average ability rose in English, mathematics, biology, French, geography and history, and concluded that this could not be explained wholly by improvements in teaching or in the support provided by parents. For mathematics, Kitchen (1999) and Gordon (2005) explain such changes by the changing nature of the syllabus and by a more modular approach to learning and assessment, shifting students' learning from more difficult topics, such as pure algebra, to easier matters, such as mathematical applications. In French, Milton (2006) found sharply declining knowledge of vocabulary in A-level students compared with the 1950s. Wolf (2002: 56–97) relates the problem particularly to the growth of vocational courses in secondary school. In short, school-leaving examinations were no longer providing evidence of those cultural attributes that had previously been thought indispensable for leadership.

On the other hand, the enormous increases in the proportion of the age group obtaining recognised certificates at school did suggest at least some minimal democratisation of access to that culture. If a standard reached by fewer than one in ten students in, say, 1960 has been replaced by a somewhat lower standard that is reached by one in three, that is a cultural decline only if the standard is now intrinsically worthless or if the top one-tenth of students no longer achieve what their predecessors did. Nevertheless, that the new situation may indeed have been worse than the old for the population as a whole is shown by further evidence that the level of scientific awareness among children in primary and secondary school was much lower at the turn of the century than in the 1970s (Shayer *et al.* 2007; Shayer and Ginsburg 2009).

However we resolve this, there is no doubt that controversy about educational standards has been a recurrent issue in debate since the 1970s, partly drawing upon this research evidence (Green and Cackett 2005), partly on more impressionistic analysis of syllabuses by teachers and others (Whelan 2007) and partly on critical comments by formerly influential insiders who believed that their efforts to maintain standards had been thwarted (Woodhead 2002). One plausible resolution is offered by Ryan (2005), in the phrase 'dumbing into the middle': in order to cater for more, and more intellectually varied, students than previously, syllabuses and criteria of assessment had to be specified in ever greater detail, rendering the experience of being examined more predictable but perhaps detracting from the quality of the learning that examination is meant to signify. The question about leadership then remains: are students who have been prepared in this somewhat more dependant way really able to exercise the discernment and judgement of their elite predecessors?

The collapse of organised Christianity, too, was both a symptom and a cause of the crisis of cultural value (Brierley 2000). Churches were not only sources of ethical guidance, but also places where citizens learnt about the social order, whether their place in it was to be influential or subordinate. But in presupposing stability and coherence, and to an extent also deference, their place became problematic in an era when moral codes had come to be seen as matters of personal choice, not fate. Belief in various spiritual precepts remained strong (Glendinning and Bruce 2006; Wadsworth and Freeman 1983); what had declined was their institutional expression. That then shifted the churches to the margins of social life, acutely anachronistic, especially when compared with the much greater commitment of the growing numbers of people attached to other organised faiths, notably Islam.

It sometimes seemed then that the old unwritten contract between rulers and ruled had decayed into what Marquand (1988) called 'an unprincipled society' in which a sense of mutual though hierarchical, or even corporate, governance had been replaced, not by a democratic community of equal citizens – as the founders of the welfare state had hoped – but by rampant individualism and aggressive ambition in which there was no longer any basis of a common culture. Nevertheless, in the same way as the increasingly demanding citizens provoked the political response, so the manner in which that assertiveness expressed itself took forms other than those sanctioned by the government in the 1980s and 1990s. We look at some of the trends in social participation in the next section, but the main point here is that these new freedoms were embraced even by people who did not vote for the Conservatives and who were in no sense at all selfishly individualistic. The aim of increased freedom from imposed constraints had been at the heart of the social democratic project: this has often been described as creating positive liberty, and so takes us back to Marshall's ideas again. To enable people to exercise choice and influence, it was necessary that they be relieved of the impositions of the five giant evils. If that had been a founding aim, then it is hardly surprising that the healthier, longer-living, generally wealthier and probably better-educated citizens of the last couple of decades of the century took advantage of any freedoms that were on offer.

Social participation and social attitudes

Changes in the nature of the state and of citizenship have been accompanied by changes in the ways in which citizens contribute to shaping society. The relations and influences through which this happens are sometimes referred to as social capital, and we may describe its shifting character through trends in participation and social attitudes; the birth cohorts themselves provide rich evidence on these and their explanations.

Analysis of social participation has been shaped in the last couple of decades by the writings of the American social scientist R. D. Putnam, whose provocative claims, though not straightforwardly true about Britain, do help to explain what has happened here in the last half-century (Putnam 2000). Putnam argued that social capital has collapsed in the United States. People, he said, are increasingly isolated, choosing to spend more time in front of electronic screens than actively with other people outside the home. When they do venture out, it is for instrumental reasons – such as keeping fit – rather than to contribute to the public good. He attributed all this to structural changes in society, the most important of which were the growth of what he called a suburban lifestyle, the increasing tendency for people to live alone, the financial pressure on families that requires both parents to earn money outside the home and – more nebulously – a shift over time from dominant social mores that celebrated civic culture to an ethos of hedonism.

These claims have not gone unchallenged for the United States itself, and for Britain even those who see them as having some relevance – such as Grenier and Wright (2003) – are much more interested than Putnam seems to be in the social distribution of participation; it may be relevant to note that Putnam is a political scientist, not a sociologist. Broadly put, the conclusion is that decline of social engagement is more marked in some social groups than others, with the result that the ostensibly more individualised, demanding and participative society of which writers such as Giddens and Beck have made so much in their theories may in fact be rather better described as one in which new modes of dominance have been exercised by a much expanded class of well-educated professionals.

The most searching critique of Putnam's thesis as it might relate to Britain has come from Hall (1999). He points out that Britain has a long tradition of active civic organisation: it provided the precursor to the welfare state, and indeed continued to be an important part of welfare provision from its foundation (Harris 1992). When Almond and Verba (1963) compared national civic cultures at the turn of the 1960s, they found Britain to have a high level of engagement, second only to the United States in their sample of countries and ahead of the rest of Europe. The social world in which the members of the 1958 cohort were born, and in which their 1946 predecessors were entering secondary school, was still one of strong social bonds.

At that time, this would have been true of the United States also. Hall's rejoinder was that it remained true in Britain despite Britain's having experienced many of the social changes to which Putnam attributes the decline of social participation. In Britain as in the United States there has been a growth in the tendency for both parents to work outside the home, a shift to the suburbs, an increase in the proportion of people who live on their own and an expansion of those factors to which Putnam attributes a more individualised style of life, such as levels of watching television. Yet, according to Hall's figures, there has not been a fall in general levels of social engagement, either formal or informal. As late as the 1997 general election, electoral turnout remained high. Overall membership of many kinds of civic organisation generally rose in the second half of the twentieth century: this was true of his categories of youth organisations, outdoor recreational organisations and (though data are available only from the 1970s) service organisations and environmental organisations. The main exception is what he calls 'traditional women's organisations', but this decline may be taken as an indirect indicator of the much greater participation by women in the social networks of paid work outside the home.

Hall notes, too, no drop in what he calls 'charitable endeavour', measured either by volunteering or by money donated. There also did not seem to have been any fall in the amount of informal sociability: while most people had more time off work in the 1980s than in the 1960s, 'most groups chose to use this leisure time outside, rather than inside, the home' (Hall 1999: 427). The growth of watching television was at the expense of listening to the radio, not of going out. Indeed, the only point on which Hall finds British trends agreeing with those in the United States is in the decline of social trust.

Putnam had also suggested that the generations born after the Second World War, when compared with those born during the 1930s economic depression and earlier, had been particularly prone to disengagement. Hall finds no evidence of this for Britain. People born in the 1940s and 1950s – thus including the members of the first two of the British birth cohort studies – were not any less socially engaged than those born earlier, once the stage in the life cycle had been taken into account. We return to this point below when we consider evidence from the birth cohorts themselves.

Hall then offered three explanations for the persistently high levels of social engagement in Britain. The first is growing amounts of education, long associated with social participation. As secondary and higher education have expanded enormously since 1945, there has been a growth in the tendency for the average level of participation to rise. The second explanation is the changing class structure, as the middle class has grown and the working class has shrunk. Social engagement has generally been higher in the middle class, although there has also been a decline in working class social engagement through trade unions and workers' social clubs. The third reason is that voluntarism was newly encouraged by government in the 1980s and later. Voluntary organisations came increasingly to depend on state funding, but those that received most state subsidy had the most volunteers.

Nevertheless, Hall's optimism has been questioned, and he himself notes at least three reasons not to be so sanguine as his main analysis might allow. The first is that the decline in working class organisations has led to a greater polarisation of social engagement (Grenier and Wright 2003; Li *et al.* 2003; Johnston and Jowell 1999). Li *et al.* (2003) comment that there has been no growth in participation by the service class (professionals and semi-professionals) but a sharp fall in that by the working class, especially those who have no informal ties of friendship to people in the service class; therefore only the growth in the size of the service class has prevented a fall in participation overall. Even if there is more social activism than before, it no longer has the same implications for the structure of social power. Social capital exercised only by the already powerful might actually be a form of social exclusion rather than underpinning democracy (Granovetter 1973).

The second caveat is a change in the nature of participation. As in the United States, there has been a growth in instrumental reasons for joining organisations, the paradigm being fitness clubs. The argument would then be that experience of this kind provides less training in civic activism or leadership than might, for example, a trade union, a church or a political party, all of which have shrunk in Britain since the 1950s (Gallie 2000: 308–11; Brierley 2000: 654–5; Crewe *et al.* 1995: 121–6). Even the growth of new organisations tended to be more for personal interest than for campaigning. For example, in the environmental area, membership of Greenpeace and of Friends of the Earth fell in the 1990s, and the growth was in the Royal Society for the Protection of Birds and in the National Trusts (Harrison and Webb 2000: 610–11).

If some of the kinds of membership that people now hold are no longer providing a training ground for democracy, then this might in turn explain the third reason for pessimism, the decline in social trust. Hall attributes these trends to uncertain economic conditions, to a society that is less socially integrated (which is another way of putting the point about the decline of truly civic membership) and to the general revolt against authority that we noted earlier.

The 1946, 1958 and 1970 birth cohorts provide relevant evidence here (details from Bynner and Parsons 2003; see also Wadsworth 1991: 153–6). There were sharp falls in various measures of participation across the three cohorts, recording this at approximately the same age in each. For example, at ages in the early thirties, the proportion of men who had ever been a member of an organisation fell from 59 per cent in the 1946 cohort, through 14 per cent in the 1958 cohort to 8 per cent in the 1970 cohort. The trend for women was similar although shallower (46 per cent, 25 per cent, 12 per cent). This was true also of each social class. Some kinds of membership showed slightly different patterns from this. Because women of the 1946 cohort were much less likely to be in the labour market than men, their trade union membership was also very low; but, that aside, the decline across the cohorts was still evident. A less extreme version of this was true of attending a religious service. Voting in the most recent general election was highest in the 1958 cohort, whether at age thirty-three or forty-two, but once again the lowest participation was among the 1970 cohort at age thirty. By allowing us to hold approximately constant the age at which these measures are taken, the birth cohorts generally tend to show that the late-twentieth-century decline in participation is not explained away, as Hall hopes we might be able to do, by any tendency for young people to become active as they age.

Much the same may be said of the change in attitudes towards politics. The proportion having no interest in politics grew between the 1958 and 1970 cohorts, again holding age approximately constant at the early thirties (Bynner and Parsons 2003: 276), and the later cohort was cynical about politics and less willing to challenge existing structures of social authority (pp. 281–2). Park (2004), likewise, using data in the British Social Attitudes Survey on people aged from twelve to nineteen years, found young people to be far less interested in politics than those aged over thirty, the gap growing to such an extent between the mid-1980s and 2003 that it was unlikely that it could be overcome when these young people aged.

Once again, it seems clear that there is a long-term decline of interest in politics that is related to period rather than age. Moreover, because the 1958 cohort also retained rather more interest in politics in 2000 than did the 1970 cohort in that same year, it is unlikely that the period effect that is most relevant is the date at which the surveys were undertaken: it is more likely to be a matter of the period of socialisation into adult life, the 1990s contrasted with the late 1970s and early 1980s. These changes are all the more striking when considered in the context of the rising levels of education in the population, because at any particular moment the more educated tend to be more politically engaged. The explanation is likely to be a version of that offered for similar trends in the United States by Nie *et al.* (1996). They noted that a more educated society was more liberal but not more participative. They explained this by pointing out that, whereas there is no intrinsic ceiling on how liberal people can be, there are limits on how many people may be politically active. So the increment in participation associated with any specified increment of education will depend on how common that level of education is. This is a more general version of the consequences for social leadership of educational expansion: if half the population has a university degree, then that educational level is no longer such a mark of distinction as to entice those who reach it into positions of power, or even into being interested in its exercise.

The shift to the right politically is also shown in the cohort studies, and here the change relates to current influences rather than the period of upbringing: the 1958 cohort moved to the right over the 1990s (Paterson 2009: 88). That change reflects evidence from the British Social Attitudes Survey, in which there was a slow rise during the 1990s in the proportion of people opposed to increases in public expenditure and taxation and also a fall in the proportion believing that government should redistribute income in favour of the poor (Taylor-Gooby 2005).

The cohort studies cast light on the explanations that Hall and others have offered for these changes. They confirm, first, that part of the explanation is the changing class structure, because people who have been upwardly mobile move closer to attitudes and levels of social engagement more typical of their destination class than of their origin class (Paterson 2008). Hence the large amounts of upwards mobility since 1945 – just under 50 per cent of adults' having moved upwards at the end of the century (Goldthorpe and Jackson 2007; Paterson and Iannelli 2007) – will have reinforced those attitudes and patterns of behaviour that are characteristic of non-manual groups. This tendency to acquire the characteristics of the destination class may have become stronger over time, contrasting with the 'unease' that Hoggart (1957: 292) described among the mobile in the 1960s (confirmed statistically by Goldthorpe *et al.* 1987: 208). The cohort studies show also the importance of what Nieuwbeerta *et al.* (2000) call 'acculturation' – that the longer a person spends in a new class the closer her or his views move to those typical of that class (Paterson 2008: 426).

The cohorts show that educational courses taken during adulthood can influence people's attitudes and civic engagement (Bynner *et al.* 2003; Feinstein and Hammond 2004). On the other hand, it is not the case that all kinds of education are straightforwardly associated with more participation or with social attitudes that are more liberal or more conducive to democracy (Paterson 2009). What matters is whether people have learned to think critically for themselves: for example, those who have acquired a habit of reading books for pleasure are more liberal, more opposed to racism and more interested in politics. More fundamental than any educational matter, however, may be people's basic intelligence: Deary *et al.* (2008), using the 1970 cohort, found that tests of general intelligence taken at age ten better predicted people's attitudes (more liberal attitudes being associated with higher scores on the test) than the respondents' own social class or education, or than their paternal social class.

A rather different way of analysing social cohesion is in patterns of crime, in which there was a very large increase starting in the 1950s and reaching a plateau by the 1990s (Hood and Roddam 2000; Maguire 2007; Scottish Government 2009). The birth cohorts reflect this, the crime levels in the 1970 sample being higher than those in the 1958 and 1946 cohorts (Bynner and Parsons 2003: 285–91). There was then much concern politically in the 1980s and later as to whether this rise might indicate a more general breakdown of social order: the left tended to attribute it to the consequences of the free market, the right to the selfish individualism that they perceived as having started in the 1960s. So the late-century concern with the status of childhood, whether with poverty or with moral education, may be traced to these sources, because criminological research (some using the cohort studies) showed that many of the precursors of crime were laid down early in life.

Thus Britain has not experienced any critical social breakdown during the past half-century, but there has been erosion of some of the essential norms of civility and social responsibility. There has been some shift in the character of social participation, away from that kind which encourages debate and which offers experience of civic leadership towards more instrumental benefits that might even be quite solitary. There has been a decline of general social trust and, much more sharply, of trust in and respect for the political system. There have, however, been some countervailing trends – a growth in support for women's rights and in opposition to racism. Part of the explanation of the greater liberalism, and part of the explanation of why there has not been much of a decline in participation, has been the growth in the amount of education that people have, especially higher education. There has also, however, been a growth in social polarisation in these respects, as the residual working class loses its characteristic social institutions and falls far behind the burgeoning professional class in its levels of social engagement. Social capital thus becomes not so much the foundation of democracy as a new way in which power is exercised.

The relevance to the birth cohort studies

Many of the topics dealt with in this chapter cannot be investigated using the birth cohorts because the relevant questions were not asked in the early waves. It would have been interesting to have had data on the political attitudes and voting habits of the parents of sample members, but we do not (except for information in the

1946 cohort about the political attitudes of the parents of cohort members). We also do not have anything on their wider social attitudes, or on their social participation (except, to a limited extent, around children themselves), or even on any aspects of their own education that might have influenced their attitudes or their inclination to participate: we have nothing, for example, on what the parents read, on whether they paid attention to current affairs, or on whether they discussed politics with their friends. There is some information on the social participation of the sample members when they were children, and about their and their parents' educational aspirations, but there is nothing on their social and political attitudes at ages under their early twenties. The absence of such early information reflects the essentially medical origins of the cohorts. It has only been more recently that these surveys have been used to study the topics we have looked at here.

Nevertheless, the cohorts are valuable because such questions have been asked of their members in adulthood. Even before that, however, it is also true that the aspirations of post-war politics shaped the context in which the cohorts grew up. If one of the aims of the reforms inaugurated by Beveridge was to extend Marshall's concept of social citizenship to a much larger proportion of the population than had enjoyed it hitherto, then the cohorts allow us to measure not only the extent to which reforms were put in place – access to health services or education, say – but also whether these experiences led, in adult life, to the exercise of those political and civil freedoms that Marshall argued depended upon the positive freedoms that came with this third stage of democratisation. What choices in life, what influence on events, what freedom of speech and belief, what access to property were afforded to these cohorts, and to what extent were these political and civil liberties dependent on the welfare services that the post-1945 state brought into being? How have the answers to such questions been changing not only as the cohorts age but also as the world changes: who, indeed, will care for them as they age, and shall their ageing escape the scourges that Beveridge hoped would never again be experienced? The topics of such research would not be so much the levels of access to services, although the cohorts do give us information about that, but rather whether, having had historically unprecedented levels of access because of the post-war reforms, the sample members then did lead the civic lives that the advocates of these reforms had hoped they would. Investigating these kinds of questions using the cohorts would be a large research project that has not yet been undertaken.

More specifically, the cohorts may be used to examine long-term influences on adult attitudes and social participation. There are rich bodies of data now on the extent to which the cohort members have engaged with society and also on their views of social development, and for the 1958 and 1970 cohorts we have such measurements at several ages. So we can ask what, if anything, in the members' early lives influenced these adult characteristics. Did a divided secondary-school system – as experienced by all of the 1946 cohort and about half of the 1958 cohort – add to inequalities of the inheritance of power when these children grew up, or was the family still the main channel by which social capital is passed on between the generations? Are there ways in which people in higher social classes at one point in time are able to use their social participation to enhance that status even further at a later age? Are the theories of individualisation correct, in the sense that the freedom to participate might have become less restricted by social origins during the period that the cohorts cover? To what extent can any of these adult influences overcome the effects of childhood ability, which Deary *et al.* (2008) found to be a stronger influence on social attitudes than anything else? Investigating such questions would get to the heart of whether Bourdieu's (1997) concept of the various kinds of capital is more than merely a suggestive metaphor: is it really the case, as he argues, that financial capital and cultural capital can be converted into social capital in the form of access to power?

This then also points to the importance of comparing the cohorts. The scope for doing so is, again, somewhat limited by the absence of relevant data from periods earlier than the 1990s. Thus, for the 1946 cohort we have some basic information on participation (voting, various kinds of membership), but not before the 1970s; and even for the 1958 cohort we have almost nothing until they were aged thirty-three. However, that still leaves rich scope for assessing the influences on participation and on attitudes in the couple of decades since the early 1990s, some of which have been discussed in the previous section. We might add to these many more. Did the members of the 1958 cohort, who entered adulthood on the threshold of the new right's access to political power, have more social-democratic attitudes than the children of the chaotic 1970s? Was the increasing spatial variation in political behaviour during the 1970s and 1980s a greater influence on the younger cohort than on the older one? How did attitudes to social cohesion vary among cohorts, and was there varying propensity to take socially responsible action? How, if at all, were any of these characteristics affected by the large rise in educational participation and attainment of the last couple of decades of the century? If there were these differences between the cohorts, then we might conclude that early socialisation mattered more than current events in shaping political behaviour and attitudes. If not, then we would have further confirmation of the conclusion reached by Heath *et al.* (1985) and by Evans *et al.* (1999) that what political parties do matters.

These potential research questions are merely examples. They illustrate two methodological points in conclusion. One is that, even in the absence of data on a certain topic from earlier sweeps, we may still find cohorts valuable, because we can at least ask about the social aetiology of civic life. If, as a society, we want to make things better in this respect, then that matters independent of whether we know whether people who have active parents tend to be active: politics can not do much to change the characteristics of parents, but it might be able to affect those social institutions (such as schools) which might influence people's later activism, even if all that that influence does is provide a channel through which some of the parental influence is felt.

The final point is about human development in adulthood. Although knowing about the ultimate origins of an adult characteristic is always interesting, it should not deter us from investigating influences over a shorter range. It remains of great importance to learn, from Bynner *et al.* (2003), that educational courses taken in adult life have an influence on people's attitudes even over as short a period as a decade. That civic engagement can indeed change quite quickly, and can do so in response to experiences such as education over which politics itself has some influence, is perhaps one of the more hopeful political lessons that the cohort studies have to teach us.

Acknowledgements

I am grateful to the editors for many helpful suggestions, and to Susan McVie of Edinburgh University for advice on crime statistics.

References

Aldrich, R. (2000) 'Educational standards in historical perspective', in H. Goldstein and A. Heath (eds) *Educational standards*, pp. 39–56, Oxford: Oxford University Press.

Almond, G.A. and Verba, S. (1963) *The civic culture*. Princeton: Princeton University Press.

Andersen, R. and Heath, A. (2002) 'Class matters: the persisting effects of contextual social class on individual voting in Britain, 1964–97', *European Sociological Review*, 18: 125–38.

Atkinson, A. B. (2000) 'Distribution of income and wealth', in A. H. Halsey and J. Webb (eds) *British social trends*, pp. 348–81, London: Macmillan.

Beck, U. (1992) *Risk society*. London: Sage.

Bogdanor, V. (2006) 'Oxford and the mandarin culture: the past that is gone', *Oxford Review of Education*, 32: 147–65.

Bourdieu, P. (1997) 'The forms of capital', reprinted in A. H. Halsey, H. Lauder, P. Brown and A. S. Wells. (eds) *Education: culture, economy, society*, pp. 46–58, Oxford: Oxford University Press.

Brierley, P. (2000) 'Religion', in A. H. Halsey and J. Webb (eds) *British social trends*, pp. 650–74, London: Macmillan.

Brown, G. (2004) British Council annual lecture, obtained from the website of *The Guardian* newspaper. Available at http://www.guardian.co.uk/politics/2004/jul/08/uk.labour1 (last accessed 13 December 2010).

Bulpitt, J. (1983) *Territory and power in the United Kingdom*, Manchester: Manchester University Press.

Butler, D. and Butler, G. (1985) *British political facts, 1960–1985*, London: Macmillan.

Butler, D. and Kavanagh, D. (1997) *The British General Election of 1997*, London: Macmillan.

Bynner, J. and Parsons, S. (2003) 'Social participation, values and crime', in E. Ferri, J. Bynner and M. Wadsworth (eds) *Changing Britain, changing lives*, pp. 261–94, London: Institute of Education.

Bynner, J., Schuller, T. and Feinstein, L. (2003) 'Wider benefits of education: skills, higher education and civic engagement', *Zeitschrift für Pädagogik*, 49: 341–61.

Calder, A. (1969) *The people's war*, London: Cape.

Clarke, P. (1996) 'The Keynesian consensus', in D. Marquand and A. Seldon (eds) *The ideas that shaped post-war Britain,* pp. 67–87, London: Fontana.

Coe, R. (1999) 'Changes in examination grades over time: is the same worth less?', paper for the British Educational Research Association Annual Conference, Durham: Curriculum, Evaluation and Management Centre.

Crewe, I., Fox, A. and Day, N. (1995) *The British electorate, 1963–1992*, Cambridge: Cambridge University Press.
Crick, B. (1991) 'The English and the British', in B. Crick (ed.) *National identities*, pp. 90–104, Oxford: Blackwell.
Curtice, J. and Steed, M. (1982) 'Electoral choice and the production of government: the changing operation of the electoral system in the United Kingdom since 1955', *British Journal of Political Science*, 12: 249–98.
Curtice, J. and Steed, M. (1997) 'Appendix 2: the results analysed', in D. Butler and D. Kavanagh, *The British General Election of 1997*, pp. 295–325, London: Macmillan.
Deary, I., Battey, G. D., and Gale, C. R. (2008) 'Bright children become enlightened adults', *Psychological Science*, 19: 1–6.
Dilnot, A. and Emmerson, C. (2000) 'The economic environment', in A. H. Halsey and J. Webb (eds) *British social trends*, pp. 324–47, London: Macmillan.
Dorling, D. and Rees, P. (2003) 'A nation still dividing: the British census and social polarisation 1971–2001', *Environment and Planning*, 35: 1287–313.
Dunleavy, P. and Hood, C. (1994) 'From old public administration to new public management', *Public Money and Management*, July–September: 9–17.
Evans, G., Heath, A. and Payne, C. (1999)'Class: Labour as the catch-all party?', in G. Evans and O. Norris (eds) *Critical elections*, pp. 87–101, London: Sage.
Farnham, D. and Horton, S. (eds) (1996) *Managing the new public services*, London: Macmillan.
Feinstein, L. and Hammond, C. (2004) 'The contribution of adult learning to health and social capital', *Oxford Review of Education*, 30: 199–21.
Gallie, D. (2000) 'The labour force', in A. H. Halsey and J. Webb (eds) *British social trends*, pp. 281–323, London: Macmillan.
Gamble, A. and Wright, T. (eds) (1999) 'The new social democracy', *Political Quarterly*, 70 (S1): 1–9.
Giddens, A. (1994) *Beyond left and right*, Cambridge: Polity.
Glendinning, T. and Bruce, S. (2006) 'New ways of believing or belonging: is religion giving way to spirituality?', *British Journal of Sociology*, 57: 400–14.
Goldthorpe, J. (1999) 'Modelling the pattern of class voting in British elections, 1964–1992', in G. Evans (ed.) *The end of class politics?*, pp. 59–82, Oxford: Oxford University Press.
Goldthorpe, J. and Jackson, M. (2007) 'Intergenerational class mobility in contemporary Britain: political concerns and empirical findings', *British Journal of Sociology*, 58: 525–46.
Goldthorpe, J. H., Llewellyn, C. and Payne, C. (1987) *Social mobility and class structure in modern Britain*, 2nd edn, Oxford: Clarendon Press.
Gordon, N. (2005) 'Crisis, what crisis?', *MSOR Connections*, 5: 1–10.
Granovetter, M. (1973) 'The strength of weak ties', *American Journal of Sociology*, 78: 1360–80.
Green, D. and Cackett, B. (2005) *Education: better results and declining standards*, London: Civitas.
Grenier, P. and Wright, K. (2003) 'Social capital in Britain: an update and critique of Hall's analysis', International Working Paper Number 14, London: Centre for Civil Society, London School of Economics.
Hall, P. (1999) 'Social capital in Britain', *British Journal of Political Science*, 29: 417–61.
Harris, J. (1992) 'Political thought and the welfare state 1870–1940: an intellectual framework for British social policy', *Past and Present*, 135: 116–41.

Harris, J. (1996) '"Contract" and "citizenship"', in D. Marquand and A. Seldon (eds), *The ideas that shaped post-war Britain,* pp. 122–38, London: Fontana.
Harrison, B. and Webb, J. (2000) 'Volunteers and voluntarism', in A. H. Halsey and J. Webb, *British social trends*, pp. 587–619, London: Macmillan.
Harvie, C. (1994) *Fool's gold: the story of North Sea oil*, London: Hamish Hamilton.
Heath, A., Jowell, R. and Curtice, J. (1985) *How Britain votes*, Oxford: Pergamon.
Hills, J. and Stewart, K. (eds) (2005) *A more equal society?*, Bristol: Policy Press.
Hirst, P. (1995) 'Quangos and democratic government', *Parliamentary Affairs*, 48: 341–59.
Hoggart, R. (1957) *The uses of literacy*, London: Chatto and Windus.
Hood, R. and Roddam, A. (2000) 'Crime, sentencing and punishment', in A. H. Halsey and J. Webb (eds) *British social trends*, pp. 675–709, London: Macmillan.
Ipsos Mori (2009) 'Trust in doctors 2009: annual survey of public trust in professions', report of survey commissioned by the Royal College of Physicians. Available at http://www.ipsos-mori.com/researchpublications.aspx (last accessed 12 November 2010).
Johnston, M. and Jowell, R. (1999) 'Social capital and the social fabric', in R. Jowell, J. Curtice, A. Park and K. Thomson (eds) *British social attitudes: the 16th report*, pp. 179–200, Aldershot: Ashgate.
Kelsall, R. K. (1955) *Higher civil servants in Britain*, London: Routledge and Kegan Paul.
Kitchen, A. (1999) 'The changing profile of entrants to mathematics at A level and to mathematical subjects in higher education', *British Educational Research Journal*, 25: 57–74.
Li, Y., Savage, M. and Pickles, A. (2003) 'Social capital and social exclusion in England and Wales 1972–1999', *British Journal of Sociology*, 54: 497–526.
Lowe, R. (2005) *The welfare state in Britain since 1945*, 3rd edn, Basingstoke: Palgrave.
Maclennan, D. and Parr, J. (eds) (1979) *Regional policy: past experience and new directions*, Oxford: Martin Robertson.
Maguire, M. (2007) 'Crime data and statistics', in M. Maguire, R. Morgan and R. Reiner (eds) *Oxford handbook of criminology*, 4th edn, pp. 241–301, Oxford: Oxford University Press.
Marquand, D. (1988) *The unprincipled society*, London: Fontana.
Marshall, T. H. and Bottomore, T. (1992) *Citizenship and social class*, London: Pluto.
Martin, R. (1993) 'Remapping British regional policy: the end of the north–south divide?', *Regional Studies*, 27: 797–805.
Marwick, A. (1964) 'Middle opinion in the thirties: planning, progress, and political "agreement"', *English Historical Review*, 79: 285–98.
Middlemas, K. (1979) *Politics in industrial society*, London: André Deutsch.
Milton, J. (2006) 'Language lite? Learning French vocabulary in school', *French Language Studies*, 16: 187–205.
Nie, N. H., Junn, J. and Stehlik-Barry, K. (1996) *Education and democratic citizenship in America*, Chicago: University of Chicago Press.
Nieuwbeerta, P., de Graaf, N. D. and Ultee, W. (2000) 'The effects of class mobility on class voting in post-war western industrialised countries', *European Sociological Review*, 16: 327–48.
Park, A. (2004) 'Has modern politics disenchanted the young?', in A. Park, J. Curtice, K. Thomson, C. Bromley and M. Phillips (eds) *British social attitudes: the 21st report*, pp. 23–48, London: Sage.
Paterson, L. (2002) 'Is Britain disintegrating? Changing views of "Britain" after devolution', *Regional and Federal Studies*, 12: 21–42.

Paterson, L. (2003) 'The three educational ideologies of the British Labour Party', *Oxford Review of Education*, 29: 165–86.

Paterson, L. (2008) 'Political attitudes, social participation and social mobility: a longitudinal analysis', *British Journal of Sociology*, 59: 413–34.

Paterson, L. (2009) 'Civic values and the subject matter of educational courses', *Oxford Review of Education*, 35: 81–98.

Paterson, L. and Iannelli, C. (2007) 'Patterns of absolute and relative social mobility: a comparative study of England, Wales and Scotland', *Sociological Research Online*, 12 (6).

Perkin, H. (1989) *The rise of professional society*, London: Routledge.

Pierson, C. (1991) *Beyond the welfare state?*, Cambridge: Polity.

Pimlott, B. (1985) *Hugh Dalton*, London: Cape.

Poggi, G. (1978) *The development of the modern state*, London: Hutchinson.

Putnam, R. D. (2000) *Bowling alone*, New York: Simon and Schuster.

Rubinstein, W. D. (1986) 'Education and the social origins of British élites, 1880–1970', *Past and Present*, 112: 163–207.

Ryan, A. (2005) 'New Labour and higher education', *Oxford Review of Education*, 31: 87–100.

Savage, M. (2000) *Class analysis and social transformation*, Buckingham: Open University Press.

Scottish Government (2009) *Recorded crime in Scotland, 2008–9*, Edinburgh: Scottish Government.

Shayer, M. and Ginsburg. D. (2009) 'Thirty years on – a large anti-Flynn effect? II: 13 and 14 year olds. Piagetian tests of formal operational norms 1976–2006/7', *British Journal of Educational Psychology*, 79: 409–18.

Shayer, M., Ginsburg. D. and Coe, R. (2007) 'Thirty years on – a large anti-Flynn effect? The Piagetian test *Volume* and *Heaviness* norms 1975–2003', *British Journal of Educational Psychology*, 77: 25–41.

Skidelsky, R. (1996) 'The fall of Keynesianism', in Marquand and Seldon (eds) *The ideas that shaped post-war Britain*, pp. 41–66, London: Fontana.

Smith, G. (2000) 'Schools', in A. H. Halsey and J. Webb (eds) *British social trends*, pp. 179–220, London: Macmillan.

Smith, M. J. (1994) 'Understanding the "politics of catch-up": the modernisation of the Labour Party', *Political Studies*, 42: 708–15.

Taylor-Gooby, P. (2005) 'Attitudes to social justice', paper, London: Public Policy Research.

Timmins, N. (1995) *The five giants: a biography of the welfare state*, London: Fontana.

Tsoukalis, L. (1997) *The new European economy revisited*, Oxford: Oxford University Press.

Tymms, P. and Fitz-Gibbon, C. (2001) 'Standards, achievement and educational performance: a cause for celebration?', in R. Phillips and J. Furlong. (eds) *Twenty-five years of politics, policy and practice*, pp.156–73, London: Routledge.

Wadsworth, M. (1991) *The imprint of time*, Oxford: Clarendon Press.

Wadsworth, M. and Freeman, S. (1983) 'Generational differences in beliefs: a cohort study of stability and change in religious beliefs', *British Journal of Sociology*, 34: 416–37.

Webb, J. (2000) 'Social security', in A. H. Halsey and J. Webb (eds) *British social trends*, pp. 548–83, London: Macmillan.

Whelan, R. (2007) *The corruption of the curriculum*, London: Civitas.

Wolf, A. (2000) 'A comparative perspective on educational standards', In H. Goldstein and A. Heath (eds) *Educational standards,* pp. 9–30, Oxford: Oxford University Press.
Wolf, A. (2002) *Does education matter?*, Harmondsworth: Penguin.
Woodhead, C. (2002) *Class war: the state of British education*, London: Little, Brown.
Young, H. (1989) *One of us: a biography of Mrs. Thatcher*, London: Macmillan.

3 Family structure and family policy and practice

Lynda Clarke and Ceridwen Roberts

Introduction

The 1960s and 1970s marked a structural shift in demographic behaviour and societal norms, known as the 'Second Demographic Transition' (van de Kaa 1987, 2003). This major turning point in relationship behaviour, childbearing and family change was experienced in most developed countries. Increases in cohabitation, births outside marriage, divorce and family break-up as well as rising age at first birth and increasing employment of mothers had dramatically affected family structure, norms and experience since the middle of the twentieth century. The cultural shift towards 'individualism' and a post-modern society has been identified as a product of post-war welfare regimes, economic prosperity and increasing educational levels (Inglehart 1990; Beck 1992), with an increasing emphasis on self-fulfilment as opposed to a community orientation. These behavioural and attitude changes and the coincidental policy contexts had major implications for family life.

These changes in demographic behaviour are described in the first section of this chapter and the evolution of family policy in the second section. It covers the ageing of the population, changes in household composition, marriage, cohabitation and family breakdown, ages at having children, births outside marriage and lone parenthood as well as the changing attitudes to family life that have had dramatic implications for trends in family behaviour. These broad social changes influenced and altered partnership and family behaviour and created the context for policy priorities. Ideological shifts towards liberalism and less proscription of behaviour, the growth of feminism, the women's movement and gay rights all strongly influenced change. These changes in demographic behaviours and attitudes affected policy and practice developments, which affected family life.

Family policy includes social and economic policies that take 'the family' as their focal point, whatever the definition of family. Britain has only recently moved from an implicit to explicit interest in policies affecting families. Until the 1970s marriage was regarded as the cornerstone of families, but the liberalisation of attitudes that began in the 1960s led to equality legislation and the emergence of lone parenthood and child poverty as policy problems to be addressed. It was not until the 1990s that family policy became a legitimate area for government action in its own right.

Family structure and dynamics

Ageing

The population of the United Kingdom, in common with that of many other developed countries, has experienced dramatic demographic, social and economic changes since the Second World War. One of the most profound changes is an ageing of the population: people over age sixty-five were 11 per cent of the population in 1951, and 16 per cent in 2001; that is predicted to reach 23 per cent by 2031 (Office of Health Economics 2009). In contrast, the proportion of children decreased and by 2007 the percentage of people of pensionable age (sixty-five and over for men and sixty and over for women) was for the first time greater than the proportion of children under the age of sixteen (ONS 2009a).

The ageing of the population resulted from increasing longevity and a more recent decrease in fertility and family size. The baby bulge in 1947 and a drop in the fertility rate in the early 1950s was followed by the baby boom in the mid-1960s. Thereafter fertility declined to 2001 but rates have risen slightly since. The total fertility rate (the average number of children that would be born to a woman if she experienced the age-specific fertility rates for a particular year throughout life) peaked at 2.95 in 1964, reached a record low of 1.63 in 2001, but rose to 1.96 in 2008, which is still below the replacement level of 2.1. The recent increase is mainly due to increasing fertility among UK-born women. Non-UK-born women have higher fertility at all ages than UK-born women, and constitute an increasing proportion of women of childbearing age, and also contribute to the increase (Matheson 2009).

Immigration has become the predominant driver of population change (Dunnell 2007). In 1981, 6 per cent of the UK population had been born abroad whereas by 2008 this had risen to 11 per cent. There is thus increasing diversity in the ethnic mix, so that in the 2008 Annual Population Survey only 84.7 per cent of people classified themselves as 'white British' (ONS 2008a).

Households

Since the war the ageing population and falling fertility have meant that households comprising parents and dependent children became a smaller proportion of the whole population. There was a growth of one-person households, particularly among the elderly but more recently among people of working age (Table 3.1). Since 1961 families can be distinguished from households in census data, and average household size fell from 3.1 in 1961 to 2.4 in 2006 (ONS 2008b). This reflects the fall in the proportion of households comprising couples with dependent children, whereas the proportion of lone parents with dependent children and one-person households increased (ONS 2008b). Over the past three decades it has been increasingly unusual for more than two generations to live together (Table 3.1). The number of households has grown faster than the size of the population because of these changes and changes in individual preferences.

Average family size is smaller among cohorts of women born since the 1960s

Table 3.1 Percentage of households by type of household and family, Great Britain

	1961	*1971*	*1981*	*1991*	*2001*	*2008*
One-person households						
Under state pension age	4	6	8	11	14	15
Over state pension age	7	12	14	16	15	15
One-family households						
Couple						
No children	26	27	26	28	29	29
1 or 2 dependent children	30	26	25	20	19	18
3 or more dependent children	8	9	6	5	4	3
Non-dependent children only	10	8	8	8	6	6
Lone parent						
Dependent children	2	3	5	6	7	7
Non-dependent children only	4	4	4	4	3	3
Two or more unrelated adults		4	5	3	3	3
Multi-family households	3	1	1	1	1	1
All households (=100%) (millions)	16.3	18.6	20.2	22.4	23.9	25.0

Sources: ONS (2002, 2009a).

than among those born in the 1940s. Women born in 1963 had an average of 1.93 children per woman whereas those born in 1943 and 1923 had an average of 2.24 and 2.1 children per woman respectively.

Household sizes of Bangladeshi and Pakistani ethnic groups are larger than the national average because of a higher proportion of multi-family households, and they also have larger families than other ethnic groups. In 2001, 40 per cent of families in these groups had three or more dependent children compared with 20 per cent of Indian families and 17 per cent of white British families (ONS 2005).

Marriage, cohabitation and family breakdown

The number of marriages rose from 1959, reaching a peak in 1972 (Figure 3.1) and then falling as cohabitation increased. The number of marriages in 2005 was the lowest since 1895. In 1940, 91 per cent of partners were marrying for the first time, but that fell, especially after the Divorce Reform Act 1969, operative in 1972. In 1996 only 58 per cent of marriages were a first for both partners, and in 2006 39 per cent of marriages were a remarriage for one or both partners (ONS 2008b).

There has been a trend towards later ages at marriage in both sexes, partly because cohabitating before marriage increased, but also because of a tendency to remain in the family home for longer and to live independently before forming a partnership. Additionally, in 2006/7 there were four times as many students

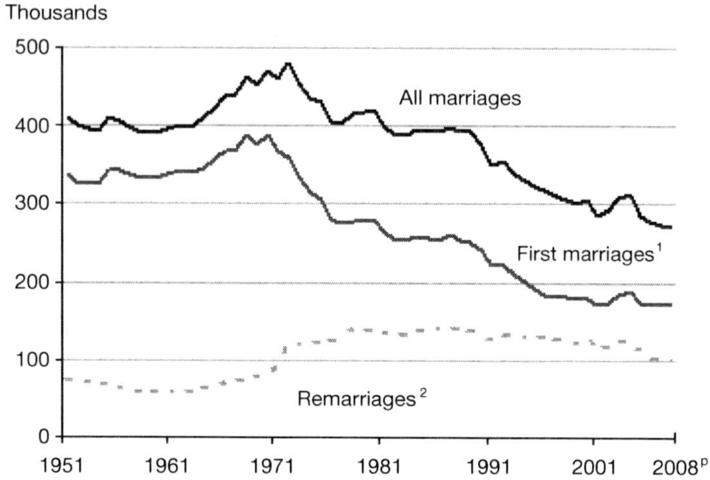

Figure 3.1 Marriages, United Kingdom, 1951–2008. 1, for both partners; 2, for one or both partners; p, figures for 2008 are provisional. Source: Office for National Statistics (2008) *Social Trends*, No. 38, Figure 2.8. London: Palgrave Macmillan.

in higher education than in 1970/1. Young people no longer follow a pattern of moving from the parental home into marriage, which was the norm in the 1950s (Young and Willmott 1957).

Cohabitation has increased, especially among cohorts born since the 1950s (Table 3.2). In 2006 24 per cent of unmarried men aged from sixteen to fifty-nine were cohabiting compared with 11 per cent in 1986 (ONS 2009a). In 1992 6 per cent of the population of England and Wales aged sixteen or older were cohabiting, rising to 10 per cent by 2007 (Wilson 2009), and this will increase to 22 per cent by 2021 (Haskey 2001). Since the 1990s the average length of cohabitation has increased and children are more likely to be born into cohabitation (Murphy 2000). Rather than a precursor to marriage it has also become an alternative.

Table 3.2 Percentage of individuals cohabiting by year of birth and age at survey, 2006, Great Britain

	15–19	*20–24*	*25–29*
1966–70	0.9	12.7	17.6
1971–5	1.5	14.9	25.6
1976–80[a]	1.8	20.0	28.2

Source: ONS (2008c).

Note

a Data are not yet complete for ages 25–29 where individuals were born between 1976 and 1980.

In 2007 divorce rates reached their lowest level since 1981, at 11.9 per thousand of the married population. Age at marriage for both sexes increased and so did age at divorce. Predictors of a high risk of divorce include low age at first marriage and an unexpected change in personal economic circumstances (Chan and Halpin 2008; Boheim and Ermisch 2001; Becker *et al.* 1977), and cohabiting couples are twice as likely to separate as married couples (Boheim and Ermisch 2001). In marriage cohorts from the 1950s to the 1990s premarital cohabitation and marriage to a previously divorced person were risk factors for divorce (Clarke and Berrington 1999), but in the 1990s this negative influence decreased, probably because of the increasing popularity of cohabitation and increased incidence of divorce. Nevertheless, cohabitation is still a much less stable union than marriage. The risk of family breakdown also increases with the number of children (Boheim and Ermisch 2001; Chan and Halpin 2008). Co-incident with increasing family breakdown has been an increase in family re-constitution through remarriage and re-partnership, leading to stepfamilies of various configurations.

The composition of the population by marital status and family structure reflects these major changes in relationship formation. The proportion of single individuals has increased, and by 2031 the proportion of never-married persons is projected to be larger than the proportion of ever-married persons (ONS 2009a). Despite the increase in the proportion who divorced and the decrease in marriage since the early 1970s, marriage is still the most common form of partnership (ONS 2009a) and the most common form of family experienced by dependent children (Table 3.3), but some of these married and cohabiting couple families will be stepfamilies for some, or all, of the children.

Family formation: having children

Changing patterns of relationship formation and increasing female participation in education and the labour market have implications for the timing of birth. The average age at birth in England and Wales fell from 28.7 for women born in 1920 to

Table 3.3 Dependent children[a] (millions) by family type, United Kingdom[b]

	1997	*2001*	*2005*	*2008*
Married couple	9.57	9.00	8.57	8.32
Cohabiting couple	1.00	1.34	1.46	1.66
Female lone parent	2.51	2.66	2.75	2.81
Male lone parent	0.23	0.24	0.25	0.24

Source: Derived from Labour Force Survey, ONS (2009a).

Notes

a Children aged under 16 and those aged 16–18 who have never married and are in full-time education. See Appendix, Part 2: Families.

b Data are at Q2 (April–June) each year and are not seasonally adjusted. See Appendix, Part 4: Labour Force Survey.

26.0 for women born in the mid-1940s. It has risen steadily since and is projected to be around 29 for women born in the early 1980s (ONS 2009a). The average age at first child was 23.7 in 1971 but 27.5 in 2007. In 2007 the average age at birth was 27.1 for unmarried women compared with 31.5 for married women (ONS 2009a), partly reflecting the higher teenage fertility rate for unmarried mothers. Childlessness has doubled in the last two decades: 23 per cent of women born in 1960 were childless at age 35, the same figure as for women born in 1920, but a lower proportion at the end of their childbearing years (20 per cent) (McAllister and Clarke 1998; ONS 2009a,b). Women born in the mid-1940s had the lowest childless rates (10 per cent). Women born in the 1930s, 1940s and 1950s were more likely to have three children than be childless (ONS 2009b,c).

Family size peaked for women born in 1934 at 2.46 children, manifest in the mid-1960s baby boom, whereas for women born in 1920 this was 2.07 children. Family size has been falling for women born since 1955, and is estimated to be 1.74 for women born in the mid-1980s (ONS 2009d). This fall is the result of an increase in childlessness, having fewer children and starting childbearing at later ages.

Postponement of births is most evident among the most educated women, and a growing proportion remain childless. The consequence is a widening gap in life cycle experience and economic prosperity between educated women and those who leave education at the minimum age.

Although smaller families have become smaller on average, the ageing of the population means that more three- and four-generation families exist, the so-called 'beanpole family'. Consequently, children are more likely to have living grandparents and great-grandparents than in the past. The growing elderly population also has implications for the need for care from younger relatives. However, families have become smaller and their structure has become more diverse because of changes in relationship behaviour.

Women's experiences of family events have changed, reflecting delayed age at marriage, increased cohabitation and delayed motherhood. Table 3.4 shows for women at age twenty-five years the increase in cohabitation and marital breakdown and the fall in marriage and births by that age.

Births outside marriage

A major implication of these changes in relationships is a dramatic increase in the proportion of children born outside marriage. In 1951 4.2 per cent of births in the UK were outside marriage but this has increased since the early 1980s to 45 per cent in 2008 (ONS 2009b,d). Younger mothers have the highest rates of births outside marriage. Most of this increase is in children being born to cohabiting parents.

Family type and lone parenthood

A consequence of the growth of cohabitation, births outside marriage and the breakdown of unions, whether married or cohabiting, has been an increase since

Table 3.4 Experience of family events (percentages) by women when aged 25 by age[a] in 2001–3, Great Britain

	Age in 2001–3[b]						
	55–59	*50–54*	*45–49*	*40–44*	*35–39*	*30–34*	*25–29*
Marriage	75	72	65	56	45	33	24
Birth of child	51	44	39	34	33	29	30
Cohabitation	1	2	4	7	12	16	21
Marriage breakdown	6	7	11	14	14	13	13

Source: General Household Surveys 2001, 2002, 2003, Office for National Statistics.

Notes
a Age at time of interview.
b Combined years: 2001, 2002 and 2003.

the 1980s in the prevalence of lone parent families and the likelihood of children living with a lone parent or in a stepfamily (Clarke 1996; Haskey 2001). In 1971 only 3 per cent of all UK households comprised a lone parent with dependent child(ren) but by 2008 this had more than doubled to 7 per cent (ONS 2009a: Table 2.2). In the 1970s and 1980s the increase in lone parent families was initially the result of divorce but later it has been a result of the breakdown of cohabitation or never-married women having children on their own.

Nevertheless the traditional family of married parents with dependent child(ren) remains the most common family type for dependent children, 64 per cent living in this type of family in 2008, 13 per cent in a cohabiting couple family and 23 per cent in a lone parent family (ONS 2009e). However, some of these couple families, married or cohabiting, will be stepfamilies. In 1972, 92 per cent of dependent children lived in a couple family but by 2008 this had fallen to 77 per cent (ONS 2009e) and much of this change can be accounted for by the increase in lone parent families. One in four dependent children lived in a lone parent family in 2008 compared with only one in fourteen in 1972 (ONS 2009f). Asian or Asian-British children are more likely than children in other ethnic groups to live with married parents (87 per cent), and nearly one-half (48 per cent) of black or black British children live with a lone parent.

Data on stepfamilies were not collected in a census until 2001, when 10 per cent of all families were stepfamilies (ONS 2005). Stepfamilies tend to be larger and the children older than in other families (McConnell and Wilson 2007).

Cohabiting couple families, on average, are more financially and socially disadvantaged than married couple families but lone mother families, on average, are the most disadvantaged (Kiernan and Wicks 1990; Clarke and Berrington 1999). Mothers in cohabiting relationships are more likely than married mothers to be socially disadvantaged, to smoke, not to breastfeed and not to attend antenatal classes (Kiernan and Smith 2003). However, both cohabiting and married mothers score higher on all health and social indices than lone mothers (Kiernan and Pickett 2006). Children of cohabiting couples are more likely to have poorer educational attainment, labour market situation and health status than children from married couple families but they fare better, on average, than children from lone parent families (Joshi *et al.* 1999; Ermisch 2001). Stepfamilies have, on average, more stressful relationships and parents have poorer mental health than those in first families (Pryor and Rodgers 2001; Feijten *et al.* 2009). Children in stepfamilies can experience more conflict and adverse later life events than those from intact families (Dunn and Deater-Deckard 2001; Pryor and Rodgers 2001).

Families and work

Mothers' employment rates have trebled since 1951 and the dual or one and a half earner family has become the norm; in 1951 around one in six mothers were employed, rising to four in six in 2008 (Hansen *et al.* 2006; ONS 2008d). This is related to expanded educational opportunities and higher aspirations for financial independence and careers among women, as well as the increased need for families to have two incomes. Thus, women are more likely to work before and return to work after childbirth, although in married couple families this is likely to be part-time employment. Women in higher occupational groups are more likely to return to full-time work than those in lower occupational groups.

Despite these changes fathers spend most time in the labour market and are the main income provider in most families with children, while mothers are still the primary domestic worker. The interdependence of parents in the care of children has developed alongside the increasing role of fathers in their children's lives. Most families have become more pressurised by competing demands on their time, so that families' leisure time together has changed.

The gap between affluent and disadvantaged families has increased because of labour market participation; it has been termed the difference between 'work-rich' and 'work-poor' families (Berthoud 2007). Mothers more likely to be in work (work-rich families) tend to be either married or cohabitating, be in owner-occupied housing, have fewer children, have older children, have higher academic qualifications and be classified as white British.

Although families have become more diverse and dispersed they are still the most important source of emotional and practical support for the great majority and a significant source of care for the sick and disabled and frail older people, given that the beanpole family of three or even four generations is more prevalent.

Attitudes to family life

In the post-war decades there was a shift from patriarchy and maternal dependence to new concepts of security, responsibility and duty. Feminist debates and the growth of gender equality issues coupled with the changing labour market position of women shaped the changing roles of mothers and fathers. There was a move away from the 'authoritarian' to the 'democratic' family and an increase in the recognition of children's rights.

These considerable changes in attitudes and behaviour have had significant implications for people's interpretations of their roles and responsibilities. In 2006 66 per cent of people in Great Britain thought there was little social difference in being married or living together but 54 per cent felt that marriage was the best form of partnership (British Social Attitudes Survey 2006). Only 29 per cent felt that married couples made better parents than cohabiting parents.

Attitudes to pre-marital sex, births outside marriage and family breakdown have became considerably more liberal with less stigmatisation of non-traditional relationships and childbearing. There has been increased tolerance towards premarital sex and contraception over the last twenty-five years, which has relevance for cohabitation, but an unchanged level of disapproval towards extra-marital sex (Duncan and Phillips 2008).

Growing awareness of gender equity, increasing employment of mothers and the recognition of the agency of the child led to changing perceptions and expectations of parental roles. The increase in paid work among mothers and fulfilment of individual goals in preference to communal ones does not necessarily negate the importance of the family but may change its manifestation (McGlone *et al.* 1998). Obtaining a comfortable lifestyle may take preference to starting a family (McAllister and Clarke 1998). The trend away from prescribed dependent family relationships and towards companionate marriage may be part of a more general move towards negotiated relationships (Finch and Summerfield 1991).

The sharing of domestic chores and caring for children and older family members has coincided with an increased role of fathers in the lives of their children (Burghes *et al.* 1997).

Family policy and practice

There have also been significant policy and practice developments over the last sixty years that have affected family life, and the majority have been a response to wider socio-economic changes and they have shaped how people think about and behave in their families.

However, only relatively recently has the UK government explicitly developed a family policy. *Supporting Families*, the first ever policy document for families, was published by the Labour government in 1998 (Home Office 1998). Yet British governments 'do have family policies . . . it's just that family policies do not get recognised in those terms' (Deakin 1988; Wynn 1972). Family life was seen as a private arena into which the state did not step. Consequently there were until recently not only no explicit policies but also no accompanying institutions in central or local government such as a minister or a lead department for families.

The 1940s to the 1970s

The importance of the family as a key societal institution with calls for policy interventions has been long recognised by social reformers (Rathborne 1940) but it was not until the establishment of the welfare state that the Family Allowance Act 1945 recognised the role of the state in fiscal support for families with children.

This was one of many key pieces of legislation in the 1940s that shaped succeeding decades, affecting life chances for all. The Education Act 1944 made full-time education compulsory and free for all children aged from five to fifteen years, and the National Health Act initiated in 1948 the free National Health Service, which, at a stroke, removed a major fear of not being able to pay for medical care. Many of the key ideas of the 1942 Beveridge Plan were embodied in the National Insurance Act 1946, which laid the foundations of the post-war welfare state.

Dominant assumptions and the importance of marriage

That act assumed that people were either unmarried and financially independent and any entitlement to benefit was based on their own contributions, or married with the husband as breadwinner and the wife financially dependent on the husband (Roll 1991). A woman's dependent status was independent of whether she had caring responsibilities for children or disabled/elderly relatives; it was a consequence of being a wife.

Until the 1960s this model of breadwinner husband and wife at home persisted and in some part reflected the majority experience. The high levels of employment for men, substantial house-building programmes and a rise in the standard of living generated a period of prosperity for many families. Prime Minister Harold Macmillan concluded in 1957 that 'most of our people have never had it so good' (from a speech by Prime Minister Harold Macmillan to a Tory Party rally on 20 July 1957). This period had policies for improving the context for family life but not for explicitly intervening in it.

But, although this was the dominant view of family life reflected in television advertisements through the 1960s, major changes were occurring that led to government enquiries and legislation. After the early post-war rise in divorce to 47,041 dissolutions in 1947, much of it accounted for by the ending of hasty wartime marriages, divorce never returned to the pre-war levels (Dominian 1980).

There was concern about the level and causes of divorce and pressure to alter the divorce laws of 1937. In 1951 the government set up the Royal Commission on Marriage and Divorce, which reported in 1956 (Smart 1999; Finch and Summerfield 1991) and recommended no changes or easing in the grounds for divorce. The report shows the early recognition that marriage was changing into the more companionate relationship favoured at the end of the twentieth century. People demanded personal fulfilment from marriage rather than seeing it as an institution with concomitant duties.

Pressure for reform was unstoppable, but reform allowing divorce on the basis of irretrievable breakdown as evidenced by, desertion, adultery or separation with consent after two years or without consent after five years or unreasonable behaviour only came in 1969. These changes were seen as strengthening marriage as they enabled people to leave unhappy marriages and make new ones. This coincided with peak numbers of first marriages in 1970.

Divorce and the growth of lone parenthood

Divorce, especially among younger couples, was accompanied by increasing levels of lone parenthood in the 1960s and 1970s. Public concern grew, particularly about the lack of financial support for lone parents from former partners and the pressures their financial support placed on supplementary benefit. Richard Crossman, Secretary of State for Social Services, established the Finer Committee in 1969 to consider the problems of one parent families and what help could be given. This was a major policy initiative.

The committee collected evidence from social scientists, practitioners, service providers and moralists and reported in 1974. It estimated that there were about 570,000–620,000 lone parents in 1971 and recognised that financial support for these families was inadequate; maintenance was frequently not paid by fathers and it was difficult for mothers to combine employment with childcare. However, the committee's recommendation that the state take over the role of father by paying a Guaranteed Maintenance Allowance to be collected from the 'liable relative' was not adopted. These debates foreshadowed those around Child Support policy from the 1990s onwards (Evans 2006).

The liberalising 1960s: birth control, abortion and homosexual reform

The changing attitudes to marriage and divorce reflected the many attitudinal and behavioural changes that impacted on family life and public policy. The 1960s saw several important developments that had an enormous impact on attitudes to sexual relations and therefore family life. First, in 1961 the oral contraceptive ('the pill') was licensed for NHS use and the 1967 Family Planning Act allowed local authorities to open family planning clinics. This revolutionised contraception and consequently people's attitudes to sex, which became increasingly separated in people's minds from a marital relationship and childbearing.

Second, the Abortion Act was passed in 1967 (effective 1968), legalising abortion under twenty-eight weeks free on the NHS. This together with the pill was to have a significant impact on women's ability to control their fertility and therefore their lives and in due course how men and women felt about sex.

Third, after a parliamentary struggle throughout the 1960s, the 1967 Sexual Offences Act legalised sexual relationships between consenting adult men thereby allowing public recognition of homosexuality. This opened up public discussions of sexuality and relationships more generally

Equality legislation and the women's movement

None of this policy and legislation was enacted with family issues in mind. Indeed, a much more dominant theme was the issue of rights for women. Labour shortages were pulling women into the labour market, and, although the 1960s were about how to encourage women into paid employment, they also saw increased agitation for the removal of discriminatory legislation, pay and practices in paid work and in the provision of goods and services (Hunt 1968; Martin and Roberts 1984).

The Labour government (1964–1970; 1974–1979) was committed to advancing women's rights, acting on pressure from the trade union movement and the emerging women's movement. The Equal Pay Act 1970 came into effect in 1975, accompanied by the Sex Discrimination Act 1975 and, importantly from a family point of view, the Employment Protection Act 1979, which gave maternity pay and job protection for the first time to some employed women. By the end of the 1970s, therefore, legislation reflected changing attitudes to men's and women's public and private roles and facilitated continuing change, all of which impacted on family life and public understanding of how families worked.

In the 1970s the Women's Liberation Movement challenged public attitudes to women as dependents of men and the role of the state in upholding this (Wilson 1977). It campaigned for increased childcare facilities so that women could enter the labour market liberated from their caring roles, and challenged the domestic division of labour and the more generalised patriarchy that underlay society in general and family life in particular (Coote and Campbell 1982). The argument that women should be seen as independent, able to enter into financial agreements in their own right, echoed the growing emphasis on individualism.

Services for families and the rediscovery of poverty

Historically family policy in Britain has been concerned with either setting the broad parameters by fiscal or benefit policy, laws on marriage and divorce, or with the protection of the vulnerable, seeing state intervention in family life as for the protection of children, but little else.

The profession of social work developed since the 1940s with key legislation encouraging public intervention in 'problem families' (Welshman 1999). Under the 1948 Children Act local authorities established children's departments and employed childcare officers. The 1970 Local Authority Social Services Act amalgamated councils' social work and care services into social services departments, to provide a unified community-based response to families' needs through casework, much of which was premised on psychological and behavioural approaches.

Concern about the circumstances of poor families grew throughout the 1960s and poverty was 'rediscovered'. Peter Townsend and Brian Abel Smith's study of family income and resources, undertaken from the mid-1960s, proved seminal, and this and associated studies, combined with Townsend's campaigning work (he founded the Child Poverty Action Group in 1964), drew public attention to the failure of the welfare state for poor families (Townsend 1979).

There were, however, competing views about the causes and consequences of poverty and family failure There were challenges to the body of thought emphasising the failings of the poor – a perspective underpinning much traditional social work and taken by Sir Keith Joseph MP, Secretary of State at the Department of Health and Social Security between 1970 and 1974, who distinguished between the deserving and undeserving poor. Academics and Labour politicians tended to focus on structural and environmental factors. Indeed, the influential Research Council and governmental research programme 'Transmitted Deprivation' challenged these behavioural assumptions with the researchers' wider structural, socio-economic approach (Welshman 2008).

By the end of the 1970s changes in how families and family policy were conceptualised fed into policy discussions. Writings of the feminist movement and social science research on families and family change were drivers of this. The independent Study Commission on the Family in the late 1970s was established to study the implications of these changes, becoming the Family Policy Studies Centre in the early 1980s (Wicks 1983). It played a seminal role in articulating the need to examine the impact of policies on different families and to explore the interplay between socio-demographic change and family life and public policy.

The 1980s onwards

From the late 1970s there was an increase in public, political and media interest in families. Prime Minister James Callaghan had criticised the lack of a family focus in policy making, and Mrs Thatcher as early as 1977 had said 'we are the party of the family' (Henwood *et al.* 1987). In the 1980s a more ideological Conservative government in difficult economic conditions saw high levels of unemployment and interest rates, considerable cuts in public expenditure and a consequent rolling back of the welfare state, which they saw as undermining family life.

Economic cuts and family crisis

In the 1980s there was increased talk of the family in crisis from all sides in politics (Segal 1983). Many social ills such as rising crime and delinquency and high levels of teenage pregnancy were attributed to the decline of the traditional family and this, coupled with increasing divorce and lone parenthood, diverse family forms and increasing levels of mothers going out to work, played to traditionalist fears. Families were also under greater stress as they dealt with unemployment, consequent financial pressures and reduced public services (Fagin and Little 1984).

Despite concern about families and public criticism of their failings there was little explicit family policy during the 1980s, although there was some major legislation that had enduring effects on family life. The 1980s is perhaps the last period when family policy was implicit. Yet unforeseen consequences of some legislation became drivers of changing circumstances, attitudes and policy concerning families.

Housing policies and families

The 1980 Conservative government's Housing Act allowed the sale of council (public) housing to tenants at discounted prices, to encourage wider home ownership. Councils were allowed to keep the receipts from sales but were forbidden to use this money to build new homes for rent until they had cleared their debts. As a consequence pressure on low-cost housing for poorer families grew, especially in high-cost areas, and some low-income families were forced to buy when they were not well placed to do so. An unintended consequence was that less good council housing was left, more prosperous tenants bought and moved out, and remaining council estates became more homogeneous, populated by the more vulnerable who were dependent on benefits, including many lone parent families. This policy was also one of the drivers of increased female labour market participation. Although popular, especially with those able to buy, this housing policy was criticised, and in 1997 the Labour government reduced the discounts allowed in areas where affordable housing was in short supply.

The Children's Act 1989

This was perhaps the most lauded and innovative legislation affecting families in this period. It brought together fragmented public and private law dealing with the state's role vis-à-vis children to provide a coherent foundation for far-ranging policies. It embodied two crucial concepts. Parental responsibility replaced parental rights and became an important theme over the next twenty years, as did the idea that the child's welfare should be central to decision making about children. This has been a key principle in courts' decisions about taking children into public care or in deciding where they live or who they see in contested parental separations. In addition, it clarified the role of local authorities, detailing their duties and powers in providing services to children and families, particularly those in need, and it argued for more cooperation between parents and statutory authorities.

Changing the unit for tax and social security assessment

The increased demands for recognition of women's financial and legal independence led to criticism of the tax structure, which treated a married couple as one unit. This was seen as increasingly outmoded as more women had their own earnings and resented their tax affairs being conducted through their husbands.

The Green Paper on the reform of personal taxation (HMSO 1986) was challenged by feminists and child poverty reformers as, although it proposed independent taxation, it argued for transferable allowances between married couples when one partner was at home. This, they argued, negated their financial independence and was not the best way to support mothers with children (Lister and Bennett 1986). The 1990 Act introduced independent taxation without transferable allowances but retained the married man's allowance, subsequently renamed the married couple's allowance, and finally abolished from 2000–1.

In the 1980s continuing reform of the social security system in part reversed some of the changes of the 1970s. The Social Security Act 1986 was both a response to the need for public expenditure cuts but also a desire to move away from a universal, comprehensive insurance approach to a more means-tested system of benefits. Despite continuing recognition of the growing numbers of lone parents, the thrust of the proposals was to encourage men as breadwinners, so much so that it was proposed to absorb child benefit into the new benefit of Family Credit and to pay it to men through their pay packets. A campaign uniting diverse sections of society reversed this proposal (Kiernan *et al.* 1998). The 1986 social security reforms continued the additional benefit support to lone parents, but over the 1980s concern about parity between married and lone parents was matched by concern about the growing inequality of treatment between married and cohabiting couples that a complex tax and benefit system was creating.

Lone parents – the emergence of a 'problem'

The number of lone parents increased throughout the 1980s, burdening the benefit system. Obtaining maintenance from former partners had been a problem for many, exacerbated by changes in financial arrangements on divorce, which the 1984 Matrimonial and Family Proceeding Act in effect encouraged. Although children's interests were to be put first, courts were to balance the interests of men's first and second families, and often put second families first. Increasingly there was a view that as far as possible there should be a clean break (Kiernan *et al.* 1998), argued for on the grounds that individuals should take responsibility for themselves, and that more women were now in employment for more of their lives. However, contemporary data showed how small a share of household income working women contributed and how their employment was constrained by their caring responsibilities (Martin and Roberts 1984; Henwood *et al.* 1987).

The availability of state benefits began to be taken into account in financial settlements although this had not been intended. By the end of the 1980s the increase in numbers of lone parents and the tendency to substitute benefit for maintenance support for children placed huge strains on the social security budget. The characteristics of lone parents were changing also. The proportion of widows was declining and, increasingly, single, never-married young women were becoming lone parents as their relationships broke up. Attitudes towards lone parents were becoming more critical. Conservative ministers began talking about the dependency culture, suggesting that the benefit system was contributing to the rise of family break-ups and 'illegitimacy' and encouraging young women into lone parenthood (Bradshaw 1989). The mood was set for a very different approach in the 1990s.

Families move up the policy agenda in the 1990s

The theme of families in crisis surfaces frequently in periods of economic or political uncertainty and may reflect a deeper societal unease (Gittins 1985). The 1990s were the decade when families excited criticism and comment from politicians and media alike. The attempt at the beginning of the decade to sort out the problems of lone parents inadequately supported by former partners grew to become the first explicit family policy developed by a British government.

The 1991 Child Support Act aimed to ensure adequate maintenance. The Conservative government argued that parents should honour their legal and moral responsibilities and set up the Child Support Agency to effect this. It was bedeviled by problems (Barnes *et al.* 1998).

Debates about family breakdown and the serious effect on children of parental separation and absent fathers increased (*Family Policy Bulletin* 1991). Proposals to reform the divorce laws led to extensive discussion about the causes and consequences of Britain's high rates of divorce. The Family Law Bill, which aimed to clarify a de facto situation of fault being used for 'quickie' divorces and reduce the costs of legal aid in contested cases, provoked enormous controversy. Traditionalists were ranged against those anxious to make divorce among couples with children less adversarial and dependent on lawyers, with settlements that would meet children's and parents' needs more realistically. The Family Law Act was eventually passed in 1996 but parts were never implemented. More importantly, perhaps, battle lines had been drawn between different sectional interests about the causes and consequences of family breakdown, which was now both high up the policy agenda and recognised as highly contentious.

In addition to the high costs of social security, politicians, the media and some social scientists blamed family breakdown for increasing anti-social behaviour and juvenile delinquency (Dennis and Erdos 1992). The links between crime, family structure and the quality of parenting attracted increasing attention (Utting *et al.* 2003). It was argued that it was not family structure per se but the quality of parent/child relationships that ensured children stayed out of trouble. These were highly contested views.

The emergence of parenting as a policy focus

British polices towards the family were predicated on 'not intervening' unless absolutely necessary and not having a family policy. Clearly issues of social security support or protecting very vulnerable children from their dysfunctional families had long been seen as legitimate concerns, as had giving parents health advice about their children. But in 1994 the International Year of the Family (IYF) widened the debate about the needs of all families, not just those who divorced or came to the attention of social services, and played a crucial role in highlighting parenting as needing public policy and support (APPG 1994).

As early as 1973, policy makers concerned with the 'cycle of deprivation' considered parenting to be a social policy issue, holding a high-level seminar to consider the role of parents, the quality of parenting and the scope for helping people in their parental role (DHSS 1974). Little came from this, but twenty years later concern about parenting was not restricted to parents who came into the ambit of social services. Middle class parents worried about their skills/knowledge, and groups of semi-professional and amateur parenting educators, and leaders/supporters, emerged to advise them, as public concern about bad parenting was fanned by stories of out of control children. The Department of Health funded a programme of research on parenting in disadvantaged communities and a parenting initiative to provide support to small programmes (Roberts

1996). The Parenting Education Support Forum was founded in 1995 as a non-governmental organisation dedicated to advancing quality parent education. This issue was to become much more prominent under the Labour government (Straw and Anderson 1996).

Family policy becomes centre stage – from the mid-1990s

Public discourse in the early 1990s was dominated by the 'Back to Basics' campaign by the Conservative government that linked crime, disorder, a lack of moral probity and lone mothers, and argued for a return to 'traditional family values'. Yet beneath this rhetoric there was a growing interest in developing a more coherent policy approach to families. After years of refusing to be explicit about family policy the Conservative government appointed the first spokesman for the family, adding this to the responsibilities of the Secretary of State for Health in 1994. But this interest was still very uneven. For example, although the Department of Health was beginning to accept the need for parenting education, the demand from working parents for more help with childcare provision was fiercely resisted by the Department of Trade and Industry on the grounds that this should be provided by employers and the market place rather than the state.

In 1997, under the Labour government, a Ministerial Group on the Family was set up under the Home Secretary, and overall responsibility for family policy was moved to the Home Office to deal with the problem of failing parents and the anti-social or delinquent behaviour of children. The first ever consultation document on family policy – *Supporting Families* (Home Office 1998) – reflected on what the government had achieved in its first year and outlined future plans (for a very comprehensive overview of the Labour government's first ten years see James 2009).

An explicit focus on families and a plethora of initiatives

This explicit family policy focused only on families with children as the policy was about 'investing in the future'. It encompassed all families with children, not just families at risk, and it ignored the issue of costs of care for frail and elderly people, which had come up the policy agenda in the 1980s and 1990s. Central to this policy was the improvement of parenting through support and advice. Advice lines for all parents were to be improved, and key to this was a new programme of intervention called SureStart, to be directed at families with young children in deprived areas (Belsky *et al.* 2007).

SureStart, a major innovation in policy for families, was premised on early intervention, which radically changed the thrust of British family policy. Its notion of 'targeted universalism' regarded all parents of young children in an area as eligible, regardless of economic status. Other aspects of the approach were equally interventionist. The focus on tackling crime and disorder emphasised parents' responsibility for their children's behaviour, and gave courts the power to require parents of children who had offended or been involved in anti-social behaviour to attend counselling sessions to help them control their child (FPSC 1998a)

Facilitating employment for parents, especially lone parents and mothers, was a major part of Labour's programme of tackling child poverty and welfare dependency and creating more equality for women. Providing more childcare was a key feature of the policy. The new National Childcare Strategy included help with the costs of childcare, funding to increase the number of out of school places and the development of a framework to improve standards of quality, as well as increased nursery places for four-year-olds, and subsequently three-year-olds (FPSC 1998b). At the same time the government's New Deal encouraged lone mothers into work, and this became an important part of the strategy to reduce child poverty and the benefit bill (FPSC 1998c).

The first few years of the Labour government saw a flurry of activity that impacted on families. European Directives on Working Time and Parental Leave were adopted and made it easier for families to balance work and family life (FPSC 1998d), and maternity and parental leave rights were extended. Other activities included a review of child support policy (Department of Social Security 1998), a report on teenage pregnancy (Social Exclusion Unit 1999), a review of the adoption system, a consultation on the physical punishment of children by their parents (Department of Health 2000), the setting up of a Royal Commission on long-term care and the development of a National Carers' Strategy (FPSC 2000). Some of these initiatives led subsequently to legislative change.

Policy towards couple relationships

The government found it most difficult to move forwards initially in the area of couple relationships. Its apparent support of marriage as the most suitable status for rearing children, as outlined in the 1998 *Supporting Families* document, was heavily criticised, particularly by those working with less traditional families. Fiscal policy also challenged the importance of marriage. As shown above the government removed tax support from married couples and gave more support to parents of young children through child tax credit and working family tax credit to help reduce child poverty. Financial support to organisations working to help families in relationship difficulties was maintained, but the government retreated from appearing to support marriage by downplaying the couple relationship in favour of the parent/child relationship, which underpinned all new initiatives.

Recently policy has begun to change. It was not until 2007 that the government publicly recognised the importance of strong couple relationships (DCSF 2007) as the starting point for an effective family policy, and pilot studies were funded to identify better ways of co-coordinating local support for separating couples (James 2009). But the most recent document moved away from this to emphasise the importance of a wider grouping of family relationships (DCSF 2010). It explicitly says that 'marriage is a personal and private decision for responsible adults with which politicians should not interfere' but goes on to argue that 'since it is the quality of relationships that is of most significance for children and families it follows that government has a real interest in all relationships within families being strong' (DCSF 2010: summary point 28, p. 21).

The government's acceptance of diversity in family forms reflected changing public attitudes as public acceptance of same-sex couples and non-traditional family forms increased. The Adoption and Children Act 2002 broke new ground in formally allowing applications for adoptions to be made by same-sex couples or a single person. Then the Civil Partnership Act 2004 (effective 2005) gave same-sex couples the right to register their partnership and be accorded the equivalent legal rights as marriage conferred on heterosexual partners with respect to recognition as 'kin' and inheritance. Subsequently, the Human Fertilisation and Embryology Act 2008 replaced the requirement to consider the 'need for a father' with the need for 'supportive parenting' and allowed the right to name both same-sex partners on a birth certificate.

Every child matters – strategies and services for children

Recurring scandals of vulnerable children being killed by their carers, and social services held to have failed them, led directly to major reorganisation. The government initiative *Every Child Matters* was first set out in 2003 (HM Treasury 2003) and enacted in the Children Act 2004. It went beyond dealing with child protection issues and identified five desired outcomes for all children: being healthy, staying safe, enjoying and achieving, making a positive contribution and economic well-being. It reflected the government's increasing emphasis on early intervention and preventive strategies, as well as the importance of parenting, as underpinning its policies towards children. It proposed major structural change by bringing together local authority education and children services under directors of children's services.

In addition, Children's Trusts were set up to bring services, including health, together in a multi-disciplinary team and a universal database holding basic data on all children was set up to include information about 'causes of concern' about individual children so as to facilitate contact between professionals. The costs have been considerable and concern about the possible misuse of confidential data has limited what is collected. There is also now concern that there are serious human rights and data protection conflicts (Anderson *et al.* 2009).

The family courts – child contact and children at risk

Family courts deal in the main with divorce and disputes between parents over, for example, child contact (Hunt and Roberts 2004) or children being taken into public care. Concern about the cost and workings of the family courts grew, and the family courts were increasingly criticised by families engaged in public or private law cases. Only about 10 per cent of separating parents resort to the courts to settle their differences. Some cases are particularly complex and costly to resolve and sometimes have led to a vocal minority of parents arguing that the courts are secretive and biased, particularly against fathers. Some parents involved in disputes with social services about the care of their children, and at risk of having them taken into care, have also criticised the workings of the courts. Various initiatives have been tried to help parents manage the arrangements for their children more satisfactorily (Hunt and Roberts 2005) and to make the workings of the court more transparent to parents and the press (George and Roberts 2009).

Combating child poverty

Faced with international evidence about the large minority of British children living in poverty the Labour government committed itself in 1999 to eradicating child poverty by 2020 and halving it by 2010. It aimed to do so by improving the employment rate of parents, especially lone mothers, and by income transfers to families through benefits and tax credits. It also tried to improve the system of child support from non-resident parents, usually fathers. Child Benefit has continued as a universal benefit for all children while the newer financial measures such as Working Tax Credit and Child Tax Credit are aimed at lower-income families, the former for families in work, the latter, aimed at the main carer, not work dependent.

Although these measures, coupled with some limited success in encouraging more lone parents into work, reduced the numbers of children living in poverty, the significant reductions in the first half of the decade have not been maintained. The number of children living in poverty has fallen from about 4.5 million in 1998/9 to about 4 million in 2007/8. The reform of the child support legislation in 2000 failed to improve the performance of the Child Support Agency and the discredited agency was finally replaced by the Child Maintenance and Enforcement Commission in 2008. As the measure of child poverty is relative it is unlikely that levels of poverty will be significantly reduced while economic inequality remains high in the UK.

Long-term care for the frail elderly

Although the Labour government from 1997 focused on helping families with children as their approach to family policy they also had to consider the social and economic costs of an ageing population. The projected large increases in the 'old old' led to concern about how the cost of care could be met. A Royal Commission on Long-Term Care for the Elderly (1999) recommended that the state should pay for all long-term personal care, but a dissenting minority report reduced the impact of its recommendations. This idea was rejected by the government, although a policy of free personal care was introduced in Scotland in 2002. In England and Wales, state-funded personal care remained means tested.

The debate about financing long-term care continued throughout this period with different options suggested for financing it. In 2008 the Department of Health urged debate about the long-term future of England's care and support system, and a 2009 Green Paper outlined proposals for the funding of adult social care. In 2010 a White Paper (Department of Health 2010) published proposals to build a comprehensive free National Care Service for adults in England with an eligible care need.

Cohort potential for analysis of family change and policy

Because the nature of family life and family-related policies was strikingly different for each of the birth cohorts, data from the studies can help in determining the effects of increasing diversity of family life on inequalities in adulthood and in evaluating the effectiveness of the developing family policies. Different types of questions could be addressed.

- To what extent are family careers and experiences, such as teenage motherhood, repeated in the following generation, and is this less true for later cohorts of young women when teenage motherhood is less common?
- Do the known long-term negative effects of childhood adversity on the trajectories, experiences and opportunities in adulthood vary between cohorts? For example, the 1970 cohort was much more likely to experience family breakdown in childhood than previous cohorts and this can be followed through to examine later life developments in psychosocial health, physical health and health-related behaviour as well as trajectories of educational development and occupation.
- To what extent did a particular family policy have the intended impact? Variation in support from the state can be examined both within and between cohorts to determine whether and how it is related to the alleviation of family inequality.
- To what extent is there evidence from the cohort studies to inform emerging family issues? For example, the recent interest in the links between criminality and family background or inter-family support between the generations, both from and to the elderly/grandparents and grandchildren.
- What underlies the changes witnessed in family life and personal relationships? For example, what are the geographical and social patterns of family change? How have family formation and childbearing patterns changed over time between the cohorts and how are these related to changes in the labour market?
- What are the consequences of the changing labour market behaviours of men and women for family life; how has this affected the domestic roles of men and women, the nature and stability of partnerships, approaches to parenting and the well-being of children, mothers and fathers?

Conclusions

Family structures and family experiences changed markedly in the post-war era. Families have become smaller on average but with more complex relationships between generations and other households. Children have increasingly experienced a variety of family settings and the family has undergone extensive change resulting from fewer marriages, more cohabitation and births outside marriage, more divorce, family breakdown and remarriage or re-partnership and a rise in lone parent families and stepfamilies. Although the nuclear family still remains the most prevalent form, for increasing numbers of people it has become only one of the family forms they will experience. However, families are still the most important source of support and care for the majority of older people and dependants. There is a growing divide, however, between people with advantageous family lives and those in unfavourable situations, linked to education, economic prosperity and secure employment.

Partly as a consequence of these changes, interest in public policy for families has grown. Over the last sixty years Britain has moved from policies that affected families – an implicit family policy – to policies that helped families. The last twenty years have been characterised by an initially slow appreciation that a more active and even explicit policy towards families was needed. Since the late 1990s this has grown apace. There is no doubt that the emphasis on early intervention, supporting parents and tackling child poverty is central to recent policy towards families. There is an economic argument for this. In an increasingly globalised world Britain needs productive citizens to remain competitive; it cannot afford for children to fail and it needs to bring women into the labour market. These reasons, as much as the aspirations and desires of family members, are drivers in the changes we have seen.

References

Anderson, R., Brown, I., Dowty, T., Inglesant, P., Heath, W. and Sasse, A. (2009) *Database state*, York: Joseph Rowntree Foundation.

Annual Population Survey (2008) Office of National Statistics. Available at http://www.ons.gov.uk/about-statistics/user-guidance/lm-guide/sources/household/aps/index.html (last accessed 17 January 2011).

APPG (All Party Parliamentary Group) (1994) Report of the All Party Parliamentary Group on Parenting and International Year of the Family, London: UK Parliamentary Hearings.

Barnes, H., Day, P. and Cronin, N. (1998) *Trial and error – a review of child support policy*, London: Family Policy Studies Centre.

Beck, U. (1992) *Risk society: towards a new modernity*, London: Sage.

Becker, G. S., Landes, E. M. and Michael, E. C. (1977) 'An economic analysis of marital stability', *Journal of Political Economy*, 85: 1141–87.

Belsky, J., Barnes, J. and Melhuish, E. C. (eds) (2007) *The national evaluation of SureStart: does area-based early intervention work?,* Bristol: Policy Press.

Berthoud, R. (2007) *Work-rich and work-poor: three decades of change*, Bristol: Joseph Rowntree Foundation, Policy Press.

Boheim, R. and Ermisch, J. (2001) 'Partnership dissolution in the UK: the role of economic circumstances', *Oxford Bulletin of Economics and Statistics*, 63: 197–208.

Bradshaw, J. (1989) *Lone parents: policy in the doldrums*, London: Family Policy Studies Centre.

British Social Attitudes Survey (2006) London: Sage.

Burghes, L., Cronin, N. and Clarke, L. (1997) *Fathers and fatherhood in Britain*, London: Family Policy Studies Centre.

Chan, T. W. and Halpin, B. (2008) 'The instability of divorce risk factors in the UK', Working Papers, Oxford: Department of Sociology, University of Oxford.

Clarke, L. (1996) 'Demographic change and the family situation of children in Britain', in J. Brannen and M. O'Brien (eds) *Children in families: research and policy*, pp. 66–83, London: Falmer Press.

Clarke, L. and Berrington, A. (1999) 'Socio-demographic predictors of divorce', in Simons, J. (ed.) *High divorce rates: the state of the evidence on reasons and remedies: reviews of the evidence on the causes of marital breakdown and the effectiveness of policies and services intended to reduce its incidence*, *Research Series Vol. 1*, pp. 1–38, London: Lord Chancellor's Department.

Coote, A. and Campbell, B. (1982) *Sweet freedom – the struggle for women's liberation*, London: Pan Books.

DCSF (Department for Children, Schools and Families) (2007) *The children's plan: building brighter futures*, London: Department for Children, Schools and Families.

DCSF (2010) *Support for all: the families and relationships Green Paper*, London: Stationery Office.

Deakin, N. (1988) 'Family and government', in N. Deakin and M. Wicks (eds) *Families and the state*, pp. 4–18, London: Family Policy Studies Centre.

Dennis, N. and Erdos, G. (1992) *Families without fatherhood*, London: Institute of Economic Affairs, Health and Welfare Unit.

Department of Health (2000) *Protecting children, supporting parents*, London: HMSO.

Department of Health (2010) *Building the national care service*, London: Stationery Office.

Department of Social Security (1998) *Children first: a new approach to child support*, Cm 3992, London: HMSO.

DHSS (Department of Health and Social Security) (1974) *The family in society: dimensions of parenthood*, London: HMSO.

Dominian, J. (1980) *Marriage in Britain, 1945–1980*, London: Study Commission on the Family.

Duncan, S. and Phillips, M. (2008) 'New families? Tradition and change in modern relationship', in A. Park, J. Curtice and K. Thomson (eds) *British social attitudes: the 24th report*, pp. 1–28, London: Sage.

Dunn, J. and Deater-Deckard, K. (2001) *Children's views of their changing families*, York: Joseph Rowntree Foundation.

Dunnell, K. (2007) 'The changing demographic picture of the UK: the National Statistician's annual article on the population', *Population Trends*, 130: 9–21.

Ermisch, J. (2001) 'Births outside marriage: the real story', *The Edge*, 8: 8–9.

Evans, T. (2006) 'Is it futile to try to get non-resident fathers to maintain their children?' Available at http://www.historyandpolicy.org/papers/policy-paper-48.html (last accessed 4 January 2011).

Fagin, L. and Little, M. (1984) *The forsaken families*, London: Penguin.

Family Policy Bulletin (1991) December issue, London: Family Policy Studies Centre.

Feijten, P., Boyle, P., Feng, Z., Gayle, V. and Graham, E. (2009) 'Step-parenting and mental health', in J. Stillwell, E. Coast and D. Kneale (eds) *Fertility, living arrangements, care and mobility*, pp.151–170, London: Springer.

Finch, J. and Summerfield, P. (1991) 'Social reconstruction and the emergence of companionate marriage', in D. Clark (ed.) *Marriage, domestic life and social change – writings for Jackie Burgoyne*, pp. 7–32, London: Routledge.

FPSC (Family Policy Studies Centre) (1998a) 'The Crime and Disorder Bill and the family', Family Briefing Paper No. 3, London: Family Policy Studies Centre.
FPSC (1998b) 'Families and childcare', Family Briefing Paper No. 6, London: Family Policy Studies Centre.
FPSC (1998c) 'Welfare to work and the family', Family Briefing Paper No. 5, London: Family Policy Studies Centre.
FPSC (1998d) 'Fairness at work and the family', Family Briefing Paper No. 7, London: Family Policy Studies Centre.
FPSC (2000) 'Long-term care and the family', Family Briefing Paper No. 16, London: Family Policy Studies Centre.
George, R. H. and Roberts, C. (2009) 'The media and the family courts – key information and questions about the Children, Schools and Families Bill', Family Policy Briefing 6, Oxford: Department of Social Policy and Social Work, University of Oxford.
Gittins, D. (1985) *The family in question*, London: Macmillan.
Hansen, K., Joshi, H. and Verropoulou, G. (2006) 'Childcare and mothers' employment: approaching the millennium', *National Institute Economic Review*, 195: 84–102.
Haskey, J. (2001) 'Cohabitation in Great Britain: having a partner who usually lives elsewhere and living apart together (LAT)', *Population Trends*, 122: 35–45.
Henwood, M., Rimmer, L. and Wicks, M. (1987) *Inside the family: changing roles of men and women*, London: Family Policy Studies Centre.
HM Treasury (2003) *Every child matters*, London: Stationery Office.
HMSO (Her Majesty's Stationery Office) (1986) *The reform of personal taxation Green Paper*, cmnd. 9756, London: HMSO.
Home Office (1998) *Supporting families: a consultation document*, London: Stationery Office.
Hunt, A. (1968) *A survey of women's employment*, London: HMSO.
Hunt, J. and Roberts, C. (2004) 'Child contact with non-resident parents', Family Policy Briefing 3, Oxford: Department of Social Policy and Social Work, University of Oxford.
Hunt, J. and Roberts, C. (2005) 'Intervening in litigated contact: ideas from other jurisdictions', Family Policy Briefing 4, Oxford: Department of Social Policy and Social Work, University of Oxford.
Inglehart, R. (1990) *Culture shift in advanced industrial society*, Princeton: Princeton University Press.
James, C. (2009) 'Ten years of family policy 1999–2009', Policy Discussion Paper, London: Family and Parenting Institute.
Joshi, H., Cooksey, E., Wiggins, R., McCulloch, A., Verropoulou, G. and Clarke, L. (1999) 'Diverse family living conditions and child development: a multi-level analysis comparing longitudinal evidence from Great Britain and the United States', *International Journal of Law, Policy and the Family*, 13: 292–314.
Kiernan, K. and Wicks, M. (1990) *Family change and future policy*, York: Joseph Rowntree Memorial Trust.
Kiernan, K. and Smith, K. (2003) 'Unmarried parenthood: new insights from the Millennium Cohort Study', *Population Trends*, 114: 26–33.
Kiernan, K. and Pickett, K. E. (2006) 'Marital status disparities in maternal smoking during pregnancy, breastfeeding and maternal depression', *Social Science and Medicine*, 63: 335–6.
Kiernan, K., Land, H. and Lewis, J. (1998) *Lone motherhood in 20th century Britain: from footnote to front page*, Oxford: Oxford University Press.

Lister, R. and Bennett, F. (1986) *Opportunity lost: a response to the Green Paper on the Reform of Personal Taxation*, London: Child Poverty Action Group.

McAllister, F. and Clarke, L. (1998) *Choosing childlessness. Family and parenthood, policy and practice*, York: Joseph Rowntree Foundation and the Family Policy Studies Centre.

McConnell, H. and Wilson, B. (2007) 'Families', in S. Smallwood and B. Wilson (eds) *Focus on families*, pp. 2–17, Basingstoke: Palgrave Macmillan.

McGlone, F., Park, A. and Smith, K. (1998) *Family and kinship*, London: Family Policy Studies Centre.

Martin, J. and Roberts, C. (1984) *Women and employment: a lifetime perspective*, London: HMSO.

Matheson, J. (2009) 'The National Statistician's annual article on the population: a demographic review', *Population Trends*, 138: 7–21.

Murphy, M. (2000) 'The evolution of cohabitation in Britain', *Population Studies*, 54: 43–56.

Office of Health Economics (2009) 'Growth in UK elderly population and projections as a percentage of UK population, 1948–2051'. Available at http://www.ohe.org/lib/liDownload/110/comp2.csv?CFID=976145&CFTOKEN=59925903 (last accessed 17 December 2010).

ONS (Office for National Statistics) (2002) *Social Trends*, No. 32, London: Office for National Statistics.

ONS (2005) 'Stepfamilies'. Available at http://www.statistics.gov.uk/CCI/nugget.asp?ID=1164&Pos=&ColRank=1&Rank=374 (last accessed 17 December 2010).

ONS (2008a) *Social Trends*, No. 38, p. 5, London: Palgrave Macmillan.

ONS (2008b) *Social Trends*, No. 38, pp. 15–28, London: Palgrave Macmillan.

ONS (2008c) 'General household survey (longitudinal)', *Social Trends*, No. 38, Figure 2.8. Available at http://www.statistics.gov.uk/downloads/theme_social/Social_Trends38/Social_Trends_38.pdf (last accessed 16 January 2011).

ONS (2008d) *Work and family: two-thirds of mums are employed*, Newport: Office of National Statistics.

ONS (2009a) *Social Trends*, No. 39, London: Palgrave Macmillan.

ONS (2009b) 'Report: births in England and Wales, 2008', *Population Trends,* No. 138, pp. 85–89, London: Palgrave Macmillan.

ONS (2009c) 'Population by age, sex and legal marital status'. Available at http://www.statisitcs.gov.uk/STATBASE/Expodata/Spreadsheets/D9532.xls (last accessed 17 December 2010).

ONS (2009d) 'Dependent population by age, United Kingdom'. Available at http://www.statistics.gov.uk/STATBASE/Expodata/Spreadsheets/D4968.xls (last accessed 17 December 2010).

ONS (2009e) 'Fewer children live in married couple families'. Available at http://www.statistics.gov.uk/cci/nugget.asp?id=2193 (last accessed 17 December 2010).

ONS (2009f) 'Percentage of dependent children living in different family types'. Available at http://www.statistics.gov.uk/STATBASE/Expodata/Spreadsheets/D7256.xls (last accessed 17 December 2010).

Pryor, J. and Rodgers, B. (2001) *Children in changing families: life after parental separation*, Oxford: Blackwell.

Rathborne, E. (1940) *The case for family allowances*, London: Penguin.

Roberts, C. (1996) 'Families and parenting: conference report', in Utting, D. (ed.) *Families and parenting: conference report*, Paper 22, pp. 6–8, London: FPSC.

Roll, J. (1991) *What is a family?*, London: Family Policy Studies Centre.

Segal, L. (ed.) (1983) *What is to be done about the family? Crisis in the eighties*, London: Penguin.

Smart, C. (1999) 'Divorce in England 1950 to 2000: a moral tale', Care, Values and the Future of Welfare (CAVA) Workshop Paper no. 2, Leeds University.

Social Exclusion Unit (1999) *Teenage pregnancy*, London: Stationery Office.

Straw, J. and Anderson, J. (1996) *Parenting: a discussion paper*, London: Labour Party.

Townsend, P. (1979) *Poverty in the UK*, London: Penguin.

Utting, D., Bright, J., and Henderson, C. (1993) *Crime and the family: improving child-rearing and preventing delinquency*, London: Family Policy Studies Centre.

van de Kaa, D. J. (1987) 'Europe's second demographic transition', *Population Bulletin*, 42, London: ONS.

van de Kaa, D. J. (2003) 'Second demographic transition', in P. Demeny and G. McNicoll (eds) *Encyclopaedia of population*, pp. 872–5, New York: Macmillan Reference USA, Thomson-Gale.

Welshman, J. (1999) 'The social history of social work: the issue of the "problem family" 1940–1970', *British Journal of Social Work*, 29: 457–76.

Welshman, J. (2008) 'The cycle of deprivation: myths and misconceptions', *Children and Society*, 22: 75–85.

Wicks, M. (1983) *Families in the future*, London: Study Commission on the Family.

Wilson, B. (2009) 'Estimating the cohabiting population', *Population Trends*, 136: 21–7.

Wilson, E. (1977) *Women and the welfare state*, London: Tavistock Press.

Wynn, M. (1972) *Family policy: a study of the economic costs of rearing children and their social and political consequences*, London: Penguin.

Young, M. and Willmott, P. (1957) *Family and kinship in East London*, London: Routledge and Kegan Paul.

4 Education policy and practice

Gary McCulloch

Introduction

The current chapter sets out to examine the changing educational and social context in Britain since the Second World War, and also to relate this to the experience and effects of education policy. The scope of the chapter includes nursery education, primary education, secondary education, further education, higher education and adult and continuing education, and the discussion will focus on England, Wales and Scotland during this period. It will summarise continuities and changes in policy for education over this time with reference to the key acts and by describing trends in aims and attitudes, for example in relation to perceptions of the role and purpose of education in relation to the economy, social stability and low crime rates, and the fostering of a caring and participant democracy. These perceptions are reflected in the many reports published on education since the 1940s. They are played out in concerns about how to match educational provision with the requirements of the economy in a time of rapid technological change, and also about wastage of talent, inequality of opportunity, selection, assessment and measurement of educational performance, improving standards, expanding higher education, choice and control.

The chapter examines education policy in three key phases of education reform since the Education Act of 1944 and the end of the Second World War, making particular reference to the principal reports and legislation bearing on the different aspects of education. Each of these periods includes political changes and shifts in emphasis, but they also have an element of internal consistency. The first period, from 1945 to 1964, was broadly one of educational partnership and expansion following the Education Act of 1944. The second, from 1964 until 1979, encompassed educational debate and further expansion in different areas of education. The third, from 1979 until 2010, witnessed extensive educational reforms influenced by the 'New Right' and 'New Labour' currents that characterised this time.

In relation to educational practice the principal concern of the chapter is with the realisation of changes in education policy, for example concern with wasted talent, standards and equality, debates around private and state education, and trends towards child-centred education, mixed ability teaching, provision for special educational needs, mass higher education and widening participation. More broadly the chapter charts the effects of changes in the social, cultural, religious and economic context over this period, including change in relation to gender, social class, ethnicity, employment and religious practices. These are examined in relation to the policy developments in each of the key phases discussed, and with examples of personal experiences of education noted in biographical and autobiographical studies. Statistical data also demonstrate for example the changing size of the population of compulsory school age and the proportions staying on at school and going into further and higher education. The concluding section will discuss opportunities for new life course studies that could take advantage of the opportunities that the cohorts offer over this period.

Continuity and change

This first section traces the general continuities and changes of educational policy over this time. In broad generational terms this encompasses the Education Act of 1944, with its emphasis on an integrated education service, partnership and citizenship, although encouraging the development of different kinds of secondary schools, and the Education Reform Act of 1988, which emphasised parental choice and diversity of provision within the framework of a national structure of curriculum and examinations. It also reflects changing political regimes, from Labour's post-war reforms to the Conservative dominance of 1951–64, further reforms under Labour from 1964 to 1970, Conservative responses from 1970 to 1974, Labour policies from 1974 to 1979, Conservative reforms from 1979 to 1997 and, most latterly, developments under Labour from 1997 until 2010 (see, for example, Aldrich 2002).

Overarching changes since 1945 in relation to demography, statistical trends and changes in attitudes will also be considered in this first section. This section will examine in detail the relevant demographic changes over the period, for example changes in school age. It will also trace relevant statistical trends since the 1940s, such as in educational attainment and training qualifications, and identify and illustrate trends in relevant attitudes, for example to educational devolution, higher education and vocational education. The statistics, however, do not always allow a clear review of changes and continuities over this period as a whole, as in some cases the basis for collection has been significantly amended over time, and the figures may relate to England only, to England and Wales, to England, Wales and Northern Ireland or to the United Kingdom as a whole.

The overarching legislation for education during this time, besides a very large amount of relatively minor amendments in particular areas and legislation affecting Scotland, Wales and Northern Ireland in particular, were the Education Act of 1944 and the Education Reform Act of 1988. The former, taken through by R. A. Butler, as the president of the Board of Education under the wartime coalition government, established secondary education for all up to the age of fifteen years (by 1947). The act itself did not specify different types of secondary schools, although the new Ministry of Education preferred local education authorities (LEAs) to support a 'tripartite' arrangement of grammar schools for a small academic elite, technical schools for those with technical ability and non-selective modern schools for the majority (McCulloch 1994). There were also to be three successive phases of education – primary, secondary and tertiary – rather than the parallel class-based systems that had existed before the war (Simon 1974). The system as a whole was to be based on partnership between the state, which was responsible for general policy, the LEAs, which provided a local service appropriate for their areas, and schools and teachers, who exercised professional judgement in the curriculum domain in the interests of the pupils and students in their care (Sharp 2002). The Act of 1988 was introduced by Kenneth Baker under Margaret Thatcher's Conservative government. It replaced the earlier partnership arrangement so that the state was in full control of the system at the expense both of LEAs, whose powers were attenuated, and of teachers, and included for the first time a National Curriculum. The interests of parents as consumers of education were also recognised through greater rights and representation in the education service (Sharp 2002; Jones 2003).

In terms of numbers of pupils in maintained schools, this was a period of substantial growth and expansion. In 1946 there were just over 5 million full-time pupils in maintained primary and secondary schools in England and Wales; by 1977 this figure had risen to nearly 9 million (Simon 1991: 576), but fell to just over 7 million by 1988 (Simon 1991: 578). Similarly, numbers of pupils in secondary schools in England and Wales were 1.2 million in 1946, rose to over 4 million by 1977, but fell back to 3.25 million by 1988. However, although no pupils were recorded as being in comprehensive schools in 1946, this figure was nearly 3 million by 1977 and was still at around that level in 1988. In 1950 there were ten comprehensive schools with under 8,000 pupils; by 1976 there were 3,387 such schools; and in 1988 there were 3,379. The percentage of all secondary pupils in maintained schools who were in comprehensive schools in 1950 was 0.3 per cent; this figure was 75.6 per cent in 1976, and well over 90 per cent by 1988 (Simon 1991: 585–7; Table 4.1). By contrast, the number of pupils in direct grant and independent schools in England and Wales in 1950 was nearly 600,000 but by 1977 had fallen to 540,000, and in 1988 (in England only) was 523,000 (Simon 1991: 591; Table 4.1). At the turn of the century there were over 600,000 pupils in such schools, less than 7 per cent of pupils in all schools, which was over 10 million (NFER 2002: 79; Table 4.1).

There was also a trend towards the use of formal examinations during this time. Before and up to the 1940s, only a small minority went forward to School Certificate and Higher School Certificate examinations. The General Certificate of Education (GCE) was introduced from 1951 at Ordinary (O) and Advanced (A) levels, followed by the Certificate of Secondary Education (CSE) from 1962 for pupils of average ability. In 1947 a total of 133,678 candidates were entered for the School Certificate and Higher School Certificate combined, compared with over 1.5 million candidates entered for CSE, O-level and A-level examinations thirty years later in 1977, and nearly 6.2 million subject entries at these different levels (Gosden 1983: 75). In 1986, O levels and CSEs were combined to form a new examination, the General Certificate of Secondary Education (GCSE), now taken by nearly all pupils. Despite this major expansion of the system, and an

Table 4.1 Full-time pupils in primary and secondary schools, United Kingdom

	School pupils (thousands) by type of school			
	1970/1	*1980/1*	*1990/1*	*2000/1*
Nursery	50	89	105	152
Primary	5,902	5,171	4,955	5,298
Secondary				
Comprehensive	1,313	3,730	2,843	3,340
Grammar	673	149	156	205
Modern	1,164	233	94	112
Other	403	434	300	260
All public schools	9,507	9,806	8,453	9,367
Non-maintained	621	619	613	626
Special schools	103	148	114	113
Pupil referral units				10
All schools	10,230	10,572	9,180	10,116

Source: *Social Trends* (2002).

increase in the numbers succeeding in these examinations, the total achieving grades equivalent to O level in 1988 remained a small minority of the age cohort and had changed little since 1964 (Lowe 1997: 13–14). Under the Education Reform Act of 1988, moreover, a new testing regime was introduced for pupils in English and mathematics at the age of seven years and English, mathematics and science at ages eleven and fourteen, in addition to the existing examinations that were taken at ages sixteen and eighteen, forming the basis for national league tables of schools and LEAs. The Qualifications and Curriculum Authority (QCA) was then established in 1997 to take further the centralisation of examinations and curriculum matters that had earlier been dispersed. At the same time, vocational qualifications were developed for a broad range of students, although the nature and purpose of these were contested, and initiatives in this area tended to be short-lived and just as quickly superseded (Wolf 2002).

In higher education the number of full-time university students in the UK was 38,000 in 1944 and 288,000 in 1978; by the latter date there were also 49,000 students in teacher training and another 150,000 in further education (Simon 1991: 497). Emphasis shifted from part-time to full-time courses. In England alone in 1964, there were seven times as many part-timers as there were full-time students, and by 1988 there were still almost twice as many (over 1.5 million in part-time further education courses compared with 800,000 full-time students) (Lowe 1997: 19–20; Tight 2009; see Table 4.2).

In Scotland, with its largely separate provision, there was also an overall pattern of growth in a range of education sectors. Educational provision was selective

Table 4.2 UK university students

Date	*Total*[a]	*Full-time undergraduate*	*Men*	*Women*	*Women (%)*
1945	49,809	36,837	32,873	16,936	34.0
1955	104,400	71,591	74,867	29,533	28.3
1965	180,820	131,796	115,460	65,360	36.2
1975	283,057	209,078	191,313	91,744	32.4
1985	345,560	254,819	208,237	137,323	39.7
1995	1,534,369	817,788	767,477	766, 892	50.0
2005	2,287,545	1,165,445	979,180	1,308,365	57.2

Source: Adapted from Tight (2009: 55–6).

Note
a Includes part-time undergraduates.

after the Second World War and most working class children left school at ten or eleven, but selection was abolished in 1965, leading to an almost universal pattern of comprehensive education. The Education (Scotland) Act of 1945 led to the growth of a youth and community service that attempted to offer a comprehensive service for young people and adults (Standish 2003). By the 1960s there was increasing demand to stay on longer at school, and the school leaving age was raised to sixteen in 1973. Post-school education also expanded both in technical colleges and universities (Anderson 2003). The Education (Scotland) Act of 1980 with its subsequent amendments was the primary educational legislation in Scotland, although the Standards in Scotland's Schools Act of 2000 was also significant in setting out a new improvement framework and a legal basis for children's rights (Jeyes 2003).

Pre-school education expanded strongly in Scotland from the 1980s, when 20 per cent of three-year-olds and 40 per cent of four-year-olds had an education authority nursery place, to the end of the century, when these figures were 80 per cent and 97 per cent respectively. Primary school pupil numbers were at their height of half a million in the late 1970s, and fell back to 430,000 in the 1980s, before returning to nearly half a million in the mid-1990s, and again falling to 432,250 by 2001. Secondary school pupil numbers peaked at over 400,000 in 1980, fell to under 300,000 by 1990, and rose again to reach 334,000 by 2001 when there were 444 secondary schools (Paterson 2003). By 2009 there were 2,151 primary schools, 375 secondary schools and 182 special schools in Scotland, with 676,760 pupils in publicly funded schools and an additional 30,507 pupils in independent schools (Scottish Government 2010). After leaving school in 1980, 35 per cent of pupils entered further or higher education, but by 2001 47 per cent of eighteen-year-olds remained in education. In 1975, 18 per cent of people entered higher education by the time they were twenty-one, compared with 26 per cent in 1990 and 50 per cent in 2000 (Paterson 2003). Both gender and social class differences in access to higher education changed over this time. The proportion of female undergraduates rose from 43 per cent in 1980 to 57 per cent by 2000. Whereas in 1980 school leavers whose fathers were in professional occupations were six times more likely to enter higher education than were leavers whose fathers were in manual occupations, by 1994 they were only twice as likely to do so (Paterson 2003 gives an overview of provision in Scotland).

These extensions in the education system and the growth in the active role of the state led to a large increase in educational expenditure over the period as a whole (see Table 4.3). In 1953–4 central government spent £46.9 million and local government £460.3 million, with educational expenditure as a whole at 3 per cent of the gross national product. Ten years later these figures were £198 million, £1,129 million and 4.3 per cent, and a decade on in 1973–4 had increased again to £670 million, £3,566 million and 5.7 per cent. This trend itself reflected a sustained period of economic growth in Britain, which averaged about 2.8 per cent a year between 1948 and 1973 (Timmins 1995: 177). The amounts continued to climb although the percentage of gross domestic product began to fall from its peak of 6.3 per cent in 1976–7 to return to less than 5 per cent by the late 1980s (Simon 1991: 599), before rising again to a level comparable to the 1970s under the Labour government at the turn of the century (Jones 2003: 144), and under the new Scottish government.

The first period: 1945–64

This is broadly a period of educational partnership and expansion following the Education Act of 1944 until the narrow election of Harold Wilson's Labour government in 1964. All sectors of education experienced further development and growth during this time, although the grammar schools that had emerged unscathed from the reforms of the 1940s came under increasing political pressure.

Table 4.3 Educational expenditure, United Kingdom

Date	*Central government (£M)*	*Local government (£M)*	*Total (£M)*
1955/6	54.6	552.4	607.0
1960/1	109.3	819.4	938.7
1965/6	278	1,358	1,636
1970/1	422	2,318	2,740
1975/6	980	6,043	7,023
1980/1	1,779	11,270	13,049
1985/6	2,398	15,041	17,439
1991/2	4,288	25,261	29,550
1996/7	11,388	26,562	37,953

Sources: Simon (1991); *Annual Abstract of Statistics* (2001).

Indeed, during this time provision for secondary education as a whole came under increasing scrutiny. Broadly, the system expanded when economic growth permitted, on the basis that it represented a significant social and economic investment for the future to reduce the high levels of wasted talent that had been permitted hitherto, while the high costs involved in this expansion became acceptable.

Attlee's Labour government from 1945 until 1951 was committed to taking forward the reforms signalled by the 1944 Act, but economic pressures made it difficult to prioritise these. It was agreed to proceed with the raising of the school leaving age to fifteen in 1947, although the school building programme was less than adequate for this. Of even greater concern for many reformers were the plans for secondary education for all, which proved to be based in many local areas on a range of systems of grammar, technical and modern schools. Under Section 11 of the 1944 Act, every LEA in England and Wales was obliged, in consultation with the Ministry of Education, to draw up a development plan that specified the nature of local provision in its area.

Among the few LEAs that championed an arrangement of multilateral or comprehensive education in its development plan was the London County Council. Swansea was another that advocated the introduction of multilateral high schools for pupils of all abilities (Jones 1990). Most LEAs opted for either a bipartite or a tripartite arrangement. Durham preferred a bipartite scheme in which 25 per cent of pupils went to grammar-technical schools and the remainder to modern schools (McCulloch 2002: 238). Others including Lancashire (the largest LEA outside London in terms of child population) and Sheffield were strong advocates of tripartism (McCulloch 2002: 241–3). A majority of LEAs in urban areas maintained at least one school that they described as technical in nature, but they were rarer in country areas. By 1950 there were still only 300 such schools, mainly for boys, with about 4 per cent of the secondary school population. This was testimony to the uncertain status of secondary technical education in England, unlike some other countries, and reflected the practical difficulties of pupil selection at age eleven, provision of equipment and accommodation, and the development of a suitable curriculum and teaching force for such schools (McCulloch 1989).

In higher education the Percy Report (1945) on higher technological education and the Barlow Report (1946) on scientific manpower both sought further expansion of and an increased emphasis on science and technology in the university sector. Demand for places in higher education increased, partly fuelled by ex-servicemen completing their courses and by larger numbers of students beginning to come from secondary education. Consequently there was demand for new universities. The University College of North Staffordshire was established in 1949 (University of Keele from 1962), an early portent of growth (Gosden 1983; Lowe 2002).

The Conservative government elected at the end of 1951 initially found little place for education, but, as the economy began to improve and social aspirations increased, education began to take on a higher public and political profile. By the final stages of the Conservative government in the early 1960s, education had been recognised as a key social and economic investment.

The selective system of secondary education came under increasing pressure during the 1950s. The eleven-plus examination, the prime instrument of selection, attracted much criticism for the unfairness and social inequality that it was held to engender, while many pupils came under strong pressure from their families to pass it (Sandbrook 2005: 395–7). For children like the young John Lennon in Liverpool, success in the eleven-plus could be rewarded with a brand-new bicycle; Lennon's own achievement in the examination in 1952 won him not only a green Raleigh Lenton but a choice between several grammar schools in central and suburban Liverpool from which he entered Quarry Bank High School. Although no fees were charged, each pupil's family was expected to supply the compulsory uniform of black blazer, cap and tie (Norman 2008: 58–9). Two years later, the future Conservative prime minister, John Major, passed the eleven-plus examination in south London and entered Rutlish School, a local boys' grammar school, where he was bullied by other pupils and left after taking his O levels (Seldon 1997: 12). Others, like the future deputy prime minister John Prescott in 1949, failed the eleven-plus examination and went to the local secondary modern school (Prescott 2008).

The Conservative government was determined to defend grammar schools and also to maintain secondary modern schools against a growing agitation for the widespread introduction of comprehensive education. There were significant differences in the social composition of grammar schools compared with the secondary modern schools. In London, for example, modern schools catered mainly for the children of manual workers, especially the semi-skilled and unskilled, while relatively few working class children were educated in grammar schools, which tended to be largely middle class in nature (Halsey and Gardner 1953; McCulloch 1998: 76–80). The social prestige of grammar schools was clearly much higher than that of technical or modern schools, which the sociologist Olive Banks attributed to the importance of examination success for upwards social mobility and occupational security. While the GCE examination, like the School Certificate before it, was prized as the passport to a better job or career, there could be no parity of esteem between different types of school (Banks 1955; McCulloch 2008).

The system of further education was also extended. In 1955, a National Council was appointed, headed by Lord Hives, chairman of Rolls-Royce, to make awards to successful technological students in technical colleges. In February 1956, a five-year programme of investment of £85 million for technical colleges was announced in a key White Paper, *Technical Education* (Ministry of Education 1956). It reflected increasing concern about international economic competition, but stressed that the expanding technical colleges should be flexible and versatile and include broader and more liberal courses, rather than remain narrowly vocational (McCulloch *et al.* 1985: 52–3). Similarly the education of boys and girls between the ages of fifteen and eighteen began to be examined by the Central Advisory Council for Education (England) from March 1956, under the chairmanship of Sir Geoffrey Crowther, the deputy chairman of Economist Newspaper Ltd. The Crowther Report, *15 to 18* (Ministry of Education 1959), recommended raising the school leaving age from fifteen to sixteen, giving this immediate priority over the provision of compulsory part-time education for all young persons of sixteen and seventeen who were not engaged in full-time education. It calculated that only one in eight young people between sixteen and eighteen years were continuing in full-time education, and recommended that this proportion should be increased to 50 per cent within twenty years (McCulloch 1989: chapter 7).

The annual cost of education in England and Wales had already increased from £280 million to £700 million in the previous ten years, but new demands arose. One concerned the education of the 'ordinary child', whose needs were examined in the Newsom Report (Ministry of Education 1963). It agreed with the Crowther Report that the school leaving age should be raised to sixteen, and argued that more support was needed for facilities and buildings especially in deprived urban areas. It also recommended that the kind of education that made most sense for the majority of pupils aged from thirteen to sixteen was practical, realistic and vocational, while also allowing opportunities for personal fulfillment.

Six days later, the Robbins Report on higher education was published (Committee on Higher Education 1963), which demonstrated the scale of the challenge that had developed in the universities. The number of university students had more than doubled since the war, while the number in training colleges and colleges of education had increased more than fourfold, and an even more marked growth had taken place in full-time students taking advanced courses in further education. Only 7.3 per cent of women in the age group entered full-time higher education in 1962, compared with 9.8 per cent of men, and if part-time education was included the figures were under 8 per cent of women and over 22 per cent of men. Moreover, only a quarter of students in British universities were women, whereas over two-thirds of the students in training colleges in England and Wales were women (Committee on Higher Education 1963: chapter 3). The committee's solution to these demands and inequalities was to expand the university system, based on the key principle that 'courses of higher education should be available for all those who are qualified by ability and attainment to pursue them and who wish to do so' (Committee on Higher Education 1963: 8).

Overall, then, education policy was receptive to growth and sought to achieve further expansion of the system over this time, seeking to promote education as an investment in what came to be described as human capital. Although it constituted a key part of the new welfare state, it also remained largely wedded to meritocratic and hierarchical approaches that maintained social differences and hierarchies. These were increasingly criticised by the later 1950s, and Michael Young's powerful satire *The Rise of the Meritocracy* reflected an emerging resentment at such inequalities (Young 1958). At the same time, education generally harboured ideals of educators as professionals who could be trusted to take care of their pupils and students without excessive involvement on the part of the state.

The second period: 1964–79

The second period is broadly one of educational debate and further expansion in different areas of education, which encouraged the state to become more actively involved. Over this time education was a key policy issue and became increasingly politicised. Moreover, during the 1970s it came to be viewed by many at least as being responsible for worsening industrial and economic problems, leading to public controversy and new calls for reform.

The debates of the 1960s and 1970s did not lead, at least initially, to major legislation of the stature of the 1944 Education Act. Instead they developed areas that had been overlooked or delayed in the 1940s, such as secondary school organisation, progressive education in primary schools, curriculum reform and higher education. From 1964 the Ministry of Education became the Department of Education and Science, reflecting the growing importance attached to scientific issues, and there was briefly also a separate Ministry of Technology. Overall this was a period of dominant emphasis on egalitarian reform and social justice in education, although the reformers' aims were by no means achieved in all cases, and as with the earlier phases of development there was an important ambiguity in terms of continuity and change (McCulloch 1994: 33).

In the early 1960s nearly 4,000 secondary modern schools in England and Wales catered for over 1.5 million pupils who had not been selected at the age of eleven either for a grammar school or for a technical school. Some modern schools gained a well-justified reputation as dumping grounds for the rejected with little hope for their futures, although others, especially those based in the more affluent suburbs, began to imitate some of the traditions of the grammar schools and introduced examinations (McCulloch 1998: chapters 6–7). However, after the election of the Labour government in 1964, there was a rapid shift in policy in favour of comprehensive schools. Circular 10/65, issued to LEAs the following year, requested them to submit plans for comprehensive reorganisation, although it did not require them to do so (DES 1965).

In primary schools, the reaction against the traditions of the old elementary schools intensified, and this led to the promotion of more child-centred and progressive methods of teaching. The Plowden Report of 1967, entitled *Children and their Primary Schools*, endorsed this general trend (Central Advisory Council for Education 1967). It sought to encourage 'positive discrimination' for schools in deprived areas, to develop educational priority areas (EPAs) and to discourage streaming of classes by ability. 'Open plan' primary schools were also intended as a movement away from the narrow and restrictive approach of the elementary schools.

In curriculum reform the 1960s also proved to be a phase of hectic activity. The 1944 Act had left the curriculum (except religious education) to the schools and LEAs, with teachers being chiefly responsible in this area. By the 1960s there was a wide range of agencies competing for influence. The Ministry of Education began to show some appetite for asserting a measure of control through the short-lived Curriculum Study Group (Dean 1997), which gave way in 1964 to the more broadly based consortium the Schools Council for Curriculum and Examinations. This new agency sponsored many curriculum projects in the 1960s and 1970s in concert with teachers in a wide range of subject areas including, for example, Project Technology and the Humanities Curriculum Project (Stenhouse 1980).

In higher education a concern to extend the range of the student clientele, combined with a perceived need for more technological skills, led to the development of polytechnics within the public sector (Sharp 1987). A binary system of universities and polytechnics was thus established, with academic degrees in polytechnics validated by the Council for National Academic Awards from 1965 until 1992. The Open University was also founded in 1969, catering for students over the age of twenty-one with few qualifications. It broadcast lectures on television, and encouraged more women, more mature students and more young people from different backgrounds to take part in higher education. By 1980 the Open University had 60,000 students (Lowe 2002: 84).

Despite this fresh activity there were many underlying continuities. The commotion of educational reform was rarely matched by fundamental change in educational practices. In primary schools, existing methods and assumptions were maintained, together with existing buildings and facilities, despite calls for a 'primary school revolution' (Simon 1991; Lowe 2007). By the end of the 1960s comprehensive reorganisation was well under way, with over 1,300 comprehensive schools including nearly one-third of secondary school age pupils, and many more were planned for the future (Benn and Simon 1972). On the other hand, this did not generally challenge the dominance of the academic curriculum of the grammar schools (Goodson 1988). It also became evident that in many cases the curriculum changes of the 1960s were not being adopted by schools, or were interpreted by teachers in ways contrary to the intentions of the reformers. Confident plans for a new curriculum soon gave way to disenchantment, especially with declining financial resources in the 1970s. Independent schools also remained highly resistant to reform, and indeed became more popular than before in direct competition with public provision. In higher education long-established universities retained a higher status than newer universities and polytechnics, while the proportion of working class students failed to rise significantly. In general, many thought that the apparent rapid change had been illusory, and that further reforms would be necessary.

To others, however, change had already gone too far and needed to be arrested and if possible reversed. There were signs of discontent with the direction of change from the early 1960s onwards. The novelist Kingsley Amis had complained of the planned increase in student numbers as early as 1960 on the grounds that 'more will mean worse' (Amis 1960: 6). By the end of the decade the self-styled 'Black Papers' declared open opposition to the social and cultural effects of current changes in primary, secondary and higher education (Cox and Dyson 1969a,b). A mixture of disillusionment with the present, fear of the future and nostalgia for the lost standards of an idealised past was also reflected in the work of the playwright Alan Bennett, in particular in 'Forty Years On' which was first performed in London in October 1968 (Bennett 1991). Bennett's play is set in Albion House, a public school on the South Downs of England, where the elderly headmaster is about to retire and give way to a young, impatient reformer, Franklin. It conveys the view that reform is futile at best and ultimately destructive of inherited traditions, with the hopes for the future doomed to disappointment and failure, in the process undermining the civilised values of English society (see also McCulloch 2007).

To some extent this conservative response represented a backlash against what were widely regarded as socially radical and subversive tendencies in education, exemplified in political protests by university students in the late 1960s and early 1970s (Crook 2006). Public controversy also arose over William Tyndale Junior School in Islington, north London, in the mid-1970s, relating to the ways in which teachers exerted undue influence over a progressive curriculum (Davis 2002). More than this, however, the overall character of educational changes symbolised by the Plowden Report and comprehensive education was often viewed with suspicion, and education policy began to reflect the antagonism that they engendered.

The Conservative government elected in 1970 continued to plan for expansion in education, as its White Paper of 1972, *Education: A Framework for Expansion* (DES 1972), made clear. The raising of the school leaving age was implemented in 1972–3. Although previous advice to LEAs to reorganise provision for secondary education on comprehensive lines was now rescinded, comprehensivisation accelerated in the early 1970s. However, growing economic and industrial difficulties began to influence the character of educational developments. In 1973, the Manpower Services Commission (MSC) was established under the aegis of the Department of Employment to help address the growing problem of unemployed youth through a Youth Opportunities Programme and a series of Youth Training Schemes. Under a Labour government from 1974, economic problems intensified, and plans for education became increasingly attuned to industrial and vocational needs while also seeking to alleviate renewed anxieties about declining educational standards.

In October 1976 the new prime minister, James Callaghan, made an unprecedented direct intervention in a speech at Ruskin College Oxford that was widely heralded as the start of a national 'Great Debate' in education. Callaghan said that, although he did not agree with those who 'paint a lurid picture of educational decline', nevertheless 'in today's world higher standards are demanded than were required yesterday and there are simply fewer jobs for those without skill'. Therefore, he concluded, 'we demand more from our schools than did our grandparents' (Callaghan 1976). In the following year a consultative Green Paper, *Education in Schools* (DES 1977), acknowledged that a major cause of criticism was the feeling that the educational system was out of touch with Britain's need to survive economically in a highly competitive world through the efficiency of its industry and commerce. These growing concerns also encouraged further direct involvement by the central state, thus undermining further the devolved partnership arrangement with LEAs and teachers that had been in operation since the 1940s.

By 1979, then, the debates about education that had developed since the early 1960s had raised important questions about the nature of educational provision and its role in preparing pupils for a changing society and for the world of work. The Conservative government elected in 1979 was presented with an opportunity to make radical changes in education in response to these demands.

The third period: 1979–2010

The period since 1979 is broadly one of protracted educational reform under Conservative governments (from 1979 to 1997) and Labour governments (from 1997 to 2010), influenced by the 'New Right' and 'New Labour' currents of the 1980s and 1990s. The 'New Right' phase under Margaret Thatcher emphasised the importance of opening up previously protected services like education and professions such as teachers and educators to the rigours of competition and demands imposed by greater consumer choice, although it also embraced neo-conservative fears about a decline in morality and support for the family. The 'New Labour' approach under Tony Blair, although continuing the thrust of Conservative education policies in the main, was more about cultivating a partnership between the public and private sectors and reforming as well as investing in services. Between them they led to a progressive centralisation that transformed the character of the education system.

One feature of educational changes in the 1980s was the need to cater more effectively for different groups in society that had hitherto been disadvantaged or largely ignored. The Education (Special Education) Act of 1981, based on the recommendations of the 1978 Warnock Report, *Special Educational Needs* (DES 1978), recommended the integration of children with special needs into mainstream schools as far as possible rather than segregation into special schools. The Swann Report of 1985 (DES 1985), following social unrest in the inner cities and increasing indications of educational inequalities faced by immigrants from overseas and their children, recommended reappraising the values and attitudes of education to promote multicultural education and meet the needs of a multiethnic society. At the same time, increasing attention was given to the educational achievements of girls in examinations and in accessing higher education (Tomlinson 2005: chapter 9). These developments reflected the wide range of patterns of social differentiation involving education, while also undermining the emphasis on social class inequalities that had been uppermost in previous decades.

Reforms in the school curriculum and examinations were designed initially to support vocational and industrial demands, but were increasingly framed in terms of enhancing standards of academic attainment. In 1982, the Technical and Vocational Education Initiative (TVEI), under the aegis of the Department of Employment and the Manpower Services Commission, sought to introduce a more technical and vocational curriculum for pupils over fourteen years who were less suited to an academic approach (McCulloch 1987). A further initiative in 1986 introduced city technology colleges (CTCs) as a 'new choice of schools' outside the influence of the LEAs, with a strong technological element in their curriculum (McCulloch 1989). However, as the economy improved, both initiatives were compromised to some extent by the more academic subject-based curriculum enforced by the Education Reform Act of 1988. As the main single legislative change in education over this period, although there were a very large number of others, this act aimed to reconcile the encouragement of parental choice with the enforcement of a national structure for curriculum, examinations and standards. It reduced the powers of LEAs and abolished the Inner London Educational

Authority, while enhancing the rights of parents to choose between schools and to take part in school governance. It also provided, for the first time, for a National Curriculum in schools, thus undermining the sphere of professional responsibility formerly associated with teachers, and established testing for all pupils at the ages of seven, eleven, fourteen and sixteen. In addition it introduced a new and stricter regime of monitoring standards in the form of the Office for Standards in Education (OFSTED), created in 1992. Its consolidation of state control was evident too in further and higher education, where it reorganised structures and funding to facilitate greater accountability.

The combined force and significance of these reforms were celebrated in the 1992 White Paper *Choice and Diversity: A New Framework for Schools* (DfE 1992). This identified the 'five great themes' of educational change in England and Wales since 1979 as being those of quality, diversity, increasing parental choice, greater autonomy for schools and greater accountability. It insisted moreover that 'Parents know best the needs of their children – certainly better than educational theorists or administrators, better even than our mostly excellent teachers' (DfE 1992: 2). This provided the basis for the Education Act of 1993, the longest Education Act ever with 308 sections, almost three times the number of the 1944 Act (McCulloch 1994: 38). Parental choice was also markedly strengthened in Scotland over this time following the Education (Scotland) Act of 1981 (Adler *et al.* 1989).

In higher education, the growing numbers of students placed increasing strains on universities, especially as funding did not keep pace with expansion. Under the 1988 Act, the University Grants Committee was superseded by a new Universities Funding Council. The binary divide that had existed since the 1960s between the new polytechnics on the one hand and the universities on the other was removed in 1992 through the Further and Higher Education Act. That created a unitary system of universities, albeit one that remained highly differentiated in terms of resources and in the scope provided for teaching and research.

The continuing problems of different phases of education were further addressed during the Conservatives' term of office in the 1990s through the establishment of three different reviews under the same person, Sir Ron (later Lord) Dearing, formerly a senior civil servant. His first brief was to consider the future of the National Curriculum following agitation by English teachers in particular over the effects of testing, leading to a report in 1994 that began to redefine and to some extent enhance the professional authority of teachers in the curriculum domain (Dearing 1994; see also McCulloch 2001). A second review, on qualifications for sixteen- to nineteen-year-olds, developed the aims of the 1991 White Paper, *Education and Training for the 21st Century* (DES 1991) to define a national framework for all young people in this age group (Dearing 1996; see also Hodgson and Spours 1997). Finally, Dearing was invited to review the purpose, shape, structure and funding of higher education. This third report recommended a shift from grants for undergraduate students to tuition fees paid for through government loans at low interest, in the context of an increasing proportion of young people reaching higher education (Dearing 1997).

Despite the extensive new policies and plans, it remained evident that educational inequalities remained highly resilient, and also that overall standards of attainment were comparatively low. An independently funded national commission on education had found that school qualifications were far lower on average than comparable qualifications in Germany, France and Japan, and that far fewer gained vocational qualifications. Large numbers of young people continued to leave school at the minimum leaving age of sixteen and often went straight into long-term unemployment (National Commission on Education 1993). League tables of examinations introduced by the Conservative government demonstrated a widening gap between those pupils who performed best in GCSEs and those who performed worst, with the independent schools taking most of the leading places in the league tables. The annual report of the chief inspector of schools in 1996 revealed that one in five secondary schools, 800 in all, suffered from poor accommodation, while 1,000 secondary schools had insufficient numbers of books. Other surveys found widespread deterioration in school facilities and inadequate resources of a kind that had been familiar in schools forty and fifty years before (McCulloch 1998: 151).

The new Labour government, sweeping to power with plans to concentrate on 'education, education, education', immediately embarked on reform. Its first White Paper on education, *Excellence in Schools* (DfEE 1997), insisted both that education would be at the heart of the government and that its policies would benefit the many rather than the few. It focused on improving standards rather than tinkering with structures, and committed itself to working in partnership with other groups seeking to raise standards. These commitments were soon followed by further interventions in particular areas of the education service; for example the Excellence in Cities programme was launched in March 1999 to raise standards and promote inclusion in urban areas, expanding from secondary schools to work closely with the Primary National Strategy.

However, a number of New Labour education policies soon proved controversial, and high hopes for reform were often frustrated. Some high-profile initiatives were soon abandoned, as in the case of the partnership-based Education Action Zones, which had echoed the EPAs of the 1960s in attempting to provide additional support for deprived urban communities (Franklin 2005). An ambitious report on the 14–19 curriculum and qualifications reform produced by Mike Tomlinson, former chief inspector of schools, recommended an overarching diploma scheme (Working Group on 14–19 Reform 2004), but this was not followed through because of anxieties about undermining the established 'gold standard' of A levels. Meanwhile, further education retained a low status and was criticised for lacking a clearly recognised and shared core purpose (Foster 2005). The Labour government also maintained the Conservative practice of 'naming and shaming' individual schools that were identified as 'failing schools' (Tomlinson 2005: 79–81). It decried 'bog standard' comprehensive schools for providing 'one size fits all' education, and increasingly favoured specialised provision catering for differences in aptitudes. Despite the government's frequent criticisms of the education service it claimed, by the beginning of its second term in 2001, to have transformed primary education and to be transforming secondary education, with teaching having been converted into a twenty-first-century profession (DfEE 2001). Sustained economic prosperity allowed additional investment in the infrastructure of education, with a large school building programme introduced under the banner of 'Building Schools for the Future', but although examination results improved there continued to be criticisms that standards were declining.

Education policy in the new century also attempted to relate education more closely to broader social and economic policy, reflecting its strategic position in government policy in general, with the Treasury taking a leading role. Innovations included the inauguration in 2003 of *Every Child Matters* (HM Treasury 2003), an integrated approach to childcare and social services set up in response to the abuse and death of Victoria Climbie, the spread of SureStart children's centres and further attention given to improving youth services (DfES 2005). Another innovation was Skills for Life, a national strategy to improve adult literacy, language and numeracy skills, launched in March 2001. This initiative had begun in 1999 with a report from the Basic Skills Agency that 20 per cent of adults lacked functional basic skills (Moser 1999). That led to the Leitch Report, which called for the country to become a world leader in skills by 2020 with 95 per cent of adults achieving the basic skills of functional numeracy and literacy (HM Treasury 2006). A further extension of this principle of joined-up services was the renaming of the central department to the Department of Children, Schools and Families (DCSF) when Gordon Brown succeeded Tony Blair as prime minister in 2007, apparently subsuming the notion of education itself. Nevertheless, educational changes continued apace, and further key legislation, the Education and Skills Act of 2008, extended the participation age in education to eighteen (as from 2015), while also requiring school governing bodies to invite and consider the views of pupils on matters affecting them.

Devolution after 1997 had permitted a more distinctive approach to be taken on educational matters in Scotland and Wales, and different national traditions were asserted, for example in the development of the Curriculum for Excellence in Scotland in 2010. Even so it was observed that 'the central dynamic of educational change in post-war Britain, especially since 1979, has been English' (Jones 2003: 3). Within this broad context, the overarching trend towards central control over education had been unmistakable in the two decades following the Education Reform Act of 1988. It was this that gave the House of Commons' Children, Schools and Families Committee (CSFC) most cause for concern in March 2010 when it reviewed the 'foundations of the education system'. It noted that the most persistent theme over that time had been a tension between central and local responsibility and control, and 'a relentless trend towards increased central control, although there are recent signs that the balance may now be starting to be redressed' (CSFC 2010: 4). The CSFC argued instead that 'governments need to provide broad frameworks rather than seeking to micro-manage the day to day work of teachers' (CSFC 2010: 3). Moreover, it discerned a loss of coherence resulting from the increased level of activity from the centre. According to the CSFC, there was a 'need to bring forward change as part of an overall vision, rather than fiddling with elements of the whole while failing to give due regard to the consequences elsewhere' (CSFC 2010: 6). Indeed, it continued, 'We also found a lack of coherence in an accountability system for schools which is of such complexity, with so many different forces and structures driving improvement, that school leaders and teachers risk becoming confused and disheartened' (CSFC 2010: 10).

Despite the large-scale investment in education over the preceding decade, educational standards remained stubbornly resistant to further improvement, and social mobility appeared at best to be stagnating. Class inequalities in educational attainment had proven to be highly resilient over the longer term (Breen 2005), with social disadvantage still a significant factor despite protracted reform (Gray 2005). The economy suffered from recession, and spending programmes faced the prospect of severe cutbacks at the end of the Labour government's third term of office. Nonetheless, the Conservative–Liberal Democrat coalition government that emerged from the general election of May 2010 committed itself to a further cycle of reform in education with the promise of extending choice and raising standards through free schools to be launched by parents and the spread of academies around the country, now to be led once more by a revived Department for Education.

Cohort-specific impact of the changing context

Over the sixty-five years covered in this general survey of educational developments there had been many changes, but also a great deal of continuity. Compared with the education service of the 1940s, the education system of 2010 was far more centralised, extended its control over a much broader age range, including pre-school services, and embraced a higher participation age as well as further, higher and adult education. Faith in education as a key social and economic investment, still in its early stages of development in the 1940s, had by the new century become a well-entrenched dogma. By then much more attention was given to issues of gender, disability, ethnicity and different types of educational disadvantage than had been evident in the 1940s. Yet many problems remained, such as the tensions between the public and private sector, concerns over wasted talent and social inequalities, the basis of fragmentation of provision between different kinds of schools, and the provision of buildings and equipment, that would have been familiar to children, parents, teachers and administrators in the years that followed the Second World War.

It is in this broader context of continuity and change that life course studies can identify, trace and analyse specific trends relating to age cohorts over this time. The general overview of social change in Britain in the second half of the twentieth century by Ferri *et al.* (2003) highlights the contrasts between the British birth cohorts of 1946, 1958 and 1970, and the Millennium Cohort Study at the end of the century. Wadsworth *et al.* (2003) note the changes in educational policy and opportunity over this period, while Makepeace *et al.* (2003) elaborate on the educational qualifications attained by these cohorts and the ways in which they entered the labour market over this time. Experiences of corporal punishment, school milk and the eleven-plus in the 1950s need to be interpreted in their historical context and in relation to broader social changes. The same is true of experiences of a more diverse school population, of failing schools and of student loans in the early years of the twenty-first century. For example, the impact of single-sex schooling on a range of academic outcomes has been recently assessed with detailed reference to the 1958 cohort (Sullivan *et al.* 2010). Birth cohort research on education to date has pursued a number of rich themes that need to be taken much further in cross-cohort analysis and as new data become available. These themes include that of educational careers, comprising the transition from one educational stage to the next and, in the longer term, engagement with education through lifelong learning. Moreover, cohort study evidence embraces three generations (cohort member, their parents and grandparents), and, when the child becomes adult, potentially a fourth generation, that of their own children. Such evidence is therefore an important source of insights into educational mobility across the generations. In relation to returns to education, too, the birth cohort studies supply a means of investigating the short-term, medium-term and long-term outcomes of education, including assessing the financial return to qualifications, taking account of other personal attributes such as social class, gender and ethnicity (see also, for example, Bynner and Joshi 2002; Hatch *et al.* 2007).

The birth cohort studies have also themselves contributed strongly to education policy over this time. For example, both the 1946 and the 1958 studies contributed to the deliberations of the Plowden committee. Each measured the ability of children in primary schools and again in the teenage years in order to show the 'wastage of talent', and its variation with pupils' gender and attitudes to school work, and also with parental socio-economic position and concern for the educational attainment of their children. They also demonstrated the crucial nature of parental concern, and showed that the influence of the home environment began in the pre-school years (Douglas 1964). The 1970 and millennium cohorts have pursued these concerns in greater depth, and also contributed to education policies in other areas such as adult basic skills, youths not in education, employment or training, social mobility, economic and social returns to education, and youth matters.

The period since the 1940s has witnessed the rise, dominance and ageing of a particular generational cohort that has exerted a strong influence on education, first as infants and children, then as youth, and then as parents, consumers, citizens and policy makers. To interpret such experience it needs to be related to the lives of specific individuals, families and groups and their diverse experiences over this time.

References

Adler, M., Petch, A. and Tweedie, J. (1989) *Parental choice and educational policy*, Edinburgh: Edinburgh University Press.

Aldrich, R. (ed.) (2002) *A century of education*, London: Falmer.

Amis, K. (1960) 'Lone voices', *Encounter*, 15: 6–11.
Anderson, R. (2003) 'The history of Scottish education, pre-1980', in T. G. K. Bryce and W. M. Humes (eds) *Scottish education*, pp. 219–28, Edinburgh: Edinburgh University Press.
Annual Abstract of Statistics (2001) No. 137, London: Stationery Office.
Banks, O. (1955) *Parity and prestige in English secondary education: a study in educational sociology*, London: Routledge and Kegan Paul.
Barlow Report (1946) *Scientific man-power*, London: HMSO.
Benn, C. and Simon, B. (1972) *Half way there*, 2nd edn, Harmondsworth: Penguin.
Bennett, A. (1991) 'Forty years on', in A Bennett, *Forty years on, and other plays*, pp. 27–96, London: Faber and Faber.
Breen, R. (2005) 'Why did class inequalities in educational attainment remain unchanged over much of the twentieth century?', in A. F. Heath, J. Ermisch and D. Gallie (eds) *Understanding social change*, pp. 55–72, Oxford: Oxford University Press.
Bryce, T. G. K. and Humes, W. M. (eds) (2003) *Scottish education*, 2nd edn, Edinburgh: Edinburgh University Press.
Bynner, J. and Joshi, H. (2002) 'Equality and opportunity in education: evidence from the 1958 and 1970 birth cohort studies', *Oxford Review of Education*, 28: 405–22.
Callaghan, J. (1976) 'Towards a national debate'. Available at http://education. guardian. co.uk/thegreatdebate/story.html (last accessed 10 December 2010).
Central Advisory Council for Education (1967) *Children and their primary schools (the Plowden Report)*, London: HMSO.
Committee on Higher Education (1963) *Higher education (the Robbins Report)*, London: HMSO.
Cox, C. B. and Dyson, A. E. (eds) (1969a) *Fight for education: a Black Paper*, London: Critical Quarterly Society.
Cox, C. B. and Dyson, A. E. (eds) (1969b) *Black Paper two: the crisis in education*, London: Critical Quarterly Society.
Crook, D. (2006) 'The Cambridge Garden House Hotel riot of 1970 and its place in the history of British student protests', *Journal of Educational Administration and History*, 38: 19–28.
CSFC (Children, Schools and Families Committee) (2010) *From Baker to Balls: the foundations of the education system*, 9th report, London: Stationery Office.
Davis, J. (2002) 'The Inner London Education Authority and the William Tyndale Junior School affair', *Oxford Review of Education*, 28: 275–98.
Dean, D. W. (1997) 'The rise and demise of the Curriculum Study Group', *Contemporary British History*, 11: 31–58.
Dearing, R. (1994) *The national curriculum and its assessment (the Dearing Report)*, London: School Curriculum and Assessment Authority.
Dearing, R. (1996) *Review of qualifications for 16–19 year-olds*, London: SCAA.
Dearing, R. (1997) *Higher education in the learning society*, London: Stationery Office.
DES (Department of Education and Science) (1965) 'The organisation of secondary education', Circular 10/65, 12 July, London: HMSO.
DES (1972) *Education: a framework for expansion*, London: HMSO.
DES (1977) *Education in schools: a consultative document*, London: HMSO.
DES (1978) *Special educational needs (the Warnock Report)*, London: HMSO.
DES (1985) *Education for all (the Swann Report)*, London: HMSO.
DES (1991) *Education and training for the 21st century*, London: HMSO.
DfE (Department for Education) (1992) *Choice and diversity: a new framework for schools*, London: HMSO.

DfEE (Department for Education and Employment) (1997) *Excellence in schools*, London: Stationery Office.

DfEE (2001) *Schools building on success*, London: Stationery Office.

DfES (Department for Education and Skills) (2005) *Youth matters*, London: Stationery Office.

Douglas, J. W. B. (1964) *The home and the school; a study of ability and achievement in the primary school*, London: MacGibbon and Kee.

Ferri, E., Bynner, J. and Wadsworth, M. (eds) (2003) *Changing Britain, changing lives: three generations at the turn of the century*, London: Institute of Education.

Foster, A. (2005) *Realising the potential: a review of the future role of Further Education Colleges*, London: DfES.

Franklin, B. M. (2005) 'Gone before you know it: urban school reform and the short life of the Education Action Zone initiative', *London Review of Education*, 3: 3–27.

Goodson, I. (1988) *The making of curriculum: collected essays*, London: Falmer.

Gosden, P. (1983) *The education system since 1944*, Oxford: Martin Robertson.

Gray, J. (2005) 'Is failure inevitable? The recent fate of secondary school reforms intended to alleviate social disadvantage', in A. F. Heath, J. Ermisch and D. Gallie (eds) *Understanding social change*, pp. 73–91, Oxford: Oxford University Press.

Halsey, A. H. and Gardner, L. (1953) 'Selection for secondary education and achievement in four grammar schools', *British Journal of Sociology*, 4: 60–75.

Hatch, S., Feinstein, L., Link, B. G., Wadsworth, M. and Richards, M. (2007) 'The continuing benefits of education: adult education and midlife cognitive ability in the British 1946 birth cohort', *Journal of Gerontology*, 62B: 404–14.

HM Treasury (2003) *Every child matters*, London: Stationery Office.

HM Treasury (2006) *Prosperity for all in the global economy: world class skills (the Leitch Report)*, London: Stationery Office.

Hodgson, A. and Spours, K. (eds) (1997) *Dearing and beyond: 14–19 qualifications, frameworks and systems*, London: Kogan Page.

Jeyes, G. (2003) 'The local governance of education: an operational perspective', in T. G. K. Bryce and W. M. Humes (eds), *Scottish education*, 2nd edn, pp. 168–83, Edinburgh: Edinburgh University Press.

Jones, G. E. (1990) '1944 and all that', *History of Education*, 19: 235–50.

Jones, K. (2003) *Education in Britain, 1944 to the present*, London: Polity.

Lowe, R. (1997) *Schooling and social change, 1964–1990*, London: Routledge.

Lowe, R. (2002) 'Higher education', in R. Aldrich (ed.) *A century of education*, pp. 75–92, London: Falmer.

Lowe, R. (2007) *The death of progressive education: how teachers lost control of the classroom*, London: Routledge.

McCulloch, G. (1987) 'History and policy: the politics of the TVEI', in D. Gleeson (ed.) *TVEI and secondary education*, pp. 13–37, Buckingham: Open University Press.

McCulloch, G. (1989) *The secondary technical school: a usable past?*, London: Falmer.

McCulloch, G. (1994) *Educational reconstruction: the 1944 Education Act and the 21st century*, London: Woburn.

McCulloch, G. (1998) *Failing the ordinary child?: the theory and practice of working class secondary education*, Buckingham: Open University Press.

McCulloch, G. (2001) 'The reinvention of teacher professionalism', in R. Phillips and J. Furlong (eds) *Education, reform and the state: twenty-five years of politics, policy and practice*, pp. 103–17, London: Routledge Falmer.

McCulloch, G. (2002) 'Local education authorities and the organisation of secondary education, 1943–1950', *Oxford Review of Education*, 28: 235–46.

McCulloch, G. (2007) 'Forty years on', *History of Education*, 36: 1–15.

McCulloch, G. (2008) 'Parity and prestige in English secondary education revisited', *British Journal of Sociology of Education*, 29: 381–9.

McCulloch, G., Jenkins, E. W. and Layton, D. (1985) *Technological revolution?: The politics of school science and technology in England and Wales since 1945*, London: Falmer.

Makepeace, G., Dolton, P., Woods, L., Joshi, H. and Galinda-Rueda, F. (2003) 'From school to the labour market', in E. Ferri, J. Bynner and M. Wadsworth (eds) *Changing Britain, changing lives*, pp. 29–70, London: Institute of Education.

Ministry of Education (1956) *Technical education*, London: HMSO.

Ministry of Education (1959) *15 to 18 (the Crowther Report)*, London: HMSO.

Ministry of Education (1963) *Half our future (the Newsom Report)*, London: HMSO.

Moser, C. (1999) *A fresh start: improving literacy and numeracy*, London: Basic Skills Agency.

National Commission on Education (1993) *Learning to succeed*, London: Heinemann.

NFER (National Foundation for Educational Research) (2002) *Education in England, Wales and Northern Ireland: a guide to the system*, London: NFER.

Norman, P. (2008) *John Lennon: the life*, London: HarperCollins.

Paterson, L. (2003) 'Educational provision: an overview', in T. G. K. Bryce and W. M. Humes (eds) *Scottish education*, pp. 19–36, Edinburgh: Edinburgh University Press.

Percy Report (1945) *Higher technological education: report of a special committee*, London: HMSO.

Prescott, J. (2008) *Prezza: my story: pulling no punches*, London: Headline.

Sandbrook, D. (2005) *Never had it so good: a history of Britain from Suez to the Beatles*, London: Little, Brown.

Scottish Government (2010) http://www.scotland.gov.uk (last accessed 17 May 2010).

Seldon, A. (1997) *Major: a political life*, London: Weidenfeld and Nicolson.

Sharp, P. (1987) *The creation of the local authority sector of higher education*, London: Falmer.

Sharp, P. (2002) 'Central and local government', in R. Aldrich (ed.) *A century of education*, pp. 93–116, London: Falmer.

Simon, B. (1974) *The politics of educational reform, 1920–1940*, London: Lawrence and Wishart.

Simon, B. (1991) *Education and the social order, 1940–1990*, London: Lawrence and Wishart.

Social Trends (2002) No. 32, London: Stationery Office.

Standish, P. (2003) 'From adult and continuing education to lifelong learning', in T. G. K. Bryce and W. M. Humes (eds) *Scottish education*, pp. 691–700, Edinburgh: Edinburgh University Press.

Stenhouse, L. (ed.) (1980) *Curriculum research and development in action*, London: Heinemann.

Sullivan, A., Joshi, H. and Leonard, D. (2010) 'Single-sex schooling and academic attainment at school and through the life course', *American Educational Research Journal*, 47: 6–36.

Tight, M. (2009) *The development of higher education in the United Kingdom since 1945*, Maidenhead: SRHE/Open University Press.

Timmins, N. (1995) *The five giants: a biography of the welfare state*, London: HarperCollins.

Tomlinson, S. (2005) *Education in a post-welfare society*, 2nd edn, Maidenhead: Open University Press.

Wadsworth, M., Ferri, E. and Bynner, J. (2003) 'Changing Britain', in E. Ferri, J. Bynner and M. Wadsworth (eds) *Changing Britain, changing lives,* pp. 1–28, London: Institute of Education.

Wolf, A. (2002) 'Qualifications and assessment', in R. Aldrich (ed.) *A century of education*, pp. 206–27, London: Falmer.

Working Group on 14–19 Reform (2004) *14–19 curriculum and qualifications reform (the Tomlinson Report)*, London: DfES.

Young, M. (1958) *The rise of the meritocracy, 1870–2033*, London: Thames and Hudson.

5 Economic policy and practice

Hugh Pemberton

Introduction

The first of the British national birth cohort studies, then entitled the 'National Survey of Health and Development', began in 1946. The babies born in that year grew up in a very different world to that we know today. In no area of life is this more true than the economy, for the post-war period saw enormous changes in both economic policy and performance that affected the lives of each of the generations studied by the five British national birth cohort studies (Appendix 1).

For much of the post-war (i.e. post-1945) period, contemporary debates about the economy tended to be couched in terms of Britain's 'decline', sometimes to a somewhat obsessive degree (Tomlinson 2000). Plainly, if one looks at Britain in terms of geo-strategic power one does see such a decline. The British Empire reached its zenith at the end of the Second World War but then almost immediately Britain began a precipitate withdrawal. In a post-war world dominated by two superpowers, Britain was a second-order power. Economically, too, as we shall see, it experienced a decline relative to other advanced economies, not least because of the post-war reconstruction of continental Europe and Japan.

It was easy, therefore, to portray the British economy in profoundly negative terms, and to blame economic policy for its apparent failure to thrive. This 'declinist' view of British economic policy and performance has proved to be remarkably enduring, and it continues to shape the views of many of the public, many journalists and many in our political elite. It is, however, in many ways a profoundly mistaken view. In this chapter I hope to demonstrate just how mistaken for in it we will explore post-war British history in much more positive terms. Put baldly, in all sorts of ways, the economic condition of Britain has improved markedly in the half-century since 1946. Today, most Britons consume many more goods and services than they did in 1946. The range of those goods and services is vastly greater than it was in 1946, and on the whole their quality is much higher. But economic well-being is about more than consumption of goods and services. Most of us work for fewer years, fewer weeks a year and fewer hours per week than our 1946 counterparts. On the whole, we are richer, we are healthier and we live longer. Anyone with memories of 1946 will confirm this. This is not to say that this transformation has been experienced equally by all. Even before the impact of the recent financial crisis and the recession that followed it was possible to find quite significant pockets of high unemployment, there was some quite notable regional patterning in terms of health and life expectancy, relative poverty was still a significant issue for many people and, despite a decade of rapidly rising public spending after 1999, there were still some notable deficiencies in the quality and quantity of the country's public infrastructure. That said, overall, the story of Britain's post-war economic development was a story of very significant economic progress.

In exploring this story in more detail, we will focus on its significant elements. In terms of economic policy, we will discuss marked shifts in thinking about what exactly the role of the state should be in promoting economic growth and well-being. But an important part of the story of government and the economy is the way in which the government became an important economic actor in its own right. Here we will highlight the way in which the growth of the state in the Second World War produced a 'ratchetting up' in the size of Britain's state, which endured despite Thatcherite attempts to 'roll back' the state in the 1980s. In the process we will examine changing patterns of government spending over time, but we will also probe big changes in the way in which the state taxed its citizens.

We will then consider developments in economic performance. We will discuss the uneven pattern of economic growth, highlighting the 1970s as the decade around which the period moved. We will explore the general rise in consumption, and in living standards. But we will also explore shifting patterns of income and wealth inequality. Likewise, we will explore significant changes in the patterns of both employment and unemployment. Part of that story is a transformation in the structure of the British economy, with a marked shift from manufacturing towards a 'service economy', and by extension a transformation in working lives. Finally, we will place Britain's economic experience since the end of the Second World War in the context of a growing and increasingly inter-linked global economy.

Demographic change

We begin, however, with a brief discussion of demographic change. For although changes in British economic policy and performance helped to shape the lives of Britons, and to shape British demography, demographic change itself had important consequences for both policy and performance. One notable change was the rise in the population, which grew from 50.2 million in the 1951 census to 60.6 million in 2006 (Office for National Statistics 2008). This was of economic importance because a growing population increased the potential for economic output, although of course it also meant that national income had to be shared out amongst more people. In both cases there were implications for living standards that should be borne in mind when we discuss economic performance.

Four features of this post-war demographic change are particularly relevant in this context: changes in the birth rate; changing gender roles; migration; and a combination of decreasing infant mortality and rising longevity. As can be seen in Figure 5.1, which shows live births in England and Wales between 1939 and 2004, the post-war period saw not one but two 'baby booms'. The first, between about 1945 and 1950, encompassed the first national birth cohort study in 1946.

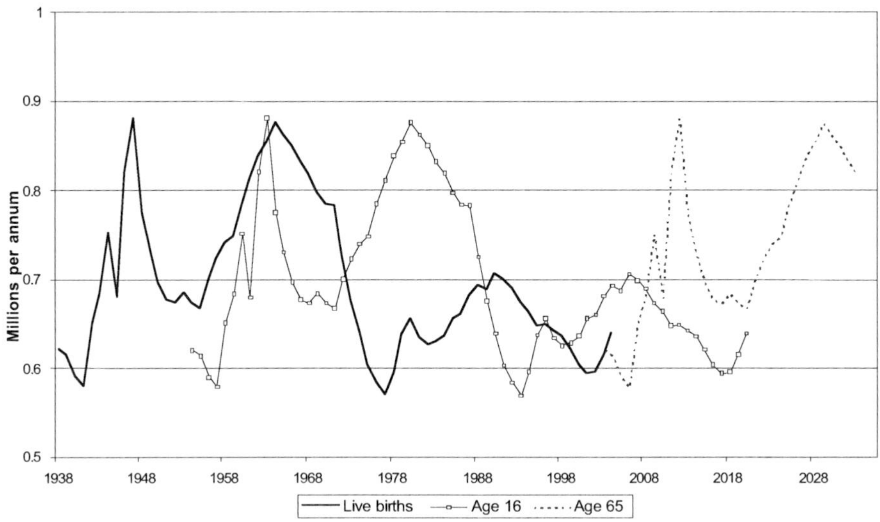

Figure 5.1 The baby boom and its ripple effect. Source: Office for National Statistics Statbase: Live births in England and Wales, 1938–2004. Available at http://www.statistics.gov.uk/statbase/.

The second occurred in the 1960s and, although peaking at a similar level as the earlier boom, represented a more sustained increase in the birth rate. The more minor upsurge in births in the 1980s pales by comparison.

Why were the baby booms economically important? Most obviously, those babies were potential workers. Figure 5.1 shows the ripple effect of the two baby booms with later peaks roughly coinciding with when these cohorts entered, and later began to leave, the labour market. The dotted line shows clearly the implications of retiring baby boomers in the near to medium term.

Nonetheless, making babies was but one of the ways in which the British labour force was able to grow in the post-war period – for grow it did, as can be seen in Table 5.1. By the end of the century the workforce was nearly half as big again as it had been in 1939. One factor behind this growth, in addition to the post-war baby booms, was a remarkable increase in the number of women in work (Johnson and Zaidi 2007). Despite rapid growth of the overall labour force, and despite a growing population, the number of men within the labour force remained stable at about 16 million. Female participation in work increased markedly, however, as Table 5.1 demonstrates.

It might be thought that immigration was also an important part of the story of Britain's growing labour force. Certainly immigration grew markedly after the passing of the 1948 British Nationality Act, but it was successfully curtailed by subsequent legislation beginning with the 1962 Commonwealth Immigrants Act (Table 5.2). Moreover, although immigration was certainly a feature of social change in post-war Britain, it was much less important economically. Between the end of the war and the end of the 1950s, immigration was only marginally

Table 5.1 UK labour force size and composition by sex, selected years 1939–2008

	1939	*1960*	*1970*	*1980*	*1990*	*2000*	*2008*
Labour force (millions)	19.8	25.2	26.5	27	28.6	29	31.2
Women (%)	26	33	36	40	44	46	46
Men (%)	74	67	64	60	56	54	54

Sources: Office for National Statistics Statbase: Labour market survey 2008; *Social Trends*, 2009. Available at http://www.statistics.gov.uk/statbase/.

greater than emigration. In the 1960s and 1970s Britain actually became a net exporter of population. It was not until the 1990s and particularly the 2000s that migration made a notable contribution to population growth and to the growth of the country's workforce.

More generally, of course, as they progressed through the life course both the baby booms and net migration affected the age profile of the country. So too did a rapid decline in infant mortality – down by nearly 75 per cent between 1940 and 1980 (Smith 1994). One obvious result was an initial rise in the ratio of young people to the working population followed by a marked contraction (see Table 5.3). Likewise, demographic change served over time to change the proportion of the population available for work in relation to the young and old people that their output supported (some sense of this can be obtained from the dependency ratios in Table 5.3).

This reference to old people is important, for the baby booms, combined with better health and rising longevity, are also part of another story: an ageing population in which the ratio between the retired and those of working age is set

Table 5.2 Population change, 1931–2007, United Kingdom

Years	*Population at start of period (millions)*	*Annual averages (thousands)*				
		Live births	*Deaths*	*Net natural change*	*Net migration*	*Overall change*
1931–61	46.04	793	603	190	22	213
1951–61	50.29	839	593	246	6	252
1961–71	52.81	962	638	324	–12	312
1971–81	55.93	736	666	69	–27	42
1981–91	56.36	757	655	103	5	108
1991–2001	57.44	731	631	100	68	167
2001–7	59.11	710	591	119	191	310

Sources: Halsey and Webb (2000: 72–3); National Statistics Statbase. Available at http://www.statistics.gov.uk/statbase/.

Table 5.3 Broad age groups as a percentage of the general population, United Kingdom, 1939–2001 and forecast up to 2021

Year	*0–14*	*15–64*	*65+*	*Overall dependency ratio*[a]	*Youth dependency ratio*[b]	*Aged dependency ratio*[c]
1931	24.3	68.3	7.4	46.4	35.6	10.8
1951	22.5	66.6	10.9	50.2	33.8	16.4
1961	23.4	64.8	11.8	54.2	36.1	18.2
	0–16	*17–64*	*65+*			
1971	25.5	61.3	13.2	63.2	41.6	21.6
1981	22.3	62.7	15.0	59.5	35.5	24.0
1991	20.3	63.9	15.8	56.5	31.8	24.7
2001	20.1	64.1	15.9	56.1	31.3	24.7
2011 forecast	18.6	64.7	16.7	54.5	28.7	25.8
2021 forecast	18.6	63.1	18.2	58.4	29.5	28.9

Sources: Halsey and Webb (2009: 75); National Statistics Statbase. Available at http://www.statistics.gov.uk/statbase/.

Notes

a The overall dependency ratio is the total of those not of working age (here assumed, for reasons of historical statistics, to be between the ages of fifteen and sixty-four) and those who are (the 'working population').

b The youth dependency ratio is here the ratio between young people and the working population.

c The aged dependency ratio is the ratio between those aged over sixty-five and the working population.

markedly to deteriorate in the near to medium term. Overall, however, it is worth remembering that, for all the panic about the 'pensions crisis', the overall dependency ratio in 2021 will still be below that experienced in the late 1960s and early 1960s, when the baby boomers were children.

Economic policy

Gross domestic product

A measure of a country's domestic economic activity (as opposed to gross national product, which measures output at home and abroad by British citizens and companies). It is calculated by adding together the annual value of the country's private consumption of goods and services, plus private and public investment, plus other public spending, plus exports (less the value of its annual imports). The result, adjusted slightly to reflect changes in the value of stocks held by firms, equals the country's annual output of goods and services. Gross domestic product per head of population serves as a useful proxy for average living standards.

The expansion of the state

The period during which the national birth cohort surveys have been running is one of both continuity and change in economic policy, not least when it comes to the role of the state in the economy. Those born in 1946 were born into a world over which the war threw a long shadow. Most notably, perhaps, the state, having expanded dramatically as Britain was rapidly converted to a virtual command economy as the country strove to cope with conditions of 'total war', then rapidly contracted. It did not, however, resume its pre-war size once the war was over. As can be seen in Figure 5.2, as in 1914–18, the 1939–45 war saw a ratchetting up in government spending as a share of gross domestic product that persisted throughout our period.

What was this larger state doing? Here we find a more complex picture of change and continuity. Of particular importance was the way in which state ownership of key industries characterised the first half of the post-war period, the ongoing importance of the welfare state set up by the 1945–51 Labour governments, and the fact that after 1945 the state accepted responsibility for managing the economy (although with considerable changes in the means by which it sought to do so). We will examine each of these factors in turn.

The ownership and control of industry

One reason why it proved so hard to reduce public expenditure in the post-war world was that the post-war state had taken on significant extra responsibilities.

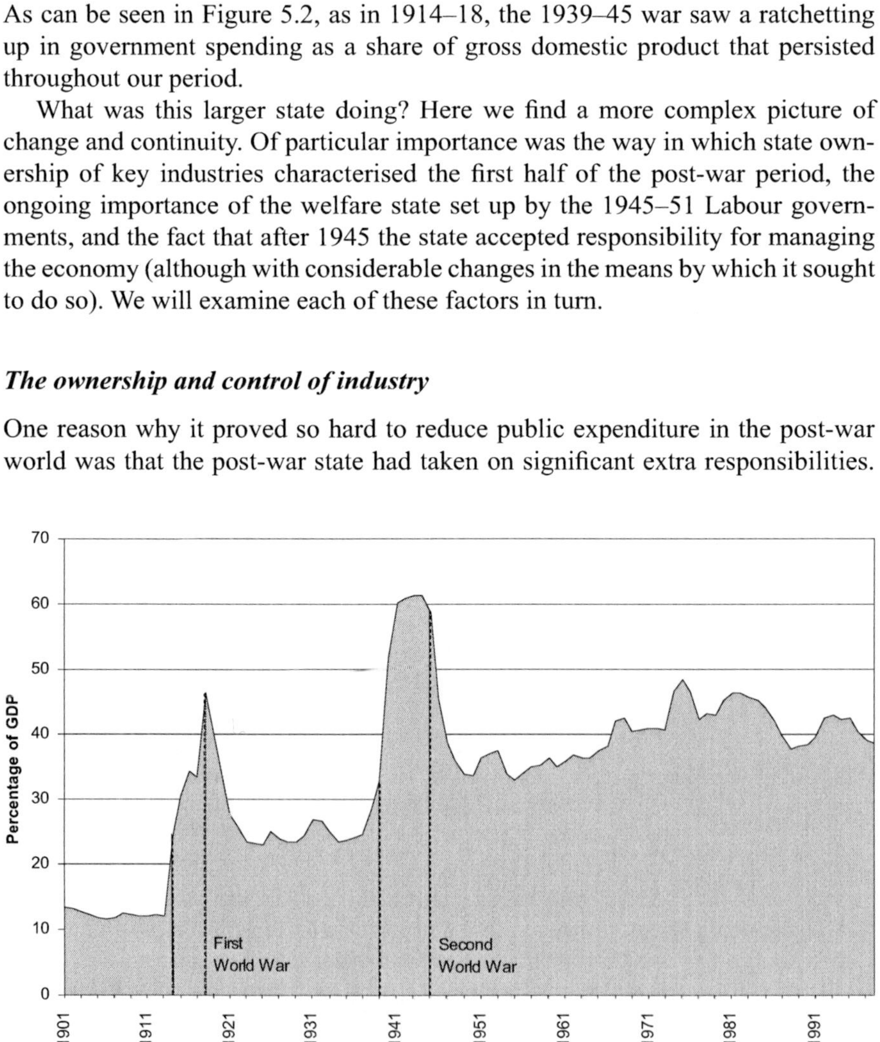

Figure 5.2 General government expenditure as a percentage of gross domestic product, 1901–98. Source: Office for National Statistics Statbase: *Social Trends*, 2000. Available at http://www.statistics.gov.uk/statbase/.

Indeed one of the most important features of post-war life was the increased role of the state in the lives of British citizens. The Second World War had almost immediately transformed economic policy as the government acted to militarise the economy to wage 'total war'. The state determined what should be imported and controlled the allocation of those imports to industry, it controlled the location and the type of new factory building and it rationed consumer goods and food supplies. In important respects, therefore, the wartime government sought to supplant the power of the market and create a 'command economy'. Many of these controls were gradually run down as part of the transition to a peacetime economy, but not all. Food rationing, for example, was actually extended in the 'austerity' years after 1945 and not abolished until 1954. Controls over industry carried on after 1945 as Labour sought rationally to plan the economy, although after the catastrophic failure of planning to maintain fuel and power supplies in the harsh winter of 1946–7 many were removed – most notably in Harold Wilson's famous 'bonfire of controls' in 1949. Nevertheless, state control over some of the 'commanding heights' of the industrial economy was perpetuated through the nationalisation of key industries such as coal, electricity, gas, rail, and iron and steel (the net cost of which is not counted in general government expenditure in Figure 5.2).

The Conservatives labelled nationalisation 'doctrinaire socialism' and dismissed it as a failure in their 1951 general election manifesto, but, with the exception of steel, which they eventually denationalised in 1961 (and which Labour renationalised in 1967), their failure to reverse much of the nationalisation project between 1951 and 1964 was notable (Burk 1988). The focus shifted somewhat after 1964 when a Labour government was elected on a promise to modernise Britain to meet the challenge of what Harold Wilson called 'the white heat of the scientific and technological revolution' (Labour Party 1963). One aspect of that promise was the institution of a 'National Plan' in 1965 in which output targets were set for a range of industries. Another was the creation of the Industrial Reorganisation Corporation in 1966, the aim of which was to encourage mergers between private sector companies in a quest for greater efficiency (Hague and Wilkinson 1983). Subsequently, Labour lost the 1970 general election and the avowed intention of the incoming Conservative government was to withdraw the state from the economy and to cease propping up 'lame ducks'. However, a famous 'u-turn' occurred in 1972 when Edward Heath took fright at the rate at which unemployment was rising and nationalised both Upper Clyde Shipbuilders and Rolls Royce. In 1974, Labour was elected on a radical manifesto that promised further nationalisations and compulsory planning agreements with major firms. Much of this was never implemented during Labour's period of office, not least because its leadership was not persuaded by the policy, but a notable exception was the new National Enterprise Board (NEB), which sought to nurture and support high-tech industries. The NEB was not without its successes, for example with Ferranti and superconductors. Too often, however, it found itself pushed into saving not just lame but dead ducks by a government determined to bring down unemployment (Morris and Stout 1985: 873). The high point of nationalisation came in 1977 when the nationalised industries accounted for 13 per cent of GDP. In this context, it is ironic that Labour undertook the first of what would become a wave of sales of state-owned industries when, as part of a package of measures required by the International Monetary Fund (IMF) in return for a loan to support sterling in 1976, the government sold off part of its stake in BP. Thereafter, 'privatisation' became the watchword of Conservative governments under Mrs Thatcher. By 1996, of the 1945–51 round of nationalisation only the Bank of England and British Waterways remained in public ownership. By the end of the century a consensus appeared to have emerged that industries were better off in the private sector, with appropriate regulation of natural monopolies (Hannah 2004). Essentially, therefore, the post-war trajectory of state ownership of industry inscribed an arc, peaking in the late 1970s.

The welfare state

The key institutions of what came to be called the 'welfare state' were created in a burst of reform, most notably under the 1945–51 Labour governments, although the roots of change lay in the 1942 report by William Beveridge entitled *Social Insurance and Allied Services*. Each of the new institutions was intended to eliminate one of the 'five giants on the road of reconstruction' – want, disease, ignorance, squalor and idleness – that had been identified by Beveridge (Timmins 2001). The new institutions were fundamental to the post-war experience of British citizens for they quite literally provided care and support 'from cradle to grave'. For this reason they are considered in many of the other chapters in this volume. Here we limit ourselves to a brief consideration of the economic dimension.

Most obviously, in this context, and as Lowe (2005: 80) points out, economic performance is an important driver of both the development and ultimate form of welfare policy. A healthy and fully employed workforce increases economic performance potential and both reduces the need to pay benefits and generates the cash to allow welfare provision to expand. The welfare state may thus be seen as both a cause and a function of post-war economic growth (Thane 2007). This relationship between welfare and economic performance can be found in almost all the major planks of the post-war welfare settlement.

In education, for example, the 1944 Education Act, passed by the wartime coalition, was followed by an explosion in spending 'probably . . . unique in the western world' (Simon 1985: 283). During the 1950s and 1960s, spending on schools grew faster than any other component of social spending, In part, the cause lay in the need to school the 'bulge' or 'baby boom' generations. But an important role was also played by the Conservatives' embracing of the idea that state education spending could have important economic benefits. Both demographic 'push' and economic 'pull' factors thus played an important role in the expansion of higher education in the 1960s and 1970s. Although political arguments raged over the form and purpose of both secondary and higher education during the whole of the post-war period, what was remarkable was the degree of consensus that a better-educated nation would be a more productive nation, that education must therefore be expanded and that the state must necessarily play an important role in its delivery (Lowe 2005: 204–45).

Likewise, one might cite the National Health Service, perhaps the most emblematic of the welfare state institutions, but one whose scope also had an economic dimension. Take the way in which post-war growth allowed the NHS to expand. In the early 1950s, for example, the Conservative government became concerned at the way in which demands, and thus nominal spending, on the NHS were rising. One factor here was that the unmet demand for health care had been underestimated but there were also important demographic 'push' factors at work, most notably the impact of the baby boom generations on the demand for pre- and post-natal health services and for paediatric services. The Conservative government's instinctive reaction was to cut back spending and it commissioned the independent Guillebaud Committee to investigate the cost of the NHS, assuming that it would provide the justification. However, when that committee reported in 1956 it demonstrated that spending on health had actually fallen both in real terms (because of inflation) and as a proportion of GDP (because of economic growth), despite a growing population. Thereafter, in large part due to the 1961 Plowden Report's recommendation that public expenditure planning decisions be taken with a view to their long-term impact, the Conservatives came to see health spending not just as benefitting from economic growth but as a potential way in which it might be increased (HM Treasury 1961). The result was the 1962 Hospital Plan, a major programme of new and refurbished hospitals that established most of the general hospitals we know today (Glennerster 2007: 88–9; Lowe 2005: 192–5).

After the mid-1970s, Conservative governments became somewhat more sceptical about the economic benefits to be derived from state spending on health. Three key factors were at work. One was that the Conservatives had rediscovered their ideological predilection for private provision. Another was the fact that health-care inflation persistently exceeded price inflation, thus creating constant pressure on health spending. The third was the financial demands of an ageing population. Given the popularity of the NHS, however, any notion that it might be privatised was seen even by Margaret Thatcher as a political step too far. Moreover, by the 1990s there was an increasing interest amongst economists in the notion of 'human capital'. In 2001, a report commissioned by the World Health Organization found a strong economic justification for health spending as a means of achieving better productivity and economic growth (Sachs 2001) With the advent of New Labour in 2007, an explicitly economic dimension became even clearer, being used to justify increasing health spending over the European average (see, for example, HM Government 2005). As Gordon Brown put it in his 2003 budget speech, 'a healthy, educated and highly skilled workforce [can allow] businesses to update products, services and working practices at the rate demanded by rapidly changing global markets and tastes' (HM Treasury 2003).

Macro-economic management

Beveridge had identified unemployment as one of his other 'five giants' and slaying that giant was to have perhaps the most extensive effect of all when it came to the economy. During the 1930s, the economist John Maynard Keynes had argued that it was possible for an economy to become stuck in a 'low output equilibrium'. In this situation, the economy would be stable, indeed might well be growing, but there would be substantial unemployment. Keynes argued forcefully that in this situation, which seemed to him to pertain in the 1930s, the state should use its powers to tax and spend to manage upwards the level of demand in the economy. By doing so, it would raise the level of economic growth, and as growth increased unemployment would fall.

Keynesianism

Keynes' (1936) *General Theory of Employment, Interest and Money* postulated two key ideas: (1) that economies can sometimes be stable even when they do not have full employment; and (2) that a government can remedy that situation by lowering taxes and/or raising its own spending, thus increasing the level of aggregate demand in the economy. After Keynes's death his ideas were developed by a younger generation of economists and taken up by politicians in the UK and abroad. By 1971, even the US Republican president Richard Nixon could remark that 'We are all Keynesians now'.

In the 1930s Keynes's ideas had relatively little impact on the Treasury. It is ironic, therefore, that 'demand management' should have been embraced in wartime not as a way of increasing consumption but as a means of holding it back. As Britain geared up its economy to wage 'total war' there was a big growth in government spending on war-related production. This fed through into higher employment and higher earnings. With very little in the shops on which to spend that money, the boom risked touching off rapid inflation and from 1941 the government began to reduce purchasing power through higher taxes and forced saving. Macro-economic demand management on Keynesian lines had arrived (Weir 1989).

In its 1944 *Employment Policy* White Paper, the coalition government accepted that after the war government should act to 'maintain a high and stable level of employment' (Minister of Reconstruction 1944: para 1). This was a decisive moment for it would require governments to intervene to sustain sufficient demand in the economy (Feinstein 1983: 13). In fact, in the very benign conditions of the post-war worldwide economic boom the commitment to unbalance the economy to maintain employment was not really tested (Matthews 1968). Nonetheless, it is generally argued that, once the war was over, 'Keynesian' demand management continued to shape policy for more than three decades (Booth 2001; Middleton 2000).

Whether Keynes would entirely have acknowledged 'Keynesian' policy in these years is debateable, however. One notable difference was the definition of 'full employment'. At the end of the war, for example, William Beveridge had equated it to an unemployment rate of 8 per cent. By the end of the 1950s, however, governments were viewing anything over 2 per cent as politically worrying, and responding by acting to raise demand. In such a fully employed economy inflationary pressures were considerable. The advent of incomes policy was fundamental to the sustenance and evolution of the Keynesian policy framework up to 1979. The jury remained out, however, on whether or not incomes policy could be effective in anything but the short term, critics arguing that short-run success was brought at the price of long-run inflation as incomes policy tended to dam up wage demands, which simply resurfaced once the brakes were off.

By the 1970s a growing body of economic opinion found post-war Keynesianism to be inherently inflationary. The 1970s saw a major challenge to the Keynesian policy paradigm, in large part induced by the collapse of the international financial system in 1972 and the quadrupling of oil prices by the Organization of the Petroleum Exporting Countries (OPEC) in 1973. The latter, in particular, served to both raise inflation and induce a severe recession (the combination of economic stagnation and inflation being dubbed 'stagflation'). Labour struggled hard to adapt the Keynesian policy model to correct its perceived shortcomings, but from 1976 the impact of the monetarists began to be apparent in British economic policy. So called 'monetarists', such as Milton Friedman, argued that action by the government to raise demand to maintain high employment had served to create inflationary pressure and to raise inflationary expectations that fed through into higher wage demands as workers sought to protect themselves against the erosion of their real incomes, thus touching off an inflationary spiral. The solution, it was argued, was for government to restrict itself to controlling the supply of money in the economy and allow market forces to operate.

Monetarism

The theory that the excessive growth of the money supply is inherently inflationary, a theory most often identified with the work of Milton Friedman. The theory argued that when the money supply expanded consumers and business would spend the extra money and that, all things being equal, inflation would rise as more money chased the same amount of goods being produced. Conversely, a contraction of the money supply would reduce idle balances, thus reducing the propensity to spend, thus reducing inflation. Highly influential on Conservatives in the 1970s, the theory implied that inflation could be driven out of the system by a government prepared to control the supply of money and accept the consequences of lower demand and higher unemployment.

In 1977, Dennis Healey, the then Labour chancellor, established monetary targets. In truth, Labour's was a half-hearted embrace of monetarism and Fforde's designation of it as 'monetarily constrained Keynesianism' sums things up well (Artis *et al.* 1992: 48). Healey himself later acknowledged that the policy had essentially amounted to political window dressing (Oliver and Pemberton 2004). His was not an intermediate target intended to control the growth in GDP (defined as 'genuine' monetarism by Pepper and Oliver 2001: xxvi–xxviii).

It was in fact only with the election of the Conservatives in 1979 that monetarism was put at the centre of British economic policy. But the 'shock therapy' instituted by the Conservatives, coming as it did on the back of another oil price increase by OPEC in 1979 and the self-inflicted raising of value added tax rates as part of a shift from direct to indirect taxation, served to create a devastating economic contraction in 1979–81 and to reignite inflation. Stagflation was thus resurrected and, ironically, the government had contrived also to make its monetary targets virtually impossible to meet. By 1985 'monetarism' was effectively dead as the government abandoned those targets.

Gradually, the framework of economic policy evolved towards a more generalised 'neo-liberal' model. This had several dimensions. First, it focused on removing supply-side bottlenecks (i.e. it aimed to make economic activity in the economy more efficient) through micro-economic policy measures such as improved education and training, use of the tax system to increase individual initiative, an emphasis on markets rather than state control, and the removal of government regulation (such as the 'war on red tape' so beloved of businesses and successive business ministers). Second, it sought to manage the economy at the macro level by manipulating interest rates rather than relying on fiscal policy as in the Keynesian framework (the latter being deemed to have produced a tendency to inflation as a consequence of fiscal stimuli persistently being both too late and too great when managing the economy in the post-war 'golden age') or on negotiation with employers and unions – the social partners as they are called on the continent (an approach seen to have conferred excessive power on the unions). The key elements of the new approach were privatisation, deregulation, the reform of industrial relations to reduce the power of trade unions, lower taxes to increase incentives to work and to invest, encouraging foreigners to invest in Britain, better control of public spending, and better investment in human capital by way of reforms of school education, expanding higher education and overhauling vocational training

This policy was not without success (Card *et al.* 2004), although the jury is still out on whether its benefits outweighed its social costs, most notably those arising from mass long-term unemployment and growing inequality, and costs arising from an increasingly degraded public infrastructure (Crafts 1997). What the policy did manage ultimately to do, however, was to drive inflation out of the system. From 1992, after Britain found itself unable to keep sterling in the European Monetary System (the latter intended to be a key step on the path to membership of an eventual euro currency), its economy seemed to enter a virtuous circle of low inflation and high growth. The neo-liberal model thus appeared to carry all before it.

In 2008, however, the world economy experienced a financial crisis greater than anything since that of 1929. Suspicions that New Labour was prepared to countenance, and was in fact practising, Keynesian demand management after 1997 (Clift and Tomlinson 2007) were succeeded by certainty in 2008 when the government responded to the worst financial crisis since 1929 with the effective nationalisation of all but one of Britain's major banks, a massive injection of liquidity in financial markets through measures such as credit guarantees and so called 'quantitative easing', the protection of nearly £600 billon of assets, and a deliberate and major unbalancing of the fiscal position (with public sector net borrowing forecast to peak at 12.4 per cent of GDP in 2009). At the time of writing, the outcome of that crisis is unclear both for the world as a whole and for Britain. Notwithstanding growing confidence by the end of 2009 that the worst was over, it is possible that the recession will be as deep and as long-lasting as that in the 1930s. What is certain is that the crisis had brought Keynesianism back into the lexicon of British economic policy makers.

Taxation

Finally, we come to taxation, the variation of which was an important part of Keynesian demand management, but the general level of which was to a large degree driven by policy decisions on the size and role of the state. Put simply, a larger state meant higher taxes to pay for it. Compared with the pre-war years, rates of tax were higher after 1945, there were a number of new taxes and more people were drawn into the tax net (most notably through the wartime invention of pay-as-you-earn income tax). Periodically, post-war governments attempted to rein in the state and to cut taxes. As Figures 5.2 and 5.3 demonstrate, however, until the late 1980s on neither score were such attempts notably successful. Most obviously, perhaps, despite Thatcherite claims to have 'rolled back the state', government spending actually rose after 1979, the 1979–81 recession requiring significant spending on unemployment benefits. Conservative successes later in the decade were then obtained by banking the proceeds of privatisation, holding down the growth in public sector salaries, cutting entitlements to welfare benefits and cutting back public capital investment. However, after 1992 all these categories of spending began to increase once more.

Economic performance

Growth and productivity

The war brought an end to the difficult economic conditions of the inter-war years but at its end many expected that the experience after the First World War would be repeated: a brief reconstruction boom would be followed by a deep and long-lasting recession. Instead, for the next quarter of a century Britain experienced what came to be seen as a 'golden age' of unprecedented peacetime growth. As can be seen in Figure 5.4, which tracks the annual performance of the British

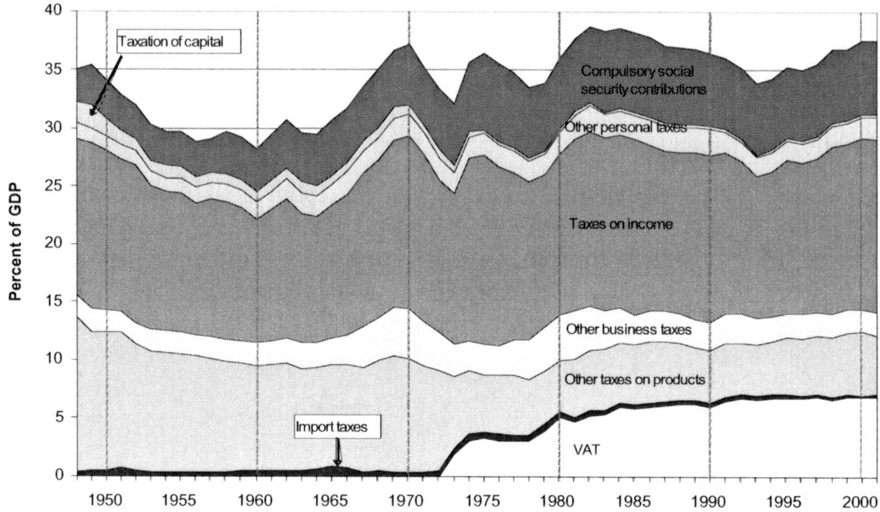

Figure 5.3 Total public sector receipts as a percentage of GDP, 1948–2001. Source: Office for National Statistics (2002).

economy from the start of 1949 (by which time the reconversion of the economy to a peacetime footing was virtually complete) to the middle of 2009, the period up to 1973 saw an average annual rate of growth of about 3 per cent. This was a remarkable performance, as was the complete absence of an economic contraction in any of these years. This is not to say that the business cycle was abolished; plainly it was not. But the trend rate of growth was more than double that needed to maintain employment in the face of productivity gains arising from technological and managerial improvement.

However, it will also be plain from Figure 5.4 that, in common with other advanced economics, the ensuing years up to 1992 were much less benign. Clearly, the economy was much more unstable in Phase 2, with serious recessions in 1974–5, 1979–81 and 1990–2. The average rate of growth was also lower – only 1.74 per cent compared with 2.98 per cent in Phase 1. A difference of little more than one percentage point might seem negligible but that difference compounded over nearly two decades had a major effect. Figure 5.5 shows both the way in which the UK economy grew and what the growth path might have looked like if the Phase 1 trend had continued. As Dow (2000) pointed out in his magisterial work on major recessions, growth foregone in such recessions was growth permanently foregone. That said, however, it is important to note that, overall, the years since 1945 have nevertheless seen a substantial increase in the size of the British economy.

Although the British economy grew during our period, its productivity performance was rather less impressive. In the early years of our period, British productivity was high by European standards, mainly because it had a relatively small number working in agriculture and a relatively productive service sector. By

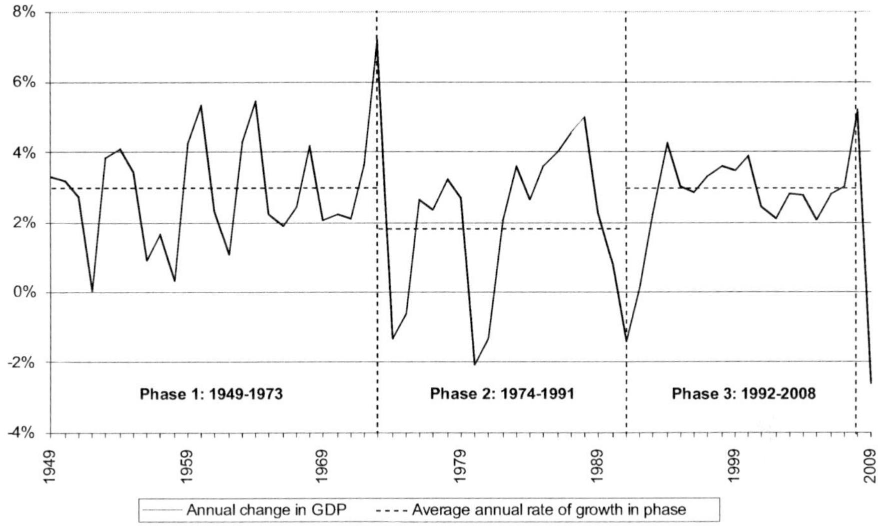

Figure 5.4 Annual growth of the UK economy, 1949–2009. Source: Office for National Statistics Statbase: UK national accounts, July 2009 (to 2007); quarterly national accounts, 1st quarter 2009 (to 2009). Available at http://www.statistics.gov.uk/statbase/.

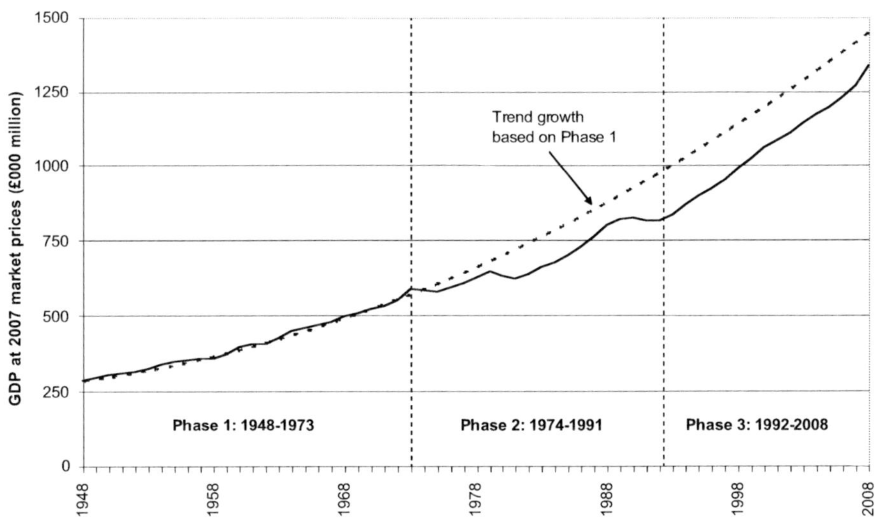

Figure 5.5 The growth of the UK economy, 1948–2008. Source: Office for National Statistics Statbase: UK national accounts, 2009 (to 2007); quarterly national accounts, 1st quarter 2009 (to 2009). Available at http://www.statistics.gov.uk/statbase/. With thanks to Roger Middleton.

the late 1960s, however, its productivity was being overtaken by European competitors. Much noise was made by the Conservative governments after 1979 about their success in increasing British productivity. Comparison with the experience of other countries is hard and subject to considerable margins of error but O'Mahony (2004) supports the finding of many analysts when she finds that, despite some improvement since 1979, Britain's relatively poor productivity performance vis-à-vis its major competitors persists. Surprisingly, perhaps, given the relative decline in Britain's system of vocational training since the 1970s, workforce skills became less important in explaining the problem. There is evidence that the growing proportion of UK school leavers entering university since the 1970s may have served to improve productivity somewhat. Rather, the problem lay in the quantity and quality of investment in infrastructure, plant and equipment, and in the way in which the country was able to manage production and introduce new technology. In this context, one notes that between 1973 and 1996 investment in the capital stock of firms and (particularly) in public infrastructure in the UK was well below that of its main competitors.

Relative economic performance

Although the story of the post-war period was one of overall economic growth, a rather different story emerges if we widen the focus to examine that performance in the context of how other advanced economies fared (see Table 5.4). As noted above, Tomlinson (2000) and others have pointed out that much of the panic about Britain's 'economic decline' was overdone, with a persistent tendency to focus on relative decline rather than absolute growth, and to ignore the welcome inevitability that other countries would catch up with the UK economy (Abramovitz 1986).

However, we should beware of Panglossianism in this analysis. As can be seen in Table 5.4, Britain was experiencing more than just a process of 'catch up and convergence'; it was being overtaken. This involved a major psychological shock – and this was a key factor in the 'declinist' mindset. However, it also produced real effects and produced real political and economic problems. Most notably, relative economic decline was an important cause of Britain's decision to liquidate its empire after 1945, although throughout our period it continued to see itself as a significant world player in global politics and strategy. To do so, it was increasingly forced to 'punch above its weight' – with higher military, intelligence and diplomatic spending than its reduced circumstances might otherwise have dictated. It might also be argued that relative economic decline, and the declinist mindset it gave rise to, drove government policy in directions that were not always beneficial. The 'monetarist revolution' after 1979 is perhaps a case in point.

There is evidence that the economic reforms begun by the Conservatives during the 1980s and 1990s, and continued by Labour after 1997, may have succeeded in halting, although not reversing, relative economic decline (Crafts 2002). Nevertheless, at the time of writing, the extent to which this was due to an improved domestic economy rather than temporarily reduced growth in

Table 5.4 Britain's economic performance relative to other OECD countries

	OECD-17 rankings					
	1950		*1973*		*1997*	
G-7 countries	*Real GDP*	*Real GDP per capita*	*Real GDP*	*Real GDP per capita*	*Real GDP*	*Real GDP per capita*
Canada	7	5	7	3	7	9
France	3	11	4	7	4	2
Germany	4	13	3	6	3	5
Italy	5	16	6	16	6	15
Japan	6	17	2	14	2	4
UK	2	6	5	11	5	14
United States	1	1	1	2	1	2

Source: Adapted from Middleton (2000: 4–5).

Note
The combined OECD rating is calculated as the average of rankings for real GDP and real GDP per capita.

competitor countries such as Germany, and thus whether it was likely to prove enduring or merely fleeting, remained to be seen. The way in which Britain was hit particularly hard by the 2008 worldwide financial crisis, and the growing realisation that the proceeds of North Sea oil are a wasting asset, might suggest that the country's relative economic decline will continue.

Income and living standards

Growth in the economy helped to raise individual living standards, although not, interestingly, to increase our happiness, as we shall see. By the early 1980s, real GDP per capita (i.e. each individual's share in the country's aggregate income from its domestic economy, adjusted for inflation) had doubled since 1945. By 2007 it had tripled.

Gini coefficient

The Gini coefficient measures income inequality by collapsing the entire income distribution into a single number between 0 and 1: the higher the number, the greater the degree of income inequality. A value of 0 corresponds to the absence of inequality, with all individuals (or households, depending on the income being measured) having the same income. In contrast, a value of 1 equates to an extreme inequality in that one individual commands all the income in the economy.

It is important to realise, however, that rising real incomes at the aggregate level do not necessarily translate into individual experiences. To understand why, we have to consider not just the level of overall income but its distribution, and doing so gives an indication of changes in the class structure and in inequalities by gender and ethnic origin. Inequality in incomes (and even more so in wealth) were a continuous feature of our period, but within this we can divide the period neatly into two. Measuring income inequality is fraught with difficulty, but one respected study (Atkinson 1995) estimated that between 1949 and 1975 the share of overall income taken by the top 10 per cent of earners fell by 4.8 percentage points. Another measure of income inequality, the Gini coefficient, fell by 4 percentage points. But much of the redistribution of income was from the top 10 per cent to the next 40 per cent (i.e. to upper middle-income earners). The share of the bottom half of the income distribution changed very little. As Table 5.5 demonstrates, since the mid-1970s, the trend has been for top-income earners (in this case the top 20 per cent) to take an increasingly large share of the cake. Alhough the bottom 20 per cent of income earners have fared somewhat better since 1992, and particularly since 1997, this has been at the expense of those in the middle of the range. What is clear, nonetheless, is that in terms of income the reduction of inequality that took place up to the mid-1970s was subsequently reversed, the Gini coefficient measured by post tax incomes rising by 4 percentage points between 1981 and 2001 (Office for National Statistics 2009a).

Consumption

The rise in both GDP and living standards eventually served to transform consumption. Initially, individual consumption was held down by post-war government 'austerity' measures, not least rationing, which were designed to maximise exports

Table 5.5 Household incomes from wages and salaries, 1977–2007

	Percentages						*Average per household (£ per year, 2006/7 prices)*
	Quintiles					*All households*	
	Bottom	*2nd*	*3rd*	*4th*	*Top*		
1977	3.3	10.9	20.7	28.2	36.9	100	13,934
1981	2.7	9.2	19.5	28.3	40.3	100	14,933
1986	2.0	6.8	17.9	29.2	44.2	100	14,792
1992	1.6	6.0	16.9	28.6	46.8	100	16,147
1996/7	1.9	6.5	16.2	28.1	47.3	100	16,785
2001/2	2.1	6.6	15.6	26.9	48.8	100	21,691
2006/7	2.6	7.3	15.4	26.6	48.0	100	23,325

Source: Office for National Statistics (December 2008) *Economic and Labour Market Review*, 2: 24.

and minimise imports. From 1951, however, individual consumption began to increase rapidly. By 1989 consumer spending had risen threefold since 1939. Consumption of food had increased by one-third. Consumption of alcohol was up by four-fifths. All other measures of spending had at least doubled. Expenditure on consumer durables such as cookers, washing machines, refrigerators and television sets was ten times higher. Spending on housing, transport and telecommunications, and most of all on services such as insurance, were all notably higher (Cairncross 1995). In the long boom of the 1990s household expenditure continued to increase – up by a further 50 per cent in real terms between 1989 and 2006 (Office for National Statistics 2008: 80).

We need to talk about increasing consumption in 'real' terms because an important feature of the post-war period was the rise and fall of price inflation (see Figure 5.6). Nonetheless, even if we strip out the effects of inflation to obtain 'real' figures for consumption, the defining feature of our period is that Britain became an increasingly affluent society. More than this, however, the defining characteristic of our period is perhaps Britain's transition to a mass consumption society. Three major factors were at work here. First, a growing economy fed into rising incomes even after inflation was taken into account. Rising real incomes allowed consumers to buy an increasing quantity of goods and services (and from a range that was both vastly wider and on the whole of considerably better quality than at the start of our period).

Second, the rising consumption of goods and services was driven by more than just real incomes. Although it has been argued that Britain would have been better to have prioritised investment for economic growth over spending on the

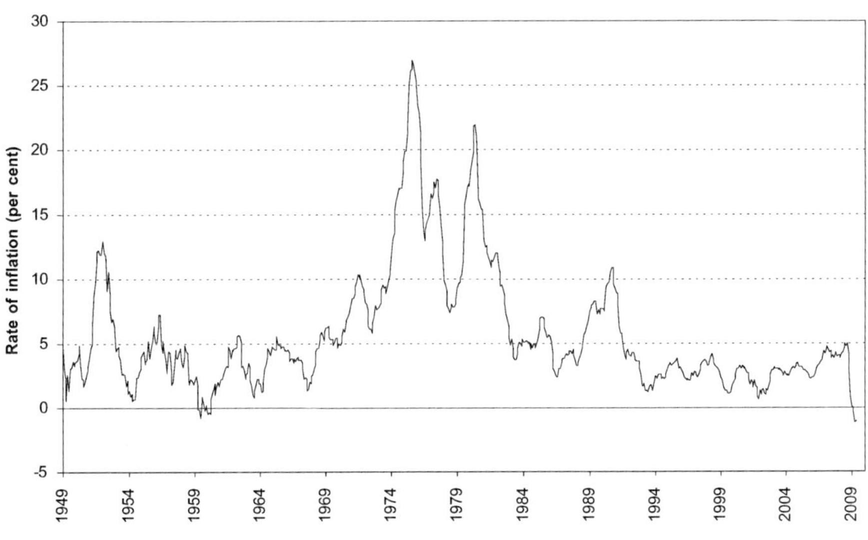

Figure 5.6 Monthly (annualised) percentage change in the retail prices index, 1949–2009. Source: Office for National Statistics Statbase: Economic trends 2009 (RPIX). Available at http://www.statistics.gov.uk/statbase/.

welfare state (Barnett 1987), and that that the taxation needed to finance the welfare state served to reduce incentives to work and thus to reduce growth (Johnson 2004), an alternative view might be that the new welfare state and the experience of full employment increased confidence, and that this allowed people to spend more. Britons no longer had to worry so much about making provision for some of the inevitable challenges experienced in the life course. Education, sickness, unemployment and old age income replacement were covered by the new national insurance system. Although government worries about the cost of national insurance emerged in the 1950s, in fact much lower unemployment than expected coupled with better social services and greater social security gave consumers the confidence to spend more and save less.

Third, the post-war period saw a veritable explosion in the preparedness of consumers to take on debt to finance immediate purchases (O'Connell 2009). From the mid-1950s credit on easy terms, initially through 'hire purchase', began to be available to working class consumers, who proved eager to take advantage of it (Gurney 2005). A subtle shift began to take place as 'debt', with all its pejorative overtones, morphed into the much more attractive sounding 'credit'. Britain's first credit card was launched in 1966 by Barclays Bank. From then on, British consumers developed an apparently insatiable demand for credit, with the result that by 2004 total consumer debt in Britain exceeded £1 trillion.

Rising debt was perhaps one reason, despite rising average incomes and an expansion in both the quantity and the quality of goods purchased, why Britons did not appear to derive much by way of happiness from their improved living standards. This might seem surprising, for politicians in particular had long pursed broadly based economic growth on the Benthamite assumption that thereby the greatest happiness of the greatest number could be obtained. However, by the end of the century economic research suggested that in advanced capitalist economies such as Britain where basic needs had been met there was in fact no correlation between economic growth and happiness (Easterlin 1974; Oswald 1997). Partly this was because individual happiness tended to be concerned much less with absolute living standards and much more with how those living standards compared with others; thus if all living standards were rising happiness could be expected to remain constant. Partly it was because the individual acquisitiveness of the consumer society carried social costs in terms, for example, of less stable families, fractured communities and a generalised loss of trust between individuals (Layard 2005). Moreover, rising real incomes brought with them their own particular problems, such as the need to make choices between an expanding range of similar goods (Offer 2006).

Employment

We have already noted that an important feature of the post-war economy was its growing labour market and that this was a function of both an expanding population and a growing tendency for women to work in the labour market. The pattern of this growth, however, was not smooth. On balance, as can be seen in Figure

5.7, the number in the workforce grew across the period, but with notable shrinkages as a result of the 1979–81 and 1990–2 recessions (though not the 1974–5 recession, something for which the then Labour government received surprisingly little credit).

What is perhaps most striking is the pattern of unemployment. For the quarter century from 1948 it moved with the business cycle, certainly, but it was extraordinarily low. Between 1948 and 1974 the unemployment rate was below 2 per cent in fourteen years, and between 2 and 3 per cent in eleven years. In only two years (1971 and 1972) did it exceed 3 per cent. The rises thereafter, initially from 1974 to 1977 as the recession took its toll, and then the spectacular increase from 1979 (to 13 per cent of the workforce), are remarkable, as is the spike upwards in the early 1990s. In this period the unemployment rate never dropped below 4 per cent. There is a wealth of human misery here, the product of a major structural shift in the British economy as the size of its manufacturing sector contracted with remarkable rapidity. Only after 1992 did an improvement begin.

A notable feature of the long boom after 1992 was the very rapid expansion of the workforce, accompanied by a marked fall in the number of unemployed. However, despite the incoming Labour government's restating of full employment as an economic objective in 1997, a much higher number were now structurally unemployed, particularly the unskilled and older men who had formerly worked in manufacturing. Labour did succeed in getting the unemployment rate below 3 per cent, but a telling criticism of this achievement was that it had been brought

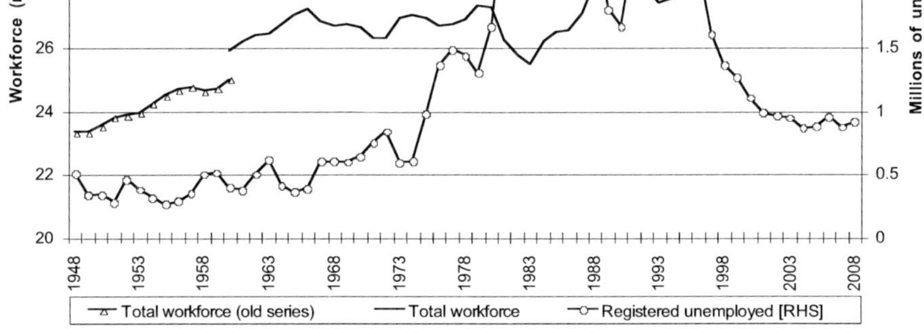

Figure 5.7 Size of workforce and number of unemployment benefit claimants. Source: Total workforce and registered unemployed from Office for National Statistics Statbase: Labour market statistics; total workforce (old series) from Annual Abstract of Statistics, 1958 and 1960. Available at http://www.statistics.gov.uk/statbase/.

about in part by the growing number of long-term sick, which by 2008 had reached 1 million.

Industrial relations

The story of industrial relations is again a game of two halves. Trade union membership rose substantially in the first half of our period. In 1939 around 31 per cent of all employees were union members. By the late 1970s the figure was nearly 55 per cent, markedly higher than competitors such as the United States, Germany and France. Subsequently it fell quickly and by the end of the century was virtually back to the level of 1939 – at which point unionisation in Britain was about the same as in Germany, but still a good deal higher than in either the United States or (particularly) France (Wrigley 2002).

The political importance of trade unions followed a similar trajectory. The Second World War saw government draw the unions into the economic waging of 'total war'. By 1945 there were high hopes that union co-operation with government and employers could help to deliver the combination of higher productivity and wage restraint demanded by a full employment mixed economy operating in a system of fixed exchange rates. However, the ability of the unions to hold their members to national collective agreements began to break down in the 1950s. Full employment both handed substantial power to union members and encouraged firms at the local level to break national bargains to secure competitive advantage. The result was a rise in the power of local union representatives, a breakdown in management control and a marked worsening of industrial relations during the 1960s and 1970s (Brown 2004; Howell 2005) with two governments arguably being brought down by trade unions – the Conservative government in 1974 and Labour in 1979. As Figure 5.8 demonstrates, days lost to strikes rose, peaking in 1984, although the peak year in terms of stoppages was actually 1970 – in other words the pattern was fewer strikes involving more workers.

A case might be made that the failure to build effective co-operative institutions, as other European countries did, was a particular problem, and that Britain's poor industrial relations discouraged investment and innovation by firms (Eichengreen 2006; Bean and Crafts 1996). More specifically, it might be argued that the unions overplayed their hand in the 1970s. After 1979, the Conservatives' analysis of the unions was profoundly antagonistic. In part this was payback for the miners' effectively bringing down the Heath government in 1974. But it also flowed from an analysis that poor industrial relations were at once degrading competitiveness and contributing to inflation. The Conservatives were prepared to countenance a much higher rate of unemployment, indeed to pursue economic policies that were actually intended to raise unemployment in order to reduce inflation, and to encourage a much higher level of competition between firms. The result was a considerable decline in unions' bargaining power. Coupled with successive legislation that limited trade unions' freedom of manoeuvre, a privatisation programme that exposed unions and union members in privatised companies to competitive pressures, the government's virtual destruction of the miners as a political force

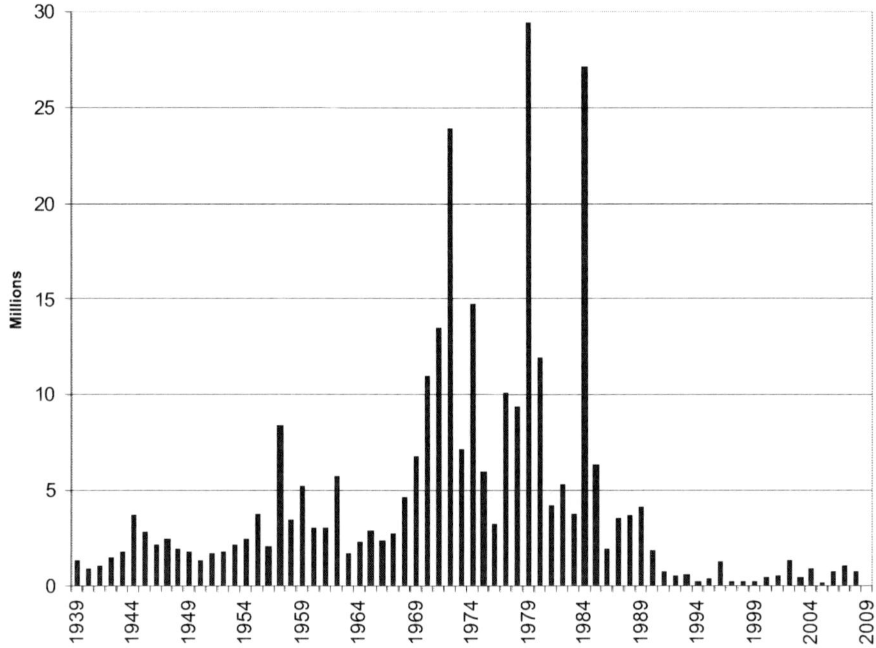

Figure 5.8 Millions of days lost in industrial disputes, 1939–2009.

in the year-long miners' strike of 1984–5 and the impact of globalisation (see, for example, Glyn 2006) the result was effectively to break the power of the unions, at least in the private sector. In the public sector, unions remained relatively strong in terms of membership, but their power was nevertheless considerably weakened by a much more difficult labour market in the 1980s and 1990s. The consequence was a marked reduction in the number of strikes and in the level of working days lost to strikes.

The changing structure of the economy

In the post-war period the structure of Britain's economy changed drastically. In part, this structural change was about a shift from labour-intensive means of production to capital-intensive production – achieved in the first half of our period mainly by automation and in the latter half by the rapid hollowing out of the manufacturing industry as jobs in heavy industry haemorrhaged in the Thatcher years and then the rise of e-businesses gave rise to assumptions that Britain was becoming a 'knowledge based' or 'weightless economy' (Coyle 1999). The most obvious feature of such change was a shift towards service sector employment. In 1939, about half of all British employees worked in the service sector. By the end of the century this had risen to about three-quarters (Millward 2004). This shift came in two stages. Between the end of the war and the 1970s employment in education and health expanded along with the welfare state. At the same time there was an increase in leisure services as disposable income rose in the 'golden age'. Beginning in the 1970s there was a further and more significant rise in the importance of the service sector, driven by the contraction of manufacturing and the growth of trade in financial and, particularly, business services such as computing, advertising, accounting, catering and cleaning that hitherto had normally been performed by companies themselves. Although traditional services such as education, health and retailing continued to be important, by 2000 the provision of such business services had grown from almost nothing to nearly 20 per cent of total service sector employment.

This change was not made without pain. As can plainly be seen in Table 5.6, the number of manufacturing jobs declined rapidly, but the rate of decline of unskilled jobs was also notable, a change that tended to affect men more than women. Increasingly, the ticket to a job was a qualification of some sort. Governments of all political complexions identified a better-educated workforce as essential in meeting the challenge of globalisation. The policy was not without its successes. Between 1975 and 1998, for example, the proportion of young women attaining two or more A levels doubled from 12 to 25 per cent, although the experience of young men was more modest with an increase from 15 to 21 per cent. However, 58 per cent of young men and 48 per cent of young women left school with less that five GCSEs graded at C or above in 1998, and 8 and 5 per cent, respectively, left with no qualification at all (Office for National Statistics 2000). For these young people the best that could be hoped for was a 'McJob' in Britain's increasingly 'flexible' labour market; the worst outcome was no job at all. In 1999, for example, after seven years of continuous economic growth, 12.5 per cent of young men and 9.3 per cent of young women aged between eighteen and twenty-four were neither in education nor economically active. By September 2009, a year after the onset of the worst financial crisis since 1929, the equivalent figures were 24.8 and 32.7 per cent, respectively, thus demonstrating the vulnerability of young people in this restructured labour market (Office for National Statistics 2009b).

Table 5.6 The structure of employment, 1950–95

Year	*Sector*	*UK (%)*	*United States (%)*	*France (%)*	*Germany (%)*
1950	Agriculture	9.8	12.4	29.3	30.5
	Manufacturing and construction	39.5	30.4	31.7	39.1
	Services	50.7	57.2	39	30.4
1995	Agriculture	2.3	2.1	4.9	3.4
	Manufacturing and construction	23.6	19	24.7	34
	Services	74.1	78.9	71	62.6

Source: Adapted from Millward (2004: Table 10.2).

Another feature of the restructuring of Britain's labour market was its distinct regional patterning. Many of the new service sector jobs were in the south, but industrial jobs were dominant in the north of England and the Celtic periphery. As can be seen in Figure 5.9, the result was an increasing north–south divide in unemployment rates that lasted for nearly two decades.

International trade

The international economy grew rapidly in the post-war 'golden age' and Britain shared in this growth. The reasons for relatively fast global economic growth between 1945 and the early 1970s are complex but owed much initially to a post-war reconstruction boom coupled with the stability afforded by new economic institutions such as the International Monetary Fund that were set up in the aftermath of the Bretton Woods Agreement in 1944. Thereafter, despite the economic difficulties experienced by advanced capitalist economies in the 1970s, and the collapse of the Bretton Woods system, the world economy continued at once to grow and to become more interlinked as a long-term process of 'globalisation' apparently accelerated and goods and capital flows increased (Tisdell and Sen 2004).

Britain's had always been an open economy, but even so the importance to it of international trade grew as world trade itself grew. For example, the share of exports within its GDP increased from 18.6 per cent in 1948 to 28.5 per cent in 1997. Within this, however, there were big changes in the direction of the country's international trade. Britain began the period as an Atlanticist economy

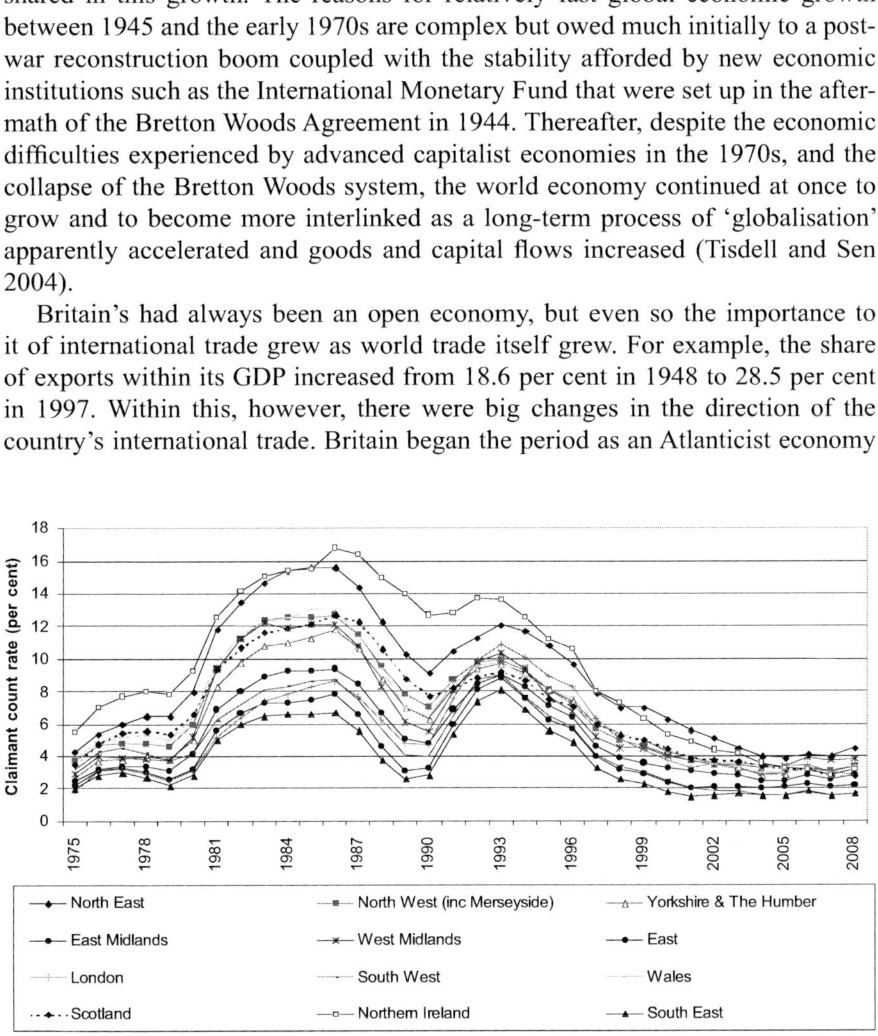

Figure 5.9 Regional unemployment rates. Source: Office for National Statistics Statbase: Labour market statistics 2008. Available at http://www.statistics.gov.uk/statbase/.

dominated by trade with its empire and with the Americas. It ended the period with an economy closely tied to the new European Union (formerly European Economic Community), which Britain joined in 1973. By the end of the century, Britain's trade with Western Europe had increased from about 40 per cent in 1973 to about 61 per cent.

We should also note, however, that, although the volume of Britain's trade with other countries grew, its share of world trade as a whole declined. This was in part an inevitable result of the reconstruction of Western Europe and Japan after the war. But it was also a function of the growth of formerly undeveloped economies. In this sense, Britain's 'loss' was others' gain. However, the process involved some painful readjustments for Britain. In particular, the increased importance of imports created some significant problems with the balance of payments (i.e. with the balance between imports and exports), as can be seen in Figure 5.10, which shows those balances measured as a proportion of total gross domestic product, with any value below zero indicating an excess of imports over exports.

There is a paradox here, though. Economically, balance of payments deficits became more serious in the second half of our period. Strangely, however, they were politically more important in the first half of the period. That was a function of the Bretton Woods system of fixed exchange rates that had been established in the wake of the Second World War. With a fixed exchange rate the outflow of funds required to finance an excess of imports over exports could not be created by an automatic devaluation of the currency. Between the first attempt to move sterling to full convertibility in 1948 and the collapse of Bretton Woods in 1971, and for a few years after, British governments were obsessed by the problem and

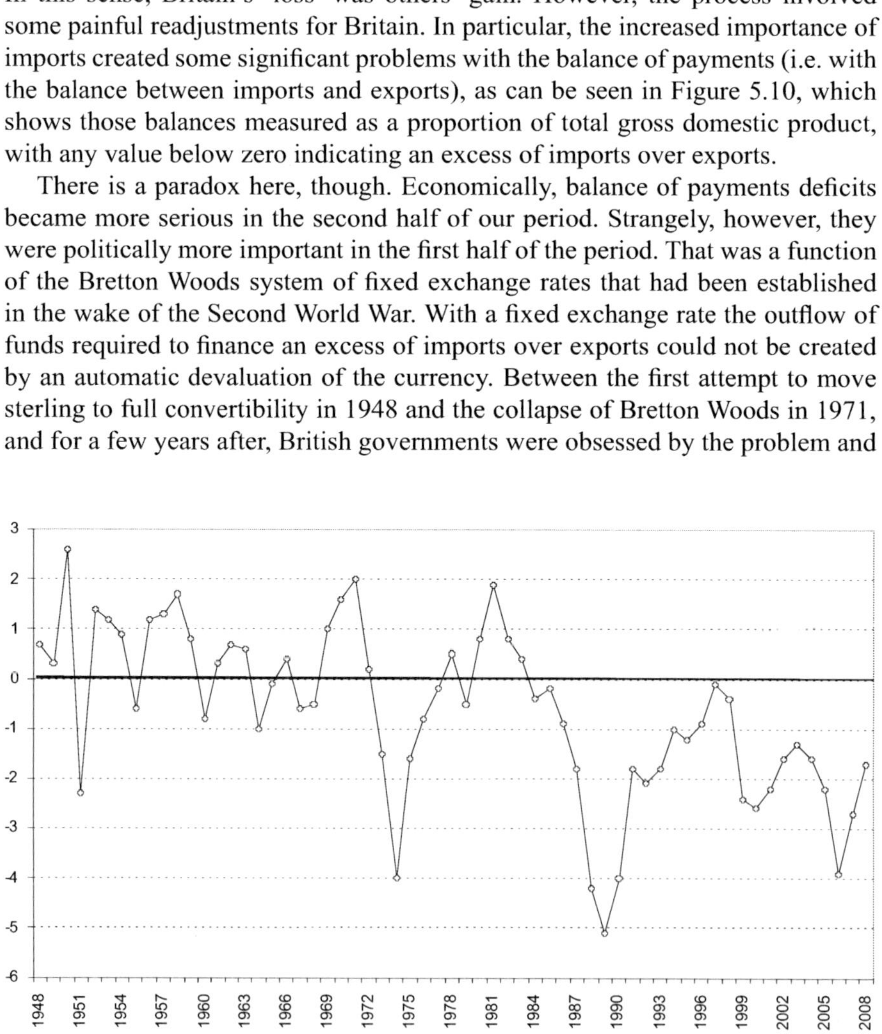

Figure 5.10 Current balance of payments as a percentage of GDP, 1948–2008. Source: Office for National Statistics Statbase: Economic trends 2008. Available at http://www.statistics.gov.uk/statbase/.

acted rapidly to address any deficit. This was the major contributor to the 'stop-go' phenomenon of the 1950s and 1960s, with strong growth generating periodic balance of payments deficits, which then caused the government to deflate to protect sterling. In retrospect, the reaction seems excessive, as for most of the 1950s and 1960s the balance of payments was actually in surplus. The reaction in the mid-1970s, most notably in 1976 when the government feared that sterling was about to 'fall through the floor' and instituted a major deflation in order to secure an IMF loan that later turned out not to have been needed, seems at first sight to have been more understandable, not least that it turned on the difficult issue of 'confidence'. But by this time the pound was floating freely on the foreign exchanges. The experience of later years, when deficits, many of a similar order or worse, were a regular feature of the economic experience but did not lead to a political reaction, is instructive. The balance of payments had ceased to be seen as a political problem, mistakenly perhaps for it may have been a harbinger of trouble ahead in that it was plainly a function of structural imbalances caused by the rapid contraction of manufacturing.

Conclusion

We have seen that the post-war British economy experienced major changes, but that there were also some important continuities. Perhaps the most notable changes were the marked growth in the British economy, the growing number of people in paid work and the general rise in living standards that took place. A growing economy allowed the country to create, and to sustain even in hard times, a welfare state that immeasurably increased people's quality of life in ways other than the merely material. Britons, it must be said, have an apparently unending ability to moan, but in these respects there was actually very little to moan about. On the whole, life really did get better, at least at the aggregate level. Probing beneath this, however, it must be acknowledged that, despite half a century of economic growth, profound inequalities in the distribution of income and wealth remained, and that whereas these inequalities had tended to narrow in the first half of our period they had widened in the second.

In policy terms, the transformation of economic policy that had occurred during the Second World War with the adoption of a Keynesian system of national accounting and the use by the state of fiscal instruments to manage aggregate demand was retained. The framework was consolidated in the 1950s and 1960s with the active management of demand deriving from the commitment to full employment. Thereafter, however, policy was subject to a major revision with the adoption of 'monetarism' after 1979, but this new framework also proved problematic, most notably failing completely to attain its targets for money supply growth, with the result that by 1986 they had been abandoned (Backhouse 2002). As a result, the new framework was itself revised in the 1980s and 1990s. The primacy of full employment as an economic objective was replaced by low inflation and there were important changes in the political priorities attached to both the balance of payments and the level of sterling. By the start of the new century, a more generalised 'neo-liberal' framework had evolved. This focused on low income tax rates, to increase incentives to work, regulation of private monopolies rather than state ownership, inflation targeting using interest rates and the pursuance of high employment through supply-side measures such as education and training rather than by managing aggregate demand on Keynesian lines.

In terms of performance, there were also important changes. The baby booms, the growing desire of women to perform paid work, migration and post-war economic growth all served to expand the workforce and to alter the experience of work. The structure of the economy was also transformed; most notably, Britain became a 'white collar' service economy and the importance of 'blue collar' industrial work declined. There was also a major change in the ownership of the economy: the rise of state ownership during the first half of our period was succeeded by successive rounds of privatisation that rolled back the nationalisation project. We have noted that, although Britain's trade with the rest of the world grew, the direction of that trade became increasingly dominated by trade with the rest of Europe. In economic, if not in political, terms Britain became less Atlanticist and more European. The membership and power of the unions rose and fell, as did the number of industrial disputes. Change was thus continuous, wide-ranging and often long-lasting, with the result that, from the economic perspective, each of the generations in the national birth cohort studies had distinct experiences (and it is worth noting here that economic researchers should make more of the studies for precisely this reason).

In terms of continuities, we have noted that the Second World War produced an apparently permanent 'ratchetting up' in the size of the state. We have also noted that the British economy experienced a continuing decline relative to other advanced economies. Nonetheless, although relative economic decline is unarguable, we should not allow that to blind us to what is perhaps the most obvious feature of the post-war British economy: its growth. A growing economy helped to raise living standards, to increase leisure, to allow greatly increased material consumption and to finance and sustain the welfare state. The first generation covered by the British national birth cohort studies was perhaps the most fortunate generation in British history. Clearly, the continuing development of economic policy and performance will continue to affect their lives, and the lives of the successor cohorts, in ways that will be unpredictable but we can hope that past performance proves to be a good guide to the future.

References

Abramovitz, M. (1986) 'Catching up, forging ahead and falling behind', *Journal of Economic History*, 46: 385–406.

Artis, M., Cobham, D. and Wickham-Jones, M. (1992) 'Social democracy in hard times: the economic record of the Labour government 1974–1979', *Twentieth Century British History*, 3: 32–58.

Atkinson, A. B. (1995) *Incomes and the welfare state*, Cambridge: Cambridge University Press.

Backhouse, R. (2002) 'The macroeconomics of Margaret Thatcher', *Journal of the History of Economic Thought*, 24: 313–34.

Barnett, C. (1987) *The audit of war: the illusion and reality of Britain as a great nation*, Basingstoke: Macmillan.

Bean, C. and Crafts, N. F. R. (1996) 'British economic growth since 1945: relative economic decline . . . and renaissance?', in N. F. R. Crafts and G. Toniolo (eds) *Economic growth in Europe since 1945*, pp.131–72, Cambridge: Cambridge University Press.

Beveridge, W. (1942) *Social insurance and allied services (the Beveridge Report)*, Cmnd. 6404, London: His Majesty's Stationery Office.

Booth, A. (2001) *The British economy in the twentieth century*, London: Palgrave.

Brown, W. (2004) 'Industrial relations and the economy', in R. Floud and P. Johnson (eds) *The economic history of Britain since 1700, Vol. 3*, pp. 399–423, Cambridge: Cambridge University Press.

Burk, K. (1988) *The first privatisation: the politicians, the city, and the denationalisation of steel*, London: The Historians' Press.

Cairncross, A. (1995) *The British economy since 1945*, Oxford: Blackwell.

Card, D., Blundell, R. and Freeman, R. B. (2004) *Seeking a premier league economy: the economic effects of British economic reforms*, 1980–2000, Chicago: University of Chicago Press.

Clift, B. and Tomlinson, J. (2007) 'Credible Keynesianism? New Labour macroeconomic policy and the political economy of coarse tuning', *British Journal of Political Science*, 37: 47–69.

Coyle, D. (1999) *The weightless world: strategies for managing the digital economy*, Oxford: Capstone.

Crafts, N. F. R. (1997) *Britain's relative economic decline: 1870–1995*, London: Social Market Foundation.

Crafts, N. F. R. (2002) *Britain's relative economic performance, 1870–1999*, London: Institute for Economic Affairs.

Dow, J. C. R. (2000) *Major recessions: Britain and the world, 1920–1995*, Oxford: Oxford University Press.

Easterlin, R. A. (1974) 'Does economic growth improve the human lot? Some empirical evidence', in P. A. David and M. W. Reder (eds) *Nations and households in economic growth: Essays in honour of Moses Abramowitz*, pp. 89–126, New York: Academic Press.

Eichengreen, B. (2006) *The European economy since 1945: coordinated capitalism and beyond*, Princeton: Princeton University Press.

Feinstein, C. H. (ed.) (1983) *The managed economy: essays in British economic policy and performance since 1929*, Oxford: Oxford University Press.

Glennerster, H. (2007) *British social policy since 1945*, Oxford: Blackwell.

Glyn, A. (2006) *Capitalism unleashed: finance, globalization and welfare*, Oxford, Oxford University Press.

Gurney, P. (2005) 'The battle of the consumer in post-war Britain', *Journal of Modern History*, 77: 956–87.

Hague, D. and Wilkinson, S. F. (1983) *The IRC – an experiment in industrial intervention: a history of the Industrial Reorganisation Corporation*, London: Allen and Unwin.

Halsey, A. H. and Webb, J. (eds) (2000) *Twentieth-century British social trends*, Basingstoke: Macmillan.

Hannah, L. (2004) 'A failed experiment: the state ownership of industry', in R. Floud and P. Johnson (eds) *The economic history of Britain since 1700, Vol. 3*, pp. 84–111, Cambridge: Cambridge University Press.

HM Government (2005) *Health, work and well-being – caring for our future. A strategy for the health and well-being of working age people*, London: Department for Work and Pensions, Department of Health, and the Health and Safety Executive.

HM Treasury (1961) *Control of public expenditure*, Cmnd. 1432, London: HMSO.

HM Treasury (2003) *2003 budget report*, Ch. 6, para. 6.1. Available at http://web.archive.org/web/20030707170306/www.hm- _bud03/budget_report/bud_bud03_repchap6.cfm (last accessed 15 December 2010).

Howell, C. (2005) *Trade unions and the state: the construction of industrial relations institutions in Britain, 1890–2000*, Princeton: Princeton University Press.

Johnson, P. (2004) 'The welfare state, income and living standards', in R. Floud and P. Johnson (eds) *The economic history of Britain since 1700, Vol. 3*, pp. 213–37, Cambridge: Cambridge University Press.

Johnson, P. and Zaidi, A. (2007) 'Work over the life course', in N. Crafts, I. Gazeley and A. Newell (eds) *Work and pay in 20th century Britain*, pp. 98–116, Oxford: Oxford University Press.

Keynes, J. M. (1936) *General theory of employment, interest and money*, Cambridge: Cambridge University Press.

Labour Party (1963) Speech at Labour Party conference, 1 October. *Annual Conference Report*, pp. 139–40.

Layard, R. (2005) *Happiness: lessons from a new science*, London: Penguin.

Lowe, R. (2005) *The welfare state in Britain since 1945*, London: Palgrave Macmillan.

Matthews, R. C. O. (1968) 'Why has Britain had full employment since the war?', *Economic Journal*, 78: 555–69.

Middleton, R. (2000) *The British economy since 1945*, Basingstoke: Macmillan.

Millward, R. (2004) 'The rise of the service economy', in R. Floud and P. Johnson (eds) *The economic history of Britain since 1700, Vol. 3*, pp. 238–66, Cambridge: Cambridge University Press.

Minister of Reconstruction (1944) *Employment policy*, Cmnd. 6527, London: HMSO.

Morris, D. J. and Stout, D. (1985) 'Industrial policy', in D. J. Morris (ed) *The economic system in the UK*, pp. 851–94, Oxford: Oxford University Press.

O'Connell, S. (2009) *Credit and community: working-class debt in the UK since 1880*, Oxford: Oxford University Press.

Offer, A. (2006) *The challenge of affluence: self-control and well-being in the United States and Britain since 1950*, Oxford: Oxford University Press.

Office for National Statistics (2000) *Social Trends 2000*, London: Office for National Statistics.

Office for National Statistics (2002) *The Blue Book*, London: HMSO.

Office for National Statistics (2008) *Social Trends 2008*, London: Office for National Statistics.

Office for National Statistics (2009a) 'Gini coefficients, 1981 to 2005/06 (per cent): the effects of taxes and benefits on household income, 2005/06'. Available at http://www.statistics.gov.uk/StatBase/ssdataset.asp?vlnk=9604&More=Y (last accessed 15 December 2009).

Office for National Statistics (2009b) 'Labour market survey 2009'. Available at http://www.statistics.gov.uk/statbase/Product.asp?vlnk=1944 (last accessed 15 December 2009).

Oliver, M. J. and Pemberton, H. (2004) 'Learning and change in 20th century British economic policy', *Governance*, 17: 415–41.

O'Mahony, M. (2004) 'Employment, education and human capital', in R. Floud and P. Johnson (eds) *The economic history of Britain since 1700, Vol. 3*, pp. 112–33, Cambridge: Cambridge University Press.

Oswald, A. (1997) 'Happiness and economic performance', *Economic Journal*, 107: 1815–31.

Pepper, G. and Oliver, M. J. (2001) *Monetarism under Thatcher*, Cheltenham: Edward Elgar.

Sachs, J. D. (2001) *Macroeconomics and health: investing in health for economic development. Report of the Commission on Macroeconomics and Health*, Geneva: World Health Organization. Available at http://whqlibdoc.who.int/publications/2001/924154550x.pdf (last accessed 3 August 2009).

Simon, B. (1985) 'The Tory government and education: background to breakout', *History of Education*, 14: 283–97.

Smith, R. M. (1994) 'Elements of demographic change in Britain since 1945', in P. Catterall and J. Obelkevich (eds) *Understanding post-war British society*, pp. 19–30, London: Routledge.

Thane, P. (2007) 'The welfare state and the labour market', in N. Crafts, I. Gazeley and A. Newell (eds) *Work and pay in 20th century Britain*, pp. 178–202, Oxford: Oxford University Press.

Timmins, N. (2001) *The five giants: a biography of the welfare state*, London: HarperCollins.

Tisdell, C. A. and Sen, R. K. (2004) *Economic globalisation: social conflicts, labour and environmental issues*, Cheltenham: Edward Elgar.

Tomlinson, J. (2000) *The politics of decline: understanding post-war Britain*, Harlow: Longman.

Weir, M. (1989) 'Ideas and politics: the acceptance of Keynesianism in Britain and the United States', in P. A. Hall (ed.) *The political power of economic ideas*, pp. 53–86, Princeton: Princeton University Press.

Wrigley, C. (2002) *British trade unions since 1933*, Cambridge: Cambridge University Press.

6 Labour market, employment and skills

David Ashton and John Bynner

Introduction

This chapter is predicated on the assumption that the major factors affecting the UK labour market over the last six decades, as well as the skills required for employment, are the twin forces of globalisation and political change within the UK. These occurred in three phases over this period: phase one, from the Second World War to 1970, one of stability and growth; phase two, from 1970 to 1990, one of restructuring; and a further phase of stability and growth from 1990 to 2008 when economic growth was abruptly halted by the financial crisis of that year.

Within each of these phases we deal first with the broader context, which means tracing the changes at the global level in the political and institutional arrangements governing economic relationships and in the organisation of production. Second we deal with the political and economic changes that occurred within the UK economy. The impact of all these changes is then traced through the labour market to the policy response of governments to these challenges.

Initially there was the establishment of a new political order following the end of the war with the world divided into two ideologically opposed blocs, namely the communist and non-communist, a division that lasted approximately three decades. This was followed by the restructuring of the economy and political relationships, which took place over the next two decades, involving the collapse of communism in Eastern Europe and the deregulation of Western economies. Finally, came a further period of stability and growth that occurred as new emergent economies, especially those of China and India, were integrated into global markets, before this was spectacularly disrupted by the banking crisis of 2008.

Within the labour market these changes have produced a radical change in the distribution of occupations, associated with the decline of manufacturing and the rise of the service industries, a shift from manual to non-manual employment, an increase in professional, technical and managerial occupations and a decline in unskilled manual work, countered by a rise in unskilled service sector work. This has resulted in a decline in male employment rates and rapid growth in female employment rates. However, these trends have also been affected by the business cycle that has created periods of boom and bust, which in turn have generated major fluctuations in the level of unemployment and political unrest. Each of these is played out in the context of the global economic and political changes that characterised the three phases.

The response of governments was to regulate the economy and labour market during and after the Second World War. During this period the government had control over a number of levers, such as interest rates and employment levels in the nationalised industries, through which it could 'manage' the level of demand for labour in the economy. When the level of economic activity fell in the private sector it could increase activity in the public sector and virtually guarantee high levels of employment. In terms of training policy it influenced the demand side of the equation by passing legislation that forced employers to train. The supply of labour and skills, the supply side, was influenced through its education and training policies.

As the UK became more closely integrated into global markets this regulatory approach was abandoned and under the guise of neo-liberalism a policy of de-regulation was instituted across both the economy and the labour market. Industries were de-nationalised and the government gave up the attempt to regulate or 'manage' the level of economic activity, the demand side, leaving this to be determined by market forces. This meant that in the labour market attempts to regulate the demand for skills were abandoned leaving the government to concentrate on influencing the supply of skills, which it continued to do through its education and training policies. These supply-side policies were pursued by governments of all political persuasions until the financial crisis of 2008 demonstrated the need for governments to extend their regulation of economic activity and pay greater attention to the demand side.

The chapter draws on a range of sources, not least the work conducted by colleagues from the Centre for Labour Market Studies at the University of Leicester over the last four decades. However, numerous other sources have been utilised to identify key trends and explain the major changes we have witnessed over this period. All this has been supplemented by hard data from the government-funded Labour Force Survey and other, one-off surveys of employers' skill requirements as well as the various cohort studies.

Stability and growth

Contextual changes

Following the end of the war the international political settlement at Bretton Woods set the parameters for international trade. Led by the United States the victorious powers established the main international institutions that would shape world trade for the next thirty years – the World Bank, the International Monetary Fund and the General Agreement on Tariffs and Trade (GATT). The World Bank provided finance to the developing world, the International Monetary Fund was to be the lender of last resort for national governments and GATT provided the framework for the gradual integration of national markets into the global market. This provided a stable economic framework within which the UK's post-war economic recovery got under way. However, there were strict limits to this emerging global market because the communist states were excluded, providing an alternative route to economic development.

Initially, this new framework worked relatively well for the UK. Some of our major competitors, such as Germany, France and Japan, had to rebuild their devastated economies, albeit with American assistance. This reduced the competitive pressure on UK employers as they too recovered from the effects of the war. However, many of the UK manufacturers were also helped by the shelter provided by their old empire markets to which they had preferential access and few competitors. The result was a period of economic growth and a consumer boom, which saw full employment established and incomes growth in real terms, thus paving the way for the 'never had it so good' society of the Macmillan years (1957–63).

Although the institutional arrangements were in place to stimulate international trade, this was still a period when trade was organised around national markets, when American industrial output was as great as that of the rest of the world combined. There was increasing trade between nations but this took the form of exports of primary and fully manufactured goods from one nation to another. Multi-national corporations (MNCs) were still in their infancy as US companies set up foreign subsidiaries abroad to get behind tariff barriers to manufacture complete products.

Politically there was a new national consensus aimed at reducing the impact of inequality on life chances, achieved through the establishment of the National Health Service, and providing employment security through policies of full employment and demand management. As Figure 6.1 shows, during this period unemployment rarely rose above 2–3 per cent (Lindsay 2003).

It appeared that the horrors of the unemployment of the 1930s had been permanently eradicated. Economically, many of the major industries, such as coal, gas, electricity, iron and steel and railways, that had been vital for the war effort were nationalised, providing effective guarantees of employment to a large part of the labour force (Ashton 1986). Others such as the banks and financial services were tightly regulated. Many of the major decisions affecting these industries were influenced by political as well as economic considerations, and the maintenance of full employment. Government influence over the economy was extensive, enabling successive governments to manage demand and keep unemployment at a low level. The trade unions played a full part in the post-war settlement. As Figure 6.2 shows membership remained stable at around 40 per cent of the labour force (Lindsay 2003). The industrial relations framework was highly centralised with the pay of many determined through national negotiations while the unions had an important say in the training arrangements for new entrants, initially at the local level and later in the 1960s at a national level with the implementation of the Industrial Training Act, which established a national system of Industry Training Boards. For the middle classes the professional associations provided a strong framework for the regulation of their work and the safeguarding of their position in the labour market.

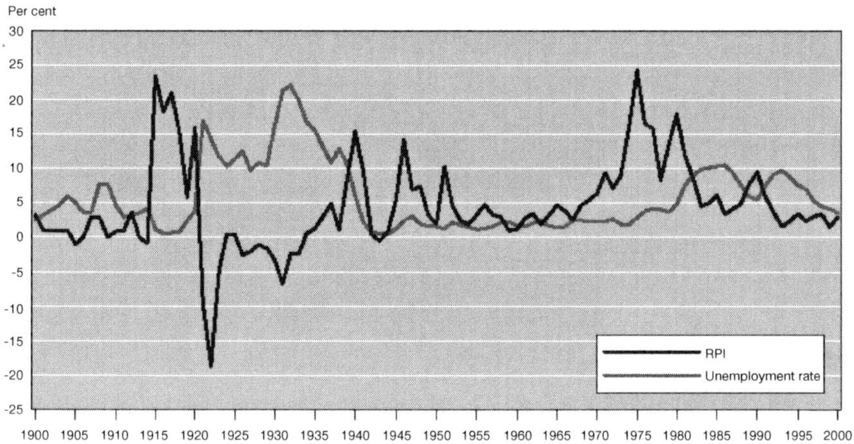

Figure 6.1 UK claimant unemployment rate over the long run. Year-on-year growth of the retail prices index (RPI) and unemployment, 1900–2000, United Kingdom. The RPI started in 1947. All figures before this date are estimated and are not official figures; they come from Layton and Crowther (1938). Unemployment data are based on register and claimant count data. Note: Data have not been adjusted to reflect the post-2001 census population estimates. UR, unemployment/labour force (LF); LF, unemployed + employed. Source: Lindsay (2003).

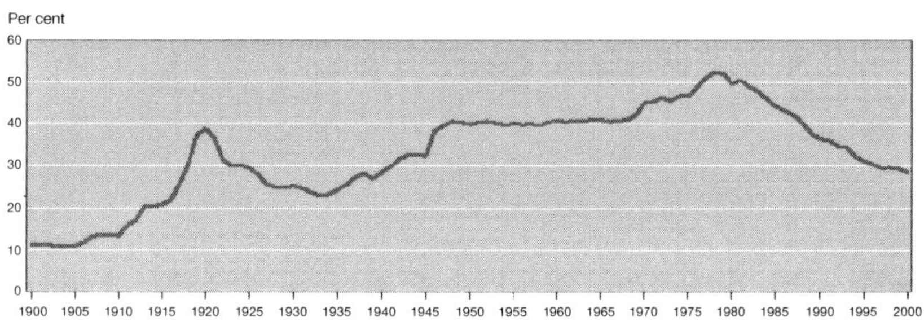

Figure 6.2 UK union density over the long run. Proportion of people in employment who are members of a trade union, 1900–2000, United Kingdom. Data since 1975 from the Certification Officer's Annual Reports are for Great Britain only. Note: Data have not been adjusted to reflect the post-2001 census population estimates. Source: Lindsay (2003).

Labour market

It was these institutional arrangements that provided the sense of stability that characterised the experience of the labour market for the post-war generation. The NHS provided security against illness; huge nationalised industries, together with centralised bargaining and economic growth, provided a regular increase in income especially for the skilled trades and professions. Women, who had stepped into the breach during the war because of the call-up of men to fight, moved back out of the labour market into the family. However, having been employed in many of the traditional male domains, in agriculture, steel making and manufacturing, they had destroyed many of the old myths surrounding the role of women – starting, as we shall see in later sections, a trend in women's rising labour market participation that has continued ever since. The demobilised military personnel joining the labour market were equipped with the skills that made employment relatively easy to find in an economy that was moving from a 'wartime' to a 'peacetime' footing aided by the Marshall Plan. At the highest tiers of industry, including the nationalised industries set up by the 1945 Labour government under Harold Wilson, ex-officers moved relatively easily into senior management positions, for example in British Rail, with somewhat mixed results. Further down the scale, ex-servicemen filled the growing number of jobs becoming available in the manufacturing industry.

Sheltered from international competition, the manufacturing industry continued to grow, with employment in manufacturing peaking at an all-time high of 48 per cent of the labour force in 1958. These jobs in mining, steel, hosiery, vehicle production and footwear, together with the new consumer goods industries based on the production of goods such as washing machines, radios, furniture and later TVs, appeared to offer a job for life. They provided the basis for large, established, working class communities – with an elite skilled male workforce and a large group of semi-skilled operatives. In the heavier industries these employees were largely men, but in the older food, hosiery and footwear, and the new consumer goods industries, women were extensively employed.

For most young people the transition from school to work was also highly structured compared with what had preceded it. Those leaving secondary school with few if any qualifications went into unskilled and semi-skilled jobs in the mines and factories. Up to the end of the 1970s, two-thirds of the population still left education at the minimum statutory age of sixteen, most without formal qualifications. Those from trade schools and the new secondary moderns with a good school record and some qualifications under their belt went into apprenticeships and those from the grammar schools went into the middle class white collar jobs. Only 5–7 per cent went to universities. The intermediate technical schools promoted in the1944 Act (the equivalent of the German *Realschule* attended by one-third of young Germans) never really took off.

For the majority, the secondary modern school curriculum was a watered down version of the old academic grammar school curriculum and offered little of relevance for many working class pupils beyond basic literacy and numeracy. However, the grammar school did provide a more relevant education for those entering the professions and other white collar jobs. When the curriculum did attempt to deliver relevant vocational instruction this was heavily gendered, with metalwork and woodwork for boys and cooking and needlework for girls. For many working class pupils school was not a very meaningful experience (Ashton and Field 1976; Willis 1977), whereas work, even in routine semi-skilled and unskilled jobs, provided a step towards adulthood and independence.

The stability characteristic of this post-war period was reflected in the fact that training was seen as a one-off activity that then provided you with the skills for life. For men entering skilled jobs this was seen to provide a virtual guarantee of a regular income. For many women work was seen as an interim period before marriage, to be followed by an exit from the labour market to bring up children. For those from the grammar schools entering white collar work training was less of a one-off activity and more of a continuous process that would be involved at every step of their movement up the career ladder. For the small percentage of each cohort (5–7 per cent) who entered university (Figure 6.3) there was a virtual guarantee of a high-level job on entering the labour market after graduation.

There is little wonder then that labour market research from this period tended to conceptualise the transitions as linear, with young people moving from a situation of dependence on the family of origin through a period of initial training into full adult status. Of course, although this was the case for many, especially those entering middle and working class careers, there were others for whom the transition was far less linear. For example, for many of those entering semi-skilled and unskilled 'career-less' factory jobs, where the work was often routine, boring and low paid, there was the temptation to continually move between jobs to obtain variety and perhaps a small increase in income. But for the majority of young people during this period the context described above provided a stable framework with full employment guaranteeing the opportunity either to progress in the job they were in or to move between jobs should they decide. Moreover, because there were opportunities within firms for those with few or no qualifications to move in the internal labour market to higher-level positions, this period provided the means for occupational and social mobility (Ashton *et al.* 1982).

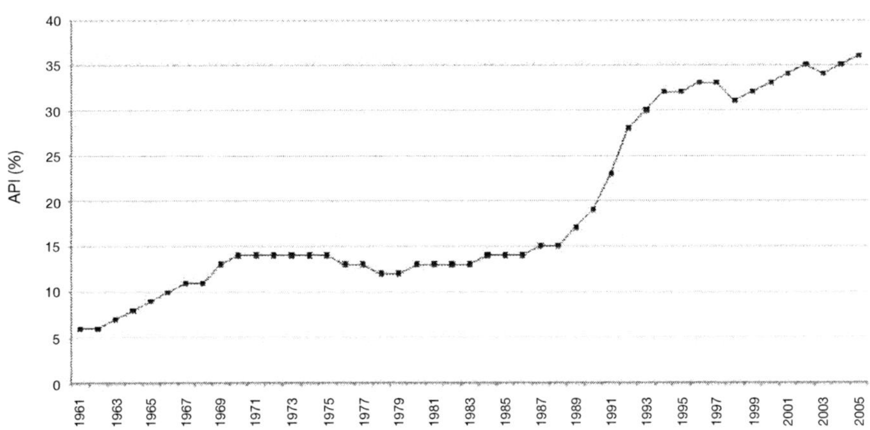

Figure 6.3 Participation by young people in higher education, Age Participation Index 2 (API), Great Britain, 1961–2005. Source: Elias and Purcell (2009).

Policy response

In terms of skills policy, the main focus tended to be directed more to the next generation – how to make the education and training system effective in sustaining and enhancing the skills base that the economy demanded. Apprenticeship was one means of doing this for the elite 120,000, mainly boys, of the 600,000 school leaver cohort who gained entry to one. Girls were more likely to enter factories or the limited number of 'female' skilled jobs obtained through apprenticeship, such as hairdressing. The other main policy initiative was the expansion of higher education reflected in the establishment of the 'new red-brick' universities and continual raising of the target numbers for university entrance. With regard to training, the major change during this period was the growing awareness on the part of the government of the inadequacy of the UK's skills base, highlighted by comparisons with international competitors, especially Germany as it rebuilt its economy after the war.

As the government had no inhibitions about using the law to rectify what it saw as employers' failings, in 1964 it passed the Industrial Training Act, which set up Industry Training Boards, steered by a tripartite grouping of employers, unions and government, with the power to impose a levy on firms and with exemptions for those that met the requisite standard of training for their industry. This provided the UK with a set of training institutions for each industry with the aim of improving the level of training, especially initial training. However, employers were never very happy with this arrangement, although they were obliged to go along with it. There was traditional resistance to firm-based training across large sections of industry because of the fear that another employer would 'poach' the trainee once their training was completed.

Restructuring

Contextual changes

By the mid-to-late-1960s the international conditions that had sustained the stability of the UK's framework were starting to change. The institutions established under the Bretton Woods Agreement were continuing to function well. The major change with regard to the UK was its position in the global division of labour. Politically, many of the nations that formed the British Empire were now seeking independence. In Africa, India and Asia, the granting of independence soon saw the new nations seeking to establish their own industries and the first to be developed were the relatively low-tech industries such as cycle production, textiles, footwear and plastics. As UK companies lost their preferential access to these markets so capital was relocated. In addition, the new 'tiger' economies of East Asia were also establishing low-tech, labour-intensive industries with the advantage of lower labour costs than in the UK. Hampered by the loss of these markets, higher wage costs, outdated technologies and long-standing reluctance to invest profits in new ones at the expense of share-holder dividends, UK-owned companies were starting to fail in the wider marketplace. The political response to this was for the government to apply for membership of the 'European Common Market', which it succeeded in joining in 1973. This symbolised the shift in focus of UK trade away from the old empire markets to the markets of Europe where most of the country's trade was to take place.

Nationally the most significant change was the election of the Conservative government under Margaret Thatcher. This marked the end of the post-war political consensus with the adoption of neo-liberal policies known as 'Thatcherism' in the UK and 'Reaganism' in the United States. In the UK this resulted in the privatisation of nationalised industries and the de-regulation of financial and business services, the so-called – with premonition in view of subsequent events – 'Big Bang'.

At the international level this period saw the radical transformation of world trade. The collapse of the Soviet Union at the end of the 1980s led to Russia and many of the newly independent satellite states rapidly adopting variants of capitalism. This was followed by a more gradual and controlled introduction of market relations by the Chinese Communist state while India abandoned its isolationist policy and integrated into the global economy. This produced a quadrupling of the global labour force (Brown *et al.* 2008) and a massive expansion of world markets. As a result, the United States lost its dominance of world markets as first Japan and then later the Asian Tigers, Brazil, Russia, India and China entered the stage. Responding to the new opportunities created by this hugely enlarged market, and facilitated by changes in technology, notably computing and later in the 1990s the internet, multi-national corporations started to globalise production across a range of industries from automobiles to financial services. From having their own secure markets, UK companies were now operating in much more intensely competitive global markets. The impact of these changes on the national economy was to accelerate job losses. One feature of the transformation was the decline in manufacturing from the 1980s onwards and its counterpart the steady and continuing rise in the service industry.

As we have seen, from the early 1970s unemployment started to rise (Figure 6.1). Operating as one manufacturing base among many in the EU, and facing tough competition from more productive Japanese, Taiwanese and Korean firms, many UK companies failed. Moreover, the UK government was no longer in a position to exercise demand management. Inflation, stimulated by the 1973 oil shortage, started to take hold. In 1976 the Wilson government abandoned full employment as a policy objective. Attempts by the same government to modernise industry through the 'white heat of the technological revolution' were only partially successful. Now, not only was the loss of manufacturing jobs starting to undermine the stability of the labour market, but the institutional structures that had sustained it, such as centralised (collective) bargaining, were also starting to be perceived as reasons why industry was slow in adapting to the new challenges of increasingly competitive global markets.

Meanwhile the unions were increasing their membership and fighting to defend the interests of their members in an increasingly hostile labour market. Industrial disputes soared in the early 1970s and the country came to be seen by some as increasingly ungovernable – the 'sick man of Europe'. In the face of threats from the miners the Heath government restricted electricity consumption by introducing the 'three day week' in December 1973. Later in the decade the attempts by the Labour government to control inflation through the use of public sector pay restraint in 1978–9 led to the 'winter of discontent' as local authority workers resisted through a series of strikes.

The incoming Conservative administration under Margaret Thatcher sought to confront the unions and reduce their power and this, together with the consequences of industrial restructuring, led to further unrest. However, social cohesion was maintained in part by the unifying effects in 1982 of the Falklands War and the extra resources available to the government by the exploitation of North Sea oil. The success of the measures that the government had taken against the unions was demonstrated when they succeeded in closing mines and defeated the mine workers in their second major strike of 1984.

Throughout this period the Conservative government created a new framework for economic activity and labour market behaviour by extending the role of market forces, freeing employers from the constraints previously imposed on their behaviour through the trade unions and government regulations. Domestically, council houses were offered for sale to tenants to encourage more private home ownership. In 1953 the proportion of home owners in England was 32 per cent, which rose to 51 per cent in 1971 and reached a peak of 85 per cent in 1981. For many of the individuals concerned this provided a sense of increasing personal wealth as house prices rose. However, back in the economy, and left to their own devices in increasingly competitive markets, many UK firms went under and manufacturing haemorrhaged jobs for a number of years. In the labour market any form of state regulation was to be dispensed with. As a result, unemployment soared to over 10 per cent in the late 1980s before falling again (Lindsay 2003), and repossessions from those unable to meet their mortgage commitments became a common occurrence.

Labour market

The combination of changes in the international division of labour reducing the competitiveness of UK firms and the powerful changes in the structure of the labour market introduced by the Thatcher government generated a radical transformation of employment. Large parts of the iron and steel and shipbuilding industries were virtually wiped out by competitors with more advanced techniques of production and lower wage costs. Whole cities with heavy dependence on single industries such as Sheffield's on light steels were placed under enormous strain with jobs disappearing and no new industries to replace them. The coal industry was destroyed by the political decision to switch electricity generation from coal to North Sea gas. Other light industries such as hosiery and textiles and footwear, and later the new consumer goods industries producing white goods, also lost out to lower-cost producers from abroad.

The social implications of this were profound as many of these industries formed the basis of traditional working class communities with strong local roots. The destruction of these industries therefore meant not only the loss of jobs but also the destruction of the community that went with them. For the heavy industries these were predominantly male jobs and male-dominated communities in which women traditionally stayed at home after childbirth. In the lighter industries, and the communities they sustained, there was more of a tradition of women continuing to work after childrearing. For the men who lost their jobs there was no longer any use for their skills in the labour market. Research into workers who experienced these changes suggests that, although a few may have moved into new careers, which offered more in the way of skill development and career prospects, many skilled workers never recovered their old status. For example, skilled engineers in the hosiery industry were obliged to take jobs as operatives in sandwich factories and hung onto their old identity, continuing to see themselves as skilled mechanics (Goodwin and O'Connor 2009). In areas of heavy industry where little job regeneration took place, some older workers were unable to secure alternative work becoming permanently excluded from the labour market. These changes in the job market carried heavy social costs.

The fact that unemployment did not rise above 10 per cent during the 1980s was due in large part to the generation of waves of new jobs in the service sector. As employment in manufacturing and mining fell, new jobs were created in financial and business services, in retail and distribution and in hotels, restaurants and the leisure industry. Some of these required professional training and high-level skills. In fact over this period there was a steady increase in the proportion of professional, technical and managerial employees. But many of these jobs were also relatively low skilled and low paid, such as check-out operators in retail, call-centre employees, security guards, bar staff, waiters and housekeeping staff in hotels and so on.

Although this transformation of the occupation structure meant severe disruptions to the lives of many of those already in the labour market, the impact was just as severe on those seeking to enter the labour market. Many of the industries that were destroyed during this phase recruited a high proportion of school leavers without any qualifications, for example mining, hosiery, footwear and steel making, the traditional routes into the labour market for the majority of sixteen-year-olds as they left school. The destruction of these jobs would not have had such a negative impact on the youth labour market had they been replaced by other jobs in the service sector that also recruited unqualified school leavers. However, as we have seen, many of these new jobs were in professional, managerial and technical occupations that required fairly high-level qualifications and were therefore not available to school leavers. Of those that did not require qualifications – and as we have seen many of the new service sector jobs were relatively unskilled – a significant proportion either were part-time, for example in retail or hotels, or had age restrictions on recruitment that precluded the employment of sixteen-year-olds, for example bar staff in hotels and drivers in distribution. This led some academic analysts to talk of the collapse of the youth labour market or 'the vanishing youth labour market' (Ashton *et al.* 1990) as the job market for sixteen-year-old school leavers dried up. The large number of young people still leaving school at the minimum age and failing to get work were seen as suffering, first from lack of skills, and second from outmoded ways of supplying them.

This collapse was particularly acute during the late 1970s and early 1980s recession when the destruction of manufacturing jobs was particularly pronounced. To compound the problem, those employers remaining in business traditionally cut recruitment, an initial reaction to any downturn in the market. Young people always suffer disproportionately during any economic downturn. The result in this case was extremely high levels of youth unemployment, with surveys revealing local unemployment rates as high as 59 per cent for males and 44 per cent for females in Sunderland (Ashton *et al.* 1990), culminating in riots in some cities. In the long run the response of young people and their families was for a higher proportion of young people to stay on at school and secure qualifications. But this sacrifice of pay for improved prospects in the labour market required not only a change in attitude among young working class school leavers, but also a change in the curriculum and qualifications systems to make appropriate qualifications available. Over time, the response of young people and their families was to raise their aspirations in relation to gaining school qualifications and also to enter higher education on an unprecedented scale. However, 50 per cent of young people still did not pursue this route up to the late 1980s, preferring to take their chances in the labour market instead.

The government's attempt to deregulate the labour market and reduce the power of trade unions provided employers with more control over the determination of wages and conditions. This led to a rapid decline in union membership with union density falling from over 50 per cent in 1980 to 28 per cent in 2006 (*Social Trends* 2008). This was particularly the case in the private sector where union density fell to less than 20 per cent in 2000 but remained much higher in the public sector at just under 60 per cent. These changes also provided employers with greater discretion enabling them to introduce new management practices such as multi-skilling and performance-related pay.

The reforms also made it easier for employers to hire and fire, enabling them to create what was sometimes referred to as the 'flexible firm' (Atkinson 1984; Atkinson and Meager 1986). This was characterised by core employees engaged on permanent contracts and a group of peripheral employees engaged on short-term or temporary contracts whose numbers could be reduced at short notice in response to changes in the demand for products or services.

The impact of these reforms was not just confined to the lower levels of the labour market. Changes were made to many of the conditions of employment for the professions. The working practices of doctors, nurses and teachers were changed. This was a period when teachers especially lost a great deal of their autonomy through the imposition of a centrally determined National Curriculum and enhanced monitoring of performance through the use of agencies such as the Office for Standards in Education, Children's Services and Skills (OFSTED). Within the public sector generally the use of outsourcing was encouraged, which meant that the conditions of many manual and service sector staff were changed as their employment was transferred from the public sector to private sub-contractors, usually on inferior terms and conditions. Taken together these changes resulted in a radical transformation of the labour market and employees' expectations of what their jobs could deliver. Whereas the first phase witnessed the collective regulation of the labour market this phase saw the individualisation of the employment relationship.

In concrete terms this resulted in the growth of self-employment, some of which was forced on workers as their old jobs were outsourced. Once largely a characteristic of the construction industry the sub-contracting of work now became much more common. It meant that the new self-employed person took on the responsibility for their own tax and insurance and holiday pay, forfeiting the security of a permanent employment contract. The other growth area was in the use of non-standard contracts, employing staff on short-term and temporary contracts to enable companies to adjust rapidly their staff numbers to changes in demand. However, the greatest change was in the use of part-time labour. This was another means by which employers could introduce greater flexibility into their use of labour as it became easier to change the number of hours worked (Felstead *et al.* 2001).

One of the consequences of these changes, both in the opportunities available in the labour market and in the ways in which employers used labour, was the decline in male employment rates (the proportion of those of working age in employment) from over 92 per cent in 1971 to just under 79 per cent in 2007 and a rapid increase in the female rate from 56 per cent in 1971 to 70 per cent in 2007. The reasons for the decline in male participation were of course the collapse of employment in the heavy industries, together with the increasing difficulty that older men in particular experienced in obtaining alternative employment. In addition, many men in their fifties, on losing jobs because of the restructuring and 'delayering' of companies, found it difficult to obtain other employment and opted for early retirement.

The most dramatic change in this phase was the increase in female participation. This was partly a consequence of changes in the demand for labour and partly a result of changes taking place in family relationships. The growth of part-time jobs provided many women with the opportunity to combine their domestic activities with paid employment at hours that were convenient for them. In the household, changes in the availability of labour-saving household devices such as washing machines and vacuum cleaners reduced the time required for household chores. In the labour market, the decline in wages that many men experienced, combined with the rise in home ownership, placed pressure on women to enter the labour market in order to meet mortgage payments or enhance living standards. However, it was not just the overall participation rates of women that changed during this period, for there was also an increase in the range of jobs that were open to them. In particular, women made inroads into traditional male professions such as medicine, pharmacy and accountancy. However, the labour market still remained segmented and women's participation in other areas remained limited.

Policy response

The structural changes taking place in the economy were placing strains on the apprenticeship with its system of time-based learning. This, together with complaints from employers, never happy with external 'interference' in what they saw as their internal affairs, led to them successfully lobbying for the closure of most of the Training Boards. As the last of the Industry Training Boards were closed down, the task of improving the country's skill levels was transferred to the Manpower Services Commission (MSC). This signalled a retreat from using the law to force employers to train and the start of what was to become an increasing reliance on supply-side measures with which to cope with the strains of restructuring. From now on public resources were to be used only for improving the supply of skills. Set up in 1974 by the Labour government under Harold Wilson following the 1973 Employment and Training Act, the MSC was charged with the task of building skill levels to enhance employability. The Training Services Agency was to be responsible for the delivery of training and the Employment Services Agency for the delivery of labour market services.

The MSC was a semi-independent agency, involving both employers and trade unions, with more powers than a traditional government department, which sought to provide nationwide programmes for helping workers make the transition that industrial restructuring required. Through its agencies it pioneered innovative programmes, especially for women returning to the labour market and for young people facing the difficulty of finding their first job (Payne 1990). Under James Callaghan the latter took the form of the Youth Opportunities Programme (YOPS), which ostensibly offered skills through work experience but was seen by critics as largely a means of keeping young people off the streets.

When it came to skills policy, the response of the new Thatcher government of 1979 was to attempt further deregulation. Any form of state 'intervention' was abhorrent and so there was pressure to get rid of centralised planning. Many of the powers of the MSC were reduced and the unions excluded from the governing body. Pioneering training programmes introduced by the MSC were abandoned as the government sought to limit any form of government intervention to instances of 'market failure'. The role of government was now seen to be restricted to dealing with failures in the operation of the market and delivering the skills that employers demanded. The market was also to be the mechanism through which training was to be delivered, served primarily by private training providers responding through the market mechanism to employers' demands.

Yet given the problems of mass (youth) unemployment (seen as a clear case of market failure) there was a need for some policy instruments inherited from the previous Labour administration to be continued. This was especially the case with regard to the youth problem so the YOPS was transformed into the Youth Training Scheme (YTS) in order to provide a better link to the labour market. YTS was also seen as a means of modernising the apprenticeship system. Thus, the 1981 New Training Initiative introduced in 1979 and delivered by the MSC was the first of a series of major reports and White Papers through which the traditional apprenticeship was to be replaced by youth training. In its place modern skills were to be imparted through YTS, which were to be available to everyone – young men and young women in equal measure. The poor quality of much of the training provided and the dislike of it by many young people and their families, who sought jobs with adult pay rather than training with an allowance – 'slave labour as some described it' (Banks *et al.* 1992) – led full circle back to the introduction by the successor Major government in 1988 of a new form of employment-based training, the modern apprenticeship, comprising a 'foundation' and 'advanced' stage and lasting up to three years.

The need to deliver a national programme to absorb unemployed youth meant that initially the MCS was saved, but as the threat of mass unemployment receded it was abolished altogether. However, there was still a need for youth and other training programmes, targeted at market failures, to be administered. In addition there was pressure from some industries such as construction and engineering for the collective provision of training. In accordance with the government policy of decentralisation and empowering employers, the government responded to these pressures by establishing Training and Enterprise Councils (TECS) and Industrial Training Organisations (ITOs). The TECs were employer-led organisations, modelled on their American counterparts, which operated at the local level and were responsible for administering the remaining government training programmes. The ITOs were also employer led and responsible for responding to employer needs for training. In this new framework for delivering skills, and helping the market respond to the structural transformation under way, there was no room for the unions or their representatives.

One of the other major changes was the introduction of new competence-based National Vocational Qualifications (NVQs), which were to provide, in place of the multitude of existing vocational qualifications, a national framework for all of them. The creation of these was meant to be employer led so that they would gain greater credence with employers. In practice, NVQs largely failed to convince and the well-regarded major accrediting agencies such as the Business and Technology Education Council (BTEC), the Royal Society of Arts (RSA) and the City and Guilds of London Institute (CGLI) offering their existing vocational qualifications survived.

Continental influence

The New Training Initiative (NTI), the YTS and the modern apprenticeship that followed it were premised on supplying training involving work-based and off-site provision over a fixed time period of initially one and then two years, compared with the five years that the traditional apprenticeship had taken to complete. The key target was to cut 'time serving' and minimise costs, drawing also on the private sector for much of the off-site provision. One important influence on its development had been continental vocational education and training (VET) systems for managing the transition from school to work. It was generally agreed that their skills acquisition and continuing high performance surpassed what had been traditionally offered on the multiple routes to skilled work in the UK's 'mixed system' (Evans 1990).

The model that attracted particular interest was the German 'dual system' of apprenticeship comprising a three-year training contract with an employer who supplied the onsite work-related training and locally run vocational education offered through a vocational school (*berufusschule).* By UK standards such schools offered a much broader VET curriculum (including general civic as well as vocational goals) as prescribed by the local Chambers of Commerce. These arrangements were central to the 'training culture' to which all sections of German society subscribed and offered qualifications that were recognised by employers throughout Germany, even those in different sectors of the labour market from the one in which the young person had been trained. Gaining an apprenticeship (or its much smaller-scale vocational school equivalent) for all those young people not proceeding to higher education was thus the essential prerequisite for getting almost any kind of proper job. Even many of those who were qualified by way of the *gymnasium* (grammar school) route for university signed up to do an apprenticeship first as a kind of 'vocational insurance' (Bynner and Roberts 1991; Evans and Heinz 1994).

Governance of the system nationally and locally was through 'the social partners' comprising employers' representatives, local policy makers and trade unions. It was this realisation that discouraged the Thatcher government at the time from following the model very far, not least because of the conviction that trade union militancy had been a major cause of the economy's problems. Basically, the YTS and even the modern apprenticeship were pale shadows of the dual system and traditional attitudes prevailed: what was needed to do most jobs was best learned on the job without any formal VET attached.

Stability and growth

Contextual changes

The political changes that we have documented as transforming the character of the UK labour mark*et als*o facilitated, but did not cause, further changes in the organisation of production. The driving force here was a mixture of the expansion of global markets, the transformation of production technologies and the globalisation of production. With the continued growth of world markets and the inclusion of countries such as Vietnam and Indonesia as major sources of manufacturing, the MNCs were now faced with even greater opportunities, new markets and new sources of low-cost, educated labour. At the same time the progress of automation, computerisation and, after the 1990s, the spread of internet technology all facilitated dramatic changes in the ways that companies organised production. What they were able to do was modularise production, that is, break down the process of production into its component parts, manufacturing separate components wherever the cost advantages were best for them. Advances in computer programming enabled companies to control the process of production in whichever geographical location they chose to locate. The internet then provided them with the means to exercise that control instantaneously across the globe while the explosion of graduate labour in countries across the world provided the human resources. It meant that production of goods and services was increasingly fragmented across the globe but centrally co-ordinated from headquarters.

This process had a number of consequences for the UK. For example, in the manufacture of cars it became more cost-effective for the new transnational corporations (TNCs) to source the more labour-intensive parts of the process such as wheels to Eastern Europe or China and some of the more high value-added activities such as R&D to India. In the service sector financial corporations outsourced many of the routine accounting and the customer service functions to countries such as India, where graduate labour was cheaper to employ. Now it was not just manufacturing jobs that were going, so too were service sector jobs. This process of modularisation of production also had the reverse effect as some MNCs sought to locate aspects of their production in the UK; this was especially the case in the financial and business services with the UK remaining one of the major destinations for foreign inward investment (UNCTAD 2005).

Much of this inward investment also brought with it the introduction of new management practices, especially those pioneered by US and Japanese companies. These introduced new and more efficient ways of organising production in the UK, sometimes referred to as high-performance working practices (HPWPs). In the automobile industry, British manufacturers of motorcycles and cars who had failed to invest in modern technology and management practices lost out and were replaced by Japanese, American and German companies with management practices that transformed the industry, with the Japanese-owned Nissan plant in Sunderland becoming the most efficient in Europe. These new management practices included team working, continuous improvement, worker involvement, performance-related pay and multi-skilling. Of course, not all companies adopted these practices and some chose to adopt some and not others. Neither was their adoption always successful, with some companies using them merely to exploit employees without providing them with any of the benefits. Other companies continued with their traditional system of management practices, usually referred to as command and control, which left employees with little discretion and subject to the arbitrary authority of their superiors.

The more widespread introduction of new management practices was also associated with further changes in the ways in which skills were acquired. From the 1980s onwards the introduction of new management practices in the private sector, and new forms of management in the public sector, meant that new skills in areas such as team working, problem solving, communication and customer service had to be acquired. This meant that more and more training was delivered on the job, aided by new techniques of training such as e-learning. Workers no longer received lifetime skills for a continuing occupation gained through their initial training as in the traditional apprenticeship. Instead for many, but not all, learning became something that was undertaken continuously within the workplace (Rainbird *et al.* 2004; Ashton and Sung 2002). The experience of formal classroom training gave way to more and more on-the-job training.

In the public sector there were also important changes taking place. The Thatcher government had sought to divest as many functions from the state machinery as possible. Almost all government departments and agencies were subject to 'market testing' the procedure that was used to see if private sector companies could deliver such functions at a lower cost than the appropriate government agency. Thus activities such as the installation and maintenance of information technology in the Inland Revenue to cleaning in hospitals were all outsourced. However, government organisations still remained huge employers and, in an attempt to improve the delivery of services ranging from health care to education and social services, they introduced a form of management by objectives. This was done through the use of performance targets that those responsible for delivering the services were obliged to meet. Although outsourcing created a downwards pressure on wages and conditions, the use of targets intensified work pressures on those responsible for service delivery.

Labour market

Not surprisingly, given the range of these sometimes contradictory pressures, their impact on the experience of employees has been a topic of some debate. With regard to skills, labour market analysts divided into two opposing camps. On the one hand there were those who interpreted the growth of professional, managerial and technical jobs, the decline of unskilled manual work in manufacturing and the increasing qualification levels among the labour force as a source of upskilling. Economists referred to this as skill-bias technological change, arguing that the introduction of new technology was increasing skill levels. Others saw in the same set of changes a process of de-skilling, arguing that what we have witnessed is a growth of more skilled jobs at the top of the labour market but a loss of intermediate skilled jobs associated with manufacturing and their replacement with routine, unskilled jobs in the service sector, sometimes referred to as 'McJobs'. Those following this interpretation spoke of the 'hollowing out' of the middle.

One of the problems with both approaches concerns the use of the term 'skills'. For those who argue for the hollowing out thesis, skill tends to be associated with the old craft occupations and their loss automatically becomes a loss of skill. Those arguing for upskilling tend to assume that skill equates with status and the growth of higher status jobs therefore implies upskilling. As Anderson (2009) has shown, if you take a more detached measure of skill then many of the new technician and service sector jobs can be realistically classified as intermediate-level skills and the hollowing out thesis starts to lack support. In fact, from the 1990s onward we have had measures of individuals skills used at work available through the Skills Survey (Ashton *et al.* 1999). This shows that on a number of measures, such as length of time taken to perform the job adequately, qualifications needed to obtain jobs, the use of computer skills and generic skills such as 'the ability to influence people', there has been a progressive increase in skills in the UK labour force (Felstead *et al.* 2007).

This progressive upskilling has had consequences for the youth labour market. It meant that, even when the economy recovered after the 1980s recession, the continuing decline of full-time unskilled jobs meant fewer opportunities for unqualified school leavers. Also, the loss of traditional manufacturing industries reduced the number of apprenticeships available while employers were demanding more in the way of qualifications for those seeking to enter the labour market. However, reforms in the qualification system associated with the introduction of NVQs in 1986 and GCSEs (in place of O levels and CSEs) in 1987 provided more opportunities for working class students to acquire certification and encouraged them to continue longer at school. After a ten-year time lag, staying on rates rose to present levels at around 70 per cent.

These developments also had ramifications in the further education sector, which throughout the 1980s had held an important role in providing the off-site component of VET and the more advanced vocational training, although this too was being transformed. Historically there has been a distinction between publically funded and locally run technical colleges (for basic business/clerical and technical education) and non-vocational adult education institutes. These gave way to an integrated system in which all publically funded courses had to enhance employability through the evidence of accreditation. At the upper end of the sector were the polytechnics offering the more advanced (degree-level) skills in specialised technical areas extending to postgraduate provision. Overlapping with them were the further education colleges that replaced the technical colleges but with a much broader brief, including academic as well as vocational courses. Although funding remained with the local education authorities, degrees were awarded nationally through the Council for National Academic Awards (CNAA), which provided a quality control mechanism to ensure that standards were being maintained.

The Thatcher government became increasingly convinced that the relatively high dropout from this provision and what they saw as patchy quality and sometimes poor management were a consequence of local education authority control. Hence, through a series of policy initiatives (e.g. *Education and Training for the 21st Century*; DES 1991), first the polytechnics in 1992 and then the further education colleges in 1998 (unchallenged by the new Labour government) were incorporated – that is, they became freestanding institutions funded directly by the government and with standards monitored by the Quality Assurance Agency (QAA). The other significant feature of the model was that the new institutions were expected to participate in a 'market' seeking to recruit students and maintain them in the system in competition with other institutions and private providers – although collaboration was also recognised as important.

A major consequence of these changes was that the intake into higher education continued to expand. At the same time, in September 1996, in recognition of the increasing labour market value of the degree, the Thatcher government introduced for the first time since the war tuition fees and a student loan system to help pay for them. The incoming 1997 Labour government, while retaining tuition fees, continued to expand the opportunities to enter higher education, setting the target for higher education entry as ultimately 50 per cent of the age cohort. Women were also major beneficiaries of the expansion with numbers entering higher education rising massively from the 1946 generation to the point at which currently A level achievement and university entrance is now higher among women than among men (Elias and Purcell 2009). By the end of the first decade of the twenty-first century, 135 higher education providers had the title of 'university' and over 35 per cent of the youth population were entering higher education. The outcome was that the average age at which young people entered the labour market was steadily rising.

In the labour market, the growth of mass higher education meant that many of those pursuing this route also sought part-time jobs to help fund their studies. The pattern of entry into work was changing dramatically, leading academic analysts to speak of 'extended transitions' and 'non-linear transitions' as more young people combined low-skilled part-time work and study before entering higher status full-time work after completing university (e.g. Furlong and Cartmel 2007). Entry into higher status skilled and intermediate-level jobs became increasingly restricted to those with qualifications

Without qualifications it became more and more difficult for those entering lower-level unskilled and semi-skilled jobs to move up, either by career progression within firms, or by moving jobs between firms (Smith 2009). This meant that there remained a group who left school at sixteen without any qualifications and who did not succeed in finding work or enter any of the available government training programmes. They became known as NEETS, defined originally as 'not in education employment or training' for six months or more over the period from sixteen to eighteen years (SEU 1999; Bynner and Parsons 2002). Such young people were likely to face continuing problems in the labour market, but were largely invisible in official figures. Various estimates suggested that they formed approximately 12 per cent of the youth population, including 15 per cent of young women, most of whom were young mothers (e.g. Payne 1999; Bynner and Parsons 2002).

Major initiatives launched to deal with this problem included a new counselling service to assist young people with educational and occupational choices. ConneXions was promoted through the government reports *Bridging the Gap* (SEU 1999) and *Young People* (SEU 2000). Such young people may often have the aspirations but not the resources to enable them to stay in education rather than seeking work. One of the more successful initiatives, Educational Maintenance Allowances, supplied financial support for staying on in education, including vocational routes to employment through further education colleges.

Although jobs were generally, but by no means universally, increasing in skill levels, there were also calls, especially from the trade union leaders, for recognition of the decline in the quality of working life. New management practices were seen as putting workers under greater pressure to perform while the new flexible labour market was seen to be creating more insecurity; the result it was argued was higher levels of stress for those in work. Green (2006, 2009) has been at the forefront of this debate and tracked changes in job quality in the UK and other countries over the two decades to 2008. He studied changes in pay, skills, worker autonomy, the effort expended at work and job security. What he found was a variable picture, with pay and skill levels increasing, but also work intensification, while worker autonomy decreased. Feelings of job security also increased over this period of economic boom but this is likely to change as a result of the 2008 financial crisis and the unemployment that followed.

Finally, it should also be noted that during this period the notion of skill has also undergone a transformation. In part this was a consequence of rising income levels, and especially two-income households, as more women entered the labour market, increasing the demand for consumer goods and services. Increased discretionary spending has resulted in a demand for more customised manufactured products and in the services sector for high standards of service in health care, restaurants, personal care and leisure services. As a result there has been less emphasis on technical skills, although these remain crucial. More and more employees are having to learn customer service skills or, as some see it, 'emotional skills'. Such skills are increasingly seen as crucial to a person's employability in a way that would not have seemed conceivable at the start of the first phase.

The policy response

The 1997 Labour government continued with a supply-side strategy, making some relatively minor changes to the framework inherited from the Conservatives. As we have seen the TECs were replaced by a central Learning and Skills Council (LSC) and local LSC partnerships, which administered government programmes, and more use was made of targets to control the use of subsidised training for NVQs. These failed to challenge the dominance of traditional academic qualifications or the well-established vocational qualifications but did succeed in providing qualifications for groups that had hitherto been denied them, such as care assistants, retail operatives and so on. Where the Blair government attempted more serious reform was in the introduction of Sector Skills Councils (SSCs), one for each major industry. These replaced the old ITOs and provided a framework through which employers were to be involved in government training programmes and supplied the means to ensure that government programmes and vocational qualifications related to employers' needs.

With the growth of professional, managerial and technical work in the 1990s, and the increasing integration of the global economy through technological change and the internet, there was a growing realisation that the outcome of competition between companies at a global level was increasingly dependent on the knowledge and expertise of their staff. Production was becoming knowledge intensive, giving rise to what many referred to as 'the knowledge economy'. In this context there was again growing concern in the UK about the skill levels of the labour force, especially when compared with other European competitors. The Blair government documented the failure of the UKs' education and skills base through a number of reports such as the 1999 Moser Report on basic skills *A Fresh Start*. The Skills for Life initiative followed – setting targets for ensuring that the proportions of the population lacking literacy and numeracy would be radically reduced and that no young person leaving the education system would lack literacy and numeracy (and subsequently IT) skills. Skills for Life was succeeded by the 2006 *Leitch Review of Skills*, broadening the aspiration further to 'world class skills' for the British population as a whole.

Within the labour market the Blair administration also maintained the deregulated framework it inherited. More employment protection was introduced but this stemmed largely from the imposition of EU regulations on the UK, apart from the introduction of the national minimum wage. Yet what will be perhaps the most radical change in the long run was the devolution of education, training and some labour market regulation powers to the three national assemblies. As a result there is a growing disparity between the countries of the UK in these areas.

It is too early to state with any certainty whether the 2008 financial crisis is the start of a new phase. It has many of the characteristics of one, namely the return of mass unemployment, a stalling of the trend for more and more of each cohort to enter university, a fall in home ownership and evidence of a growing willingness of the state to 'intervene' in the market in terms of a new industrial policy and actions aimed this time at curbing the powers of banks. In the labour market there are signs of the end of the reliance on supply-side measures and the growth of new thinking about how the state might shape employers' demands for labour in order that more highly skilled jobs can be created. Serious questions are starting to be asked of education policy as the proportion of graduates who are unemployed or 'underemployed' continues to rise, while at the same time, through the imposition of student fees and top-ups, the cost burden of paying for higher education is placed increasingly on young people and their parents. In this sense, as Willetts' (2010) argues, the preceding 'baby boomer' generation, who had free access to publically financed post-16 education, may be seen as having 'stolen' the future from the next one!

Certainly at the international level major changes have been taking place, politically in terms of the changing balance of power between the United States, Europe and China and India and economically in terms of the ability of the new emerging economies of China and India to compete at the higher end of the market with far lower labour costs than the UK. As we have shown throughout the chapter, this will no doubt have serious implications for the new cohorts in the second decade of the twenty-first century – a point worth bearing in mind as we conclude with a brief look at the impact of age and cohort changes.

Conclusion: age, period and cohort effects

The main features of economic and labour market transformation can be seen in the lives of cohort members as reported in *Changing Britain, Changing Lives* (Ferri *et al.* 2003). The comparison between cohorts at age thirty (1946, 1958, 1970) and at age forty (1946, 1958) shows most directly the general steadiness of male economic activity across the whole of the post-war period, averaging out during the thirties at around 95 per cent with periodic fluctuations in unemployment rates. Among women the picture is different, showing the steady rise in the economically active (including full-time as well as part-time work) among those in their early thirties, from 54 per cent in the 1946 cohort to 70 per cent in the 1958 cohort and 76 per cent in the 1970 cohort. The figures also dismiss what is often referred to as the growth of the 'long hours culture'. In fact, for men, hours worked declined slightly over the period, whereas among women they steadily rose. Changing patterns of family engagement with employment are also shown by the 50 per cent of the 1946 cohort households with two earners, compared with 71 per cent in the 1958 cohort and 81 per cent in the 1970 cohort. The rising affluence of individuals is thus reflected in the need to maintain living standards through family earnings to which both partners contribute.

The most striking feature of the whole period is that each new cohort experienced not only a changing economy and labour market, particularly since the 1970s, but massive technological enhancements affecting the skills base that needed to be constructed. This was coupled with periodic recession, most evident in the early 1980s and early 1990s, and now prevalent again through the collapse of the banking system. The way such periods of 'boom and bust' affect individuals in the workforce and their families depends a lot on when they were born and how old they were at the time the economic phenomena were happening. There is a risk of 'lost generations' at times when economic prospects are sparse and the key transition mechanism for entry into the labour force and continuing employment – work experience and the accumulation of human capital that goes with it – is jeopardised.

As we might expect, these concerns dominated the reports of findings at the earlier stages of each of the cohort studies and in subsequent overviews. Thus in the 1946 cohort early entry into the labour market was the striking feature, with 74 per cent of boys and 66 per cent of girls leaving school by the end of the statutory school leaving year and those staying on being overwhelmingly from non-manual families (Wadsworth 1991). Most young people who left went into jobs, and work was the dominant experience of men for most of their adult lives, whereas women spent significantly more time out of the labour market caring for children.

In the 1958 cohort apprenticeship, mainly experienced by boys, was the subject of a major report produced on the age twenty-three follow-up (Fogelman 1985). The adult work pattern was not much different from that of the 1946 cohort except that women's full-time employment was increasing. Through the early 1980s, prompted by the worldwide recession, unemployment also became a significant feature of the cohort's working lives (Ferri 1993). The advantage they had over the cohort that followed was a mainly successful transition from school to work and the acquisition of work experience and employment-related skills that went with it.

The 1970 cohort witnessed the major shift in experience when technological transformation destroyed the prospect of direct entry into work for the majority of school leavers (Bynner *et al.* 1991). The consequence was youth unemployment on an unprecedented scale, prompting the New Training Initiative and YTS, the reform of qualifications and, ten years later, a 20 per cent rise in staying on rates

The significant feature here was that this time comparable training opportunities were provided for both sexes; however the only partial success of the measures adopted is reflected by the continuing phenomenon of NEET.

Throughout this later period government played a major part in raising aspirations and opening up opportunities for achieving them through expansion of higher education and vocational education and training. Such shifts were evident across the whole population, even extending to retirees, but still tended to be heavily related to family social class and education, with, as some have argued, little solid evidence of social mobility across the generations (Erikson and Goldthorpe 1992). The most notable example of occupational mobility was the transformation of women's goals from the largely family and home-making orientations of the post-war period to occupational careers along the same lines as men's and the postponement of partnership and parenthood, especially among the most educated. At the same time class differentiation persisted for young women, with the traditional route to adulthood of early partnership and parenthood still common in working class families.

The charting of life courses that the cohort studies provides demonstrates effectively how labour market fluctuations and long-term trends can affect differentially individuals at different ages born at different times in different places to different families. Policy across the post-war period has been directed towards meeting the challenges to economic well-being of successive cohorts that these secular shifts (period effects) present. But many of the institutions and the cultural assumptions attached to them have remained impervious to current needs, remaining locked, perhaps too tightly as some would argue, to those of Britain's industrial past.

Further research

Further cohort study research will increase our understanding of how the core values and labour market behaviour associated with these ties are changing across the generations. It will also give insights into the effectiveness of policies directed at ameliorating the impact of contemporary economic conditions, including the balance between supply- and demand-side economic management, on the life course.

There are three areas of central concern to this chapter where such comparative cohort study will be particularly valuable: the timing, duration and outcomes of key transitions in working lives; the returns to human capital acquisition through education and training; and the intergenerational transfer of skills and opportunities and occupational mobility

Work transitions

The relatively early entry into the labour market of large numbers of sixteen-year-olds in the 1946 cohort contrasts with the postponement of the transition in the later cohorts, which, after stalling through the 1980s and 1990s, can be expected to continue in more recent cohorts. Similarly, later transitions, including redundancy, compulsory or encouraged early retirement and, increasingly, postponed retirement, have been changing across cohorts. As the proportion of adult life beyond official retirement increases and the pension cost burden grows, inter-cohort comparisons will show how the labour market adapted to the change, including employer strategies such as downsizing and workforce expectations and behaviour. Charting the life course changes through follow-ups throughout cohort members' lives will be the means of finding out.

Returns to human capital

The human capital acquired by individuals in the earlier cohorts through the benefit of free education extending to university will also need to be contrasted with that of the more recent cohorts for whom education costs are increasingly individually born. Close monitoring of the changing selection effects and the extent of individual and social returns to education and training should be an important feature of research, extending from monetary value to the wider benefits reflected in political and social participation, intergenerational transfer of knowledge and skills, family life and health and well-being. As education and training expand to what extent do the returns reduce and for what sections of the population? What has been the impact on the returns to human capital accumulation of technological transformation at an ever-increasing pace and the increasing demand for 'IT literacy' throughout the labour force?

Intergenerational transfers

Comparing each new generation with previous ones through the assessment of cohort effects at different life course stages should also include the study of intergenerational continuities and discontinuities within families, in order to ask to what extent children's life courses replicate those of their parents, and to what extent opportunities have increased, particularly for those who start life in adverse socio-economic circumstances. Social mobility in this broader sense of transformations of opportunities, careers and identities from one generation to the next includes the long-standing research interest in social mobility. Is there evidence of increased or reduced movement up and down the occupational structure? What social and educational factors drive such mobility and what is the role of personal agency? How can we best model the processes involved?

All these questions require more work in mapping current shifts in the contemporary labour market and collecting the data needed to model their effects on individual and collective experience. The overall picture that the cohort studies can reveal is how our changing society impacts and interacts with the dynamics of individual cohort members' lives in a rapidly changing society.

References

Anderson, P. (2009) 'Intermediate occupations and the conceptual and empirical limitations of the hourglass economy thesis', *Work Employment and Society*, 23: 169–80.

Ashton, D. N. (1986) *Unemployment under capitalism*, Brighton: Wheatsheaf Books.

Ashton, D. N. and Field, D. (1976) *Young workers*, London: Hutchinson.

Ashton, D. N. and Sung, J. (2002) *Supporting workplace learning for high performance working*, Geneva: ILO.

Ashton, D. N., Maguire, M. J. and Garland, V. (1982) 'Youth in the labour market', Research Paper No. 34, London: Department of Employment.

Ashton, D. N., Maguire, M. and Spilsbury, M. (1990) *Restructuring the labour market. The implications for youth*, London: Macmillan.

Ashton, D. N., Davies, D., Felstead, A. and Green, F. (1999) *Work skills in Britain*, Oxford: Centre for Skills, Knowledge and Organisational Performance.

Atkinson, J. (1984), 'Manpower strategies for flexible organizations', *Personnel Management*, 16: 28–32.

Atkinson, J. and Meager, N. (1986) *Changing working patterns: how companies achieve flexibility to meet new needs*, London: National Economic Development Office.

Banks, M., Bates, I., Breakwell, G., Bynner, J., Emler, N., Jamieson, L. and Roberts, K. (1992) *Careers and identities*, Buckingham: Open University Press.

Brook, K. (2002) 'Trade union membership: an analysis of data from the autumn 2001 Labour Force Survey', *Labour Market Trends*, 110, 343–53.

Brown, P., Ashton, D., Lauder, H. and Tholen. G. (2008) *Towards a high-skilled, low-waged workforce? A review of global trends in education, employment and the labour market*, SKOPE Monograph No. 10, Cardiff: Cardiff University.

Bynner, J. and Roberts, K. (eds) (1991) *Youth and work: transition to work in England and Germany*, London: Anglo German Foundation.

Bynner, J. and Parsons, S. (2002) 'Social exclusion and the transition from school to work: the case of young people not in education, employment or training NEET', *Journal of Vocational Behaviour*, 60: 289–309.

Bynner, J., Ferri, E. and Shepherd, P. (1997) *Twenty-something in the 1990s: getting on, getting by, getting nowhere*, Aldershot: Ashgate Press.

DES (Department of Education and Science) (1991) *Education and training for the 21st century*, London: HMSO.

Elias, P. and Purcell, K. (2009) *Occupational change and the expansion of higher education in the UK: the impact on graduate earnings*, University of Warwick, Institute for Employment Research.

Erikson, R. and Goldthorpe, J. (1992) *The constant flux: study of class mobility in industrial societies*, Oxford: Clarendon Press.

Evans, K. (1990) 'Post-16 education, training and employment', *British Journal of Education and Work*, 3: 41–59.

Evans, K. and Heinz, W. R. (eds) (1994) *Becoming adults in England and Germany*, London: Anglo German Foundation.

Felstead, A., Ashton, D. and Green, F. (2001) 'Paying the price for flexibility? Training, skills and non-standard jobs in Britain', *International Journal of Employment Studies*, 9: 25–59.

Felstead, A., Gallie, D., Green, F. and Zhou, Y. (2007) *Skills at work, 1986–2006*, Oxford: Centre for Skills, Knowledge and Organisational Performance (SKOPE).

Ferri, E. (1993) *Life at 33*, London: National Children's Bureau.

Ferri, E., Bynner, J. and Wadsworth, M. (2003) *Changing Britain, changing lives*, London: Institute of Education Press.

Fogelman, K. (1985) *After school: the education and training experience of the 1958 cohort*, London: Further Education Unit.

Furlong, A. and Cartmel, F. (2007) *Young people and social change: individualization and risk in late modernity*, Maidenhead: Open University Press.

Goodwin, J. and O'Connor, H. (2009)'Whatever happened to the young workers? Change and transformation in 40 years at work', *Journal of Education and Work*, 22: 417–31.

Green, F. (2006) *Demanding work: the paradox of job quality in the affluent economy*, Princeton: Princeton University Press.

Green, F. (2009) *Job quality in Britain*, London: UKCES.

Layton, W. R. Sir and Crowther, G. (1938) *An introduction to the study of prices*, London: Macmillan.

Leitch Review of Skills (2006) *Prosperity for all in the global economy – world class skills, final report*, December 2006, London: HMSO.

Lindsay, F. (2003) 'A century of labour market change: an overview of labour market conditions in the previous century', *Labour Market Trends*, 111, 133–44.

Moser Report (1999) *A fresh start – improving literacy and numeracy*, London: Department for Education and Employment.

Payne, J. (1990) *Adult off-the-job skills training. An evaluation study*, London: Policy Studies Institute.

Payne, J. (1999) *Young people not in education, training or employment: data from the England and Wales Youth Cohort Study (cohorts 8 and 9)*, London: Policy Studies Institute.

Rainbird, H., Fuller, A. and Munro, A. (2004) *Workplace learning in context*, London: Routledge.

SEU (Social Exclusion Unit) (1999) *Bridging the gap: new opportunities for 16–18-year-olds not in education employment or training*, London: Stationery Office.

SEU (2000) *Report of Policy Action Team 12: young people*, London: Social Exclusion Unit.

Smith, D. (2009) 'Changes in transitions: the role of mobility, class and gender', *Journal of Education and Work*, 22: 369–90.

Social Trends (2008) No. 38, Basingstoke: Palgrave Macmillan.

UNCTAD (United Nations Conference on Trade and Development) (2005) *World investment report*, New York: United Nations.

Wadsworth, M. (1991) *The imprint of time*, Oxford: Clarendon Press.

Willets, P. (2010) *The pinch: how the baby boomers took their children's future*, London: Atlantic Books.

Willis, P. (1977) *Learning to labour*, London: Saxon House.

7 Health policy and health care

Michael Wadsworth

Introduction

The period from the Second World War until the present includes the development of most effective forms of diagnosis, treatment and preventive care. These, together with great improvements in living standards, changed the pattern of illness from short term to long term, and increased the years of life likely to be lived without illness. The health changes, together with other social change, significantly helped to reduce the proportion of the national population at younger ages and increase the older proportion.

In the post-war years research began to show the importance for health of the interrelationship of the individual with society, of growth in the early years, of the pattern of health throughout life and the health impact of the nature of society. The delivery of health care became increasingly responsive to patients, and new ideas developed about responsibility for maintaining good health. New understanding of how risk of illness develops, together with technological and pharmaceutical innovations, brought new concepts of individual and collective responsibility for health and new thinking about health practice. In consequence, health-care policy evolved as a result of these changes and of political will.

The aim of this chapter is to describe the social changes brought by changes in health during the years since the Second World War, the implications of new directions in health care during that time for the nature of social and individual responsibility for health, and the role that the British large-scale birth cohort studies played and could in future play in these processes.

Demographic change associated with health

The profound impact of the rapid growth in effectiveness and understanding of health care, improvements in living standards and changes in health policy since the Second World War can be seen in changes in the chances of survival, expectation of years of life and disability-free years of life. Table 7.1 shows the striking changes brought about in survival of the first year of life during the period studied.

Despite the marked decline in infant mortality rates, and the increasing similarity in rates between the sexes and countries, there remain persistently greater risks

Table 7.1 Death rates aged under 1 year per thousand live births

	England and Wales		*Scotland*	
	Boys	*Girls*	*Boys*	*Girls*
1940–2	62	48	87	66
1950–2	33	25	42	32
1960–2	24	19	30	22
1970–2	20	15	22	17
1980–2	13	10	13	10
1990–2	8	6	8	6
2000–2	6	5	6	5
2007	5.3	4.3	5.2	4.2

Source: *Annual Abstract of Statistics* (2007) Table 5.20, p. 58, London: Palgrave Macmillan.

for infants living in areas of socio-economic deprivation and for infants whose parents are in poor socio-economic circumstances, whose mothers are not married, whose mothers had low or no educational attainment and whose mothers had been born in new Commonwealth countries, particularly Pakistan (Macfarlane and Mugford 2000: 129, 132–134, 138).

There are increases in expected years of life both in those born since the end of the Second World War in terms of age cohort as defined in Table 7.2 (the later the cohort the greater the expected years of life) and with increasing age within age cohort.

Data derived from the longitudinal study based on census data, which began with the census of 1971, show an increase in social class differences in expected years of life at birth. Boys born into non-manual social class families in 1972–6 could expect 2.1 more years of life than those born into manual social class families, and the comparable figure in 2002–5 was 3.3 years. In girls the non-manual social class advantage at birth in 1972–6 was 2.5 years and in 2002–5 it was 2.9 years (Office for National Statistics 2007; all means)

Expectation of healthy and disability-free years of life from age sixty-five years onwards also shows improvements and persistent gender and geographical differences (Table 7.3; Office for National Statistics 1997).

Changes in the quality of life

The extensive changes in population structure and in health were influenced by improvements in living standards. In the early post-war years families re-assembled as fathers returned from military service and children returned from evacuation. Many fathers were mentally and/or physically damaged (Grafton 1981). Women were reluctant to give up wartime paid employment (Sheridan 1990). Daily life was one of scarcity and discomfort, with food rationing and shortages of fuel and

Table 7.2 Projections of expected years of life at birth and expected age at death at ages 30 and 50 years in age cohorts in the UK born since the end of the Second World War

Birth years	*Expectation of years of life at birth*	*Expectation of age at death when aged 30 years*	*Expectation of age at death when aged 50 years*
Men			
1950–2	66.42	75.90	77.37
1960–2	68.09	76.80	77.95
1970–2	69.00	77.28	78.34
1980–2	71.04	78.67	79.61
1990–2	73.41	80.64	81.61
2000–2	75.60	82.90	83.91
Women			
1950–2	71.54	74.68	81.66
1960–2	74.00	76.23	82.98
1970–2	75.25	77.13	83.80
1980–2	77.00	78.34	84.89
1990–2	78.96	79.94	86.43
2000–2	80.59	81.37	87.84

Source: Office for National Statistics (2005) *Mortality statistics: general*. Expectation of Life Series DH1 No. 39, pp. 80–1, London: Office for National Statistics.

Table 7.3 Healthy life expectancy and disability-free life expectancy at age 65 years in 2001

	Life expectancy in years	*Healthy life expectancy in years*	*95% confidence interval*	*Disability-free years of life expectancy*	*95% confidence interval*
Men					
England	16.1	12.0	11.7–12.2	8.9	8.7–9.2
Wales	15.7	11.1	10.2–12.1	7.3[a]	6.4–8.3
Scotland	14.9	11.5	10.9–12.2	8.7	7.9–9.5
Women					
England	19.2	14.2	14.0–14.4	10.4	10.2–10.7
Wales	18.7	12.8[a]	11.8–13.8	8.5[a]	7.4–9.5
Scotland	18.0	13.5	12.8–14.2	10.0	9.2–10.8

Source: Breakwell and Bajekal (2006).

Note

a Significantly different from England at the 95% confidence level.

housing. Although wartime food surveys showed great improvements in nutrition, and considerable equity in getting a nourishing diet (Burnett 1989: 295–7), there were still social gradients in intakes of fruit and vegetables among four-year-olds in 1950 (Prynne *et al.* 2002). Food rationing continued until 1954, and free milk was provided for all schoolchildren up to age eleven years from 1946 until 1980.

Material standards also improved greatly. Britain's housing stock was in a poor condition immediately after the war. In the 1946 birth cohort study, in 1948, 49 per cent of families in that representative sample did not have running hot water (Wadsworth 1991). In total, 22 per cent of households in the general population were still without a hot water supply in 1961, and by 1971 that had fallen to 6 per cent (*Social Trends* 1970, 1980). Other indicators of improvement include the rise in households with central heating (from 34 per cent in 1971 to 59 per cent in 1981 and 90 per cent in 1998; *Social Trends* 1980, 1990; General Household Survey 2000) and the rise in the proportion of owner occupiers from 27 per cent in 1950 (in the 1946 birth cohort sample) to 53 per cent in 1978 and 71 per cent in 2007 (*Social Trends* 2009).

Since the war alcohol consumption has risen consistently (Plant and Plant 2006: 28–9), with unprecedented increases in high levels of consumption, particularly in young adults. Between 1988 and 2000 the proportion of young adult men who drank more than the recommended weekly limit rose from 12 to 14 per cent; and the proportion of women of the same age who drank more than recommended rose from 10 to 17 per cent (Plant and Plant 2006: 41–2). Between 1980 and 2007 alcohol became 69 per cent more affordable (Public Accounts Committee 2009), and currently 31 per cent of men and 20 per cent of women in Britain regularly drink more than the recommended guidelines (Public Accounts Committee 2009).

The consumption of tobacco has a very different history. Cigarette smoking began in earnest among men during the First World War and peaked during the Second World War. Women took up smoking between the wars and their peak smoking was in 1974 (Doll 2004). Attitudes to what had seemed a normal and harmless habit reversed during the period studied and the prevalence fell. In 1948 82 per cent of men and 41 per cent of women in Britain were smokers and in 2007 22 per cent of men and 20 per cent of women smoked (Forey *et al.* 2002; *Social Trends* 2009). Although Doll and Hill published their findings about smoking risks in 1950 and on deaths in a cohort of British doctors in 1954 and 1956, the steep decline in smoking did not begin until the 1970s and 1980s. Smoking is now highest in those between the ages of twenty and twenty-four and in households with income derived from routine or manual work (26 per cent smokers) compared with professional or non-manual households (15 per cent smokers) (*Social Trends* 2009).

Leisure time was scarce at the beginning of our period, and, although holidays with pay had become statutorily available before the Second World War, car ownership did not expand much above the pre-war figure until 1955, when foreign holidays also began gradually to increase (Marwick 1982). By 1971 there were 6.7 million holiday trips abroad, increasing to 45.4 million in 2007 (*Social Trends* 1970, 2009).

Exercise in the early post-war period was a compulsory part of the school curriculum and has gradually decreased since. For adults there were then fewer reasons for leisure exercise because physical activity was an integral part of life at home and at work. Approximately 75 per cent of occupations were manual, there were only 2 million car owners (petrol rationing continued until 1950) and in 1948 40 per cent of households had a vacuum cleaner and only 4 per cent had a washing machine (Howarth 1985: 56–7). Since then the nature of work has changed greatly. Whereas 74 per cent of fathers of the 1946 cohort were in manual employment in 1950, only 45 per cent of their sons were in manual work in 1982 (Wadsworth 1991). In 2000 44 per cent of men in the 1970 birth cohort were in manual work.

Sport in leisure time was common in the early post-war years, and amateur team sports were a source of community cohesion (Frankenberg 1957). However, after Britain's poor showing at the 1952 Olympic Games and a consequent government inquiry, the Sports Council was set up in 1965, adult sports activity began to be professionalised and the slogan 'Sport for All' was coined. Increasing purchasing power opened up activities such as climbing and sailing, which had been mostly 'the preserve of the prosperous or the eccentric' (Marwick 1982: 156). By 1965–6 only 11 per cent of men and 4 per cent of women reported taking part in sports or physical recreation (*Social Trends* 1970). During the 1980s and 1990s local authorities began to develop sports centres, and it became fashionable to join a gym. By 2006–7, 58 per cent of men and 43 per cent of women said that they took part in sports activity in their leisure time (*Social Trends* 2009).

The health of the population

Although there have been remarkable improvements in health as a result of innovations in treatment, diagnosis and preventive health care, as well as in living standards, those improvements have not always translated equitably into improved health of the population (Black *et al.* 1980; Acheson *et al.* 1998; Marmot 2010). This section gives examples of changes in health and health care since the end of the Second World War.

Fertility

The first reliable means of fertility control became available when the oral contraceptive was introduced in 1961. Other means of contraception introduced during this period included reliable intra-uterine devices (copper-T loops) first introduced in 1962, with an improved version in the 1970s, and injected Depo-Provera methods. In 1971 sterilisation for women was first made available in the NHS on request, and NHS surgical sterilisation services were provided for men from 1972. Abortion became legally available following the Abortion Law Reform Act of 1967.

Age at menarche or physical maturity is associated with health and nutrition and, compared with girls, boys reach maturity on average a year later. However, in the 1958 birth cohort age at menarche was not strongly associated either with socio-economic circumstances or with relative weight in childhood. It was concluded that in well-nourished populations the variability in age at menarche may be the result of genetic influence (Stark *et al.* 1989), and recent evidence from the cohort studies supports that argument (Ong *et al.* 2009).

Although there is thought to be an increase in the age at menopause there is no good supportive evidence, and it has remained at about age fifty to fifty-two years since the 1960s. However, as the main risks for an earlier menopause are smoking, nulliparity and possibly also chronic stress, a change might be expected (Kuh and Hardy 2002).

Health of the newborn

Despite great reductions in infant mortality (Table 7.1), the birth cohort studies of 1946, 1958 and 1970 showed persistent socio-economic and geographic differences in health and survival during the first week of life (Joint Committee 1948; Butler and Bonham 1963; Butler and Alberman 1969; Chamberlain *et al.* 1975). They showed risks of home births associated with lack of availability of blood transfusion and other facilities required in an emergency, and so hospital deliveries were considered safer. Consequently the proportion of mothers delivered in hospital increased from 54 per cent in 1946 to 98.2 per cent in 1994 (Macfarlane and Mugford 2000: 221).

Average weight at birth fell across the first three birth cohorts as a result of increasing chances of survival (Wadsworth *et al.* 2003), but in the 2000 birth cohort average birthweight was greater than in the 1970 study, although still less than in the earlier studies (Dezateux *et al.* 2005). These authors suggest that this may be the result of an increasing proportion of first births, proportionally more ethnic minority births, improved birthweight-specific mortality and a proportionate increase in multiple and pre-term births.

Growth

In Britain height increased with each generation in the post-war years, and the range of midlife adult heights expanded downwards as well as upwards as survival of prematurity increased (Wadsworth *et al.* 2003). The trend over time of height gain is due to improved nutrition in childhood (Tanner *et al.* 1982; Gunnell 2001). Although greatest growth in height occurred in children in the higher socio-economic groups in the 1946 cohort, there was a decrease in social class differences in height in more recent-born cohorts (Wadsworth *et al.* 2003; Li *et al.* 2008).

Childhood obesity also increased. Although at age seven years 0.2 per cent of the 1946 and 2.8 per cent of the 1958 cohort were obese (Li *et al.* 2008), that seems little compared with a prevalence of obesity of 4.6 per cent in boys and 6.8 per cent in girls aged from five to ten years in 2002–3 (Stamatakis *et al.* 2005). Those authors found that the most rapid increase in childhood obesity occurred from 2000 onwards, with risks of increase greatest in the lower socio-economic groups. The risk of obesity is apparent in the birth cohorts at increasingly younger ages (Wadsworth *et al.* 2003; Li *et al.* 2008).

Infectious disease and viral illness

Although control of infections and viral illnesses was increasingly effective following the introduction of antibiotics in the mid-1940s and the first antiviral drugs in the 1980s, they have not been in steady decline. Early in the post-war period there were still significant epidemics of some major illnesses including tuberculosis, scarlet fever, diphtheria, measles and poliomyelitis. In Britain there has been a rising incidence of sexually transmitted diseases since 1996 and of HIV and AIDS since 1983.

In preventive care probably the most influential were the introduction in the early 1950s of mass miniature radiography for screening for pulmonary tuberculosis, the polio vaccine in 1958, the measles vaccine in 1968, the rubella vaccine in 1970 and the triple vaccination against measles, mumps and rubella in 1988. Anxieties about associated risks triggered a decline in uptake of the MMR vaccine, from which a recovery began in 1999 (Vyse *et al.* 2002).

In addition to known risks of disability following some childhood infectious and viral illnesses there are suggestions that early infection may constitute a risk for later neurological illness (Martyn *et al.* 1988). For example, the international epidemics of encephalitis lethargica between 1919 and 1926 have been hypothesised to influence the later onset of Parkinson's disease, as death rates from that illness increased in the age cohorts exposed to those epidemics. Martyn *et al.* (1988) also showed that the post-war poliomyelitis epidemics in Britain coincide with the rise in adult-onset motor neurone disease experienced in midlife by those born in the post-war years.

Disability

Disability is a growing problem because of increased survival in early and in later life, the periods of greatest vulnerability, and disability may bring with it social disadvantage in adulthood (Power and Li 2000; Kuh *et al.* 1994).

Care of disability improved considerably during the period studied through greater control of pain and mental and physical symptoms, new surgical treatments for the care of deformities caused by bone and joint disorders (e.g. the Charnley hip replacement was introduced in the early 1970s), new aids for better quality of everyday life (e.g. hearing and mobility aids) and improved rehabilitation after such devastating events as brain injury and stroke, as well as following broken bones and for the care of back pain.

Preventive actions now begin in the prenatal period through improved nutrition of mothers and infants, and screening in pregnancy (Macfarlane and Mugford 2000). Prevention of adult-onset disability includes increased health and safety measures at work, improved design of domestic appliances and medication to reduce risk associated with such midlife health changes as raised blood pressure.

Social rights of those with disability were greatly enhanced through the Disability Discrimination Acts of 1995 and 2005, which made it unlawful to discriminate against persons with disability, for instance in education, employment, transport and access to buildings and services.

Mental health and illness

Clinical definitions and mental health diagnoses changed fundamentally during the post-war years, making it impossible accurately to estimate how far changes in prevalence represent absolute increases or decreases. Collishaw *et al.* (2004) used findings from a number of longitudinal studies that measured adolescent mental health over twenty-five years, and found substantial increases in conduct and emotional problems, but mixed evidence for hyperactive disorder, all of which were consistent in both sexes and in all social groups and family types. Much more mental ill health is now treated than at the beginning of the period studied, and depression is now the primary burden of disease in high-income countries (World Health Organization 2008). Concepts of mental health have expanded to include studies of positive emotions, the development of personal resilience and the measurement of happiness and contentment (Kahneman *et al.* 1999; Layard 2005; Haworth and Hart 2007).

Treatment of mental illness changed greatly through innovations in drug therapy and 'talking' therapies. Anti-psychotic medication (chlorpromazine) was introduced in 1953, followed by anti-depressant prescribing from 1975. In the mid-1980s prescribing of anti-depressants 'increased exponentially' (Middleton *et al.* 2001: 263). These authors note that 'In 1998, 23.4 million prescriptions [for antidepressants] were issued by GPs in the United Kingdom. This is nearly three times the figure for 1988' (p. 262). In England in 2007, 34 million prescriptions for anti-depressants were issued (*Social Trends* 2009). There was a greater increase in prescribing for men than for women, although women continued to have higher psychiatric morbidity (Middleton *et al.* 2001). In the 1946 birth cohort study prescription of anti-depressant, anxiolytic and hypnotic drugs increased with age, from 10.6 per thousand of the sample at age thirty-one years in 1977, to 44.6 per thousand at thirty-six years in 1982, 45.2 per thousand at forty-three years in 1989 and 59.1 per thousand at fifty-three years in 1999 (Colman *et al.* 2006). Of all the 'talking' treatments, cognitive behavioural therapy is now the most commonly recognised by the National Health Service, where it began to be used in the early 1990s (Gath *et al.*1997; Rachman 1997).

Pharmaceutical innovation also made it possible to reduce dramatically the numbers of patients in hospital and their periods of stay. In addition, the Mental Health Acts of 1959, 1983 and 2007 and the Mental Capacity Act of 2005 were concerned with definitions of mental disorder, codes of practice and the restriction of liberty. The first of these acts set up (in England and Wales) mental health tribunals through which patients may request a review of their need to remain in hospital. Changes in the legal rights of those with mental illness reflect the greater understanding of and tolerance in public attitudes to these conditions that took place throughout the period since 1945. That change was probably influenced by rising levels of education and by the improvements in treatment.

A report on mental health in the first three British national birth cohort studies concludes that, in contrast to physical health, the prevalence of mental health problems is greatest at young ages (Richards *et al.* 2009). It emphasises that early emotional and conduct problems have far-reaching effects on life chances in education, work and relationships, with cost implications for the state and the community's social cohesion.

Chronic physical illness

Since the end of the Second World War the prevailing pattern of physical illness has changed from relatively short-term infectious and viral disease to longer-term and lifelong physical illness, such as diabetes, heart disease, cancer, arthritis, asthma and chronic bronchitis (now called chronic obstructive pulmonary disease or COPD). These long-term physical illnesses generally become evident in middle and later life.

Like many mental illnesses, the development of chronic physical illness has been shown to be long term and cumulative. Brunner and Marmot (2006: 28) emphasise the interactive nature of risks in the development of chronic disease, and conclude that

> Chronic anxiety, insecurity, low self-esteem, social isolation and lack of control over work appear to undermine mental and physical health. . . .These problems increase progressively down the social strata in industrialised countries. Clustering and accumulation of psychosocial disadvantage, perhaps beginning with a poor emotional environment in early childhood, is a neglected area of public health prevention and social policy.

Care of chronic disease has improved greatly over the period studied. Care of cardiovascular disease, for instance, benefitted greatly as a result of diagnostic technology and surgical techniques, as well as drug therapies. These give increased years of active life and freedom from pain, and greatly reduce the time individual patients spend in hospital, but greatly increase demand for this kind of care.

Prevention of these diseases is complicated by their long period of risk development and the wide range of risks. Social and personal lifestyle change is involved as well as public health measures, such as the control of atmospheric pollution from coal burning (Clean Air Act 1956), regulation of contents and labelling of manufactured foods (Food Labelling Regulations 1996), control of smoking through risk description on labelling, reduction of advertising and exposure to cigarette smoke (see Appendix 2 for dates). Gradually cultural change is occurring concerning risk from prolonged stress, the value of exercise and moderation of alcohol consumption and diet. Pharmaceutical prevention, for example to control blood pressure and lipids, is proving to be an expensive option. In England prescriptions for treatment of raised blood pressure and heart failure rose from about 15 million to almost 60 million between 1998 and 2008; for lipid control over the same period they rose from approximately 0.5 million to more than 50 million (National Health Service 2009).

The long-term development of risk in chronic illness means that exposure to risk in a rapidly changing society and care environment differs considerably between age cohorts.

Ageing

Inevitably, increasing life expectancy and falling fertility over the years since the end of the Second World War led to an increase in the proportion of the population aged sixty-five years and over (Morris 1967), in addition to the effects of the baby booms. In 1951 the proportion of those aged sixty-five years and over in the UK population was 10.8 per cent; this is predicted to rise to 20.4 per cent by 2026.

Positive health care of the elderly developed throughout the period. It is now intended to 'restore an ill or disabled person to a level of maximum ability and wherever possible return the person to an independent life at home' (British Geriatric Society current objectives). The original objectives of the British Geriatric Society at its foundation in 1947 were 'the relief of suffering and distress'. In Britain geriatrics originated in Dr Marjorie Warren's care for workhouse inmates at the inception of the National Health Service (Warren 1946). She 'matched care to their needs through a system of classification. She discharged many patients by providing rehabilitation . . . and initiated upgrading of the wards, thereby improving the morale of both patients and staff' (Grimley Evans 1997: 1075). Grimley Evans (1997) identified a first phase in the history of health care of the elderly, from 1948 until the early 1970s, in which geriatricians had little influence over preventive care until patients were referred to them. The second phase was when geriatricians could begin preventive and rehabilitative care before the onset of the diseases of later life. That second phase coincides with the beginnings of academic study of health in later life and of systematic medical school teaching of geriatrics (Grimley Evans 1997; Morley 2004).

Risks associated with ageing (e.g. cognitive impairment, impairment in activities of daily living, self-reported physical illness) 'rise and approximately double by 5-year age groups from 80 years in men and 75 years in women' (Brayne *et al.* 2001: 56). In many respects the diseases of later life and markers of ageing (such as deterioration in memory, balance and respiratory and cardiac function) are associated with cumulative and interacting processes of risk that considerably predate old age (Richards and Deary 2005; Richards *et al.* 2004; Kuh and Ben Shlomo 2004). Risks include insufficient physical activity and exposure to sunlight, smoking, poor diet and obesity, as well as genetic predispositions (Ebrahim and Kalache 1996).

During the period studied great improvements were made in the care of disease that is particularly prevalent in older people, for example in rehabilitation following a stroke or a fall, in increasing mobility and dexterity through hip and joint replacement and in cataract removal and intraocular implantation. Experimental preventive health care shows that some essential aspects of function can be significantly improved through regular programmes of exercise, with demonstrable benefit in bone density, balance skills and muscle strength (Svanborg 1996).

Increases in residential care for the elderly ought to be an opportunity to introduce preventive care of this kind, but as most British institutions are privately run there is a low likelihood of that happening. Feldman (2002: 105) noted that private industry 'typically has no public-service ethos or political accountability' and that 'patchy regulation [of private care facilities] and uneven democratic scrutiny left many important values (including communal solidarity, human dignity, and democracy itself) vulnerable'. Increased government spending on health care and research into the diseases of later life is recommended (House of Lords Science and Technology Committee 2006). The Wanless Report (2006) summarised concern for the care of older people since 1946, and showed the lack of integration between health, social care and benefits policies, and noted that 'the so-called baby-boomers (born 1945–54) are likely to present a cohort of more demanding social care users insisting on greater choice and quality' (p. xxiii); this is equally likely to be true for health care. Cohort differences in the processes of ageing are to be expected in view of improvements in the care of chronic illness and the cohort differences in such health-related habits as diet and exercise.

Changing concepts of cause of ill health

As the prevailing pattern of disease changed from infections to chronic physical and mental illnesses, and the socio-economic differences in illness persisted, so searches for cause began to investigate the socio-economic environment and how exposure to risk actually caused illness, and used longitudinal methods to examine the periods of life before symptoms of chronic illness became evident.

Chronic illness usually begins in midlife and many studies of cause began there (e.g. Morris *et al.* 1953; Marmot *et al.* 1984). However, it began to be suspected that causal influences, vulnerability and resilience had their origins at earlier ages (Reid 1969; Barker 1984). Greater understanding of the long-term role of growth in early life showed its lifelong influence on physical and mental health (Jones *et al.* 1994; Barker 1998; Kuh and Ben Shlomo 2004; Murray *et al.* 2007). Current research is concerned with the interaction of genetic and environmental effects with the legacy of prenatal and infant growth. For example, in chronic obstructive pulmonary disease risk elements include poor development in early life, atmospheric pollutants such as coal burning and combustion of other fuels as well as smoking, poor diet and genetic influences (Strachan and Sheikh 2004). Poor early development is a risk for respiratory performance, particularly if followed by childhood chest illness. That in turn increases vulnerability to additional risk, such as smoking and poor diet, and consequently age-related natural decline in respiratory performance will tend to begin earlier than in others (Strachan and Sheikh 2004). Risk for cardiovascular illness includes poor early life development before and after birth and subsequent smoking, poor diet, low levels of exercise, overweight and obesity, chronic psychological stress and genetic influences (Brunner and Marmot 2006). This process is sometimes described as an accumulation of risk over the life course. Studies of mental illness show a chain or cascade of risks that includes inherited predispositions, poor physical development (e.g. early life brain development), poor and inconsistent parenting, substance and alcohol abuse and poor social integration; these sources of risk interact together and with genetic factors and may protect against or precipitate one another (Jones *et al.* 1998; Maughan 2002; Moffitt 2005; Rutter 2005). Less is known about the life course interactive effects of factors clearly shown to be protective in mental and physical health, especially those that occur in adulthood, and how they reduce the long-term impact of early life effects.

In a search for an explanation of the persistent social gradient in ill health Brunner and Marmot (2006: 28) concluded that

> the power of psychosocial factors to affect health makes biological sense. The human body has evolved to respond automatically to emergencies. This stress response activates a cascade of stress hormones which affect the cardiovascular and immune systems. . . . if the biological stress response is activated too often and for too long, there may be multiple health costs. These include depression, increased susceptibility to infection, diabetes, high blood pressure, and accumulation of cholesterol in blood vessel walls, with the attendant risks of heart attack and stroke.

Their observation that persistent exposure to psychological stress is more common in lower socio-economic groups offers an explanation for the persisting socio-economic difference in illness.

A valuable replication of these conclusions was shown in studies of societies with failing social cohesion, for instance after the collapse of the Soviet Union. There, significant increases in premature mortality, accidental injury and chronic illness were seen as the chronic stress of social insecurity increased (Wilkinson 2006; Wilkinson and Pickett 2010).

New ideas are being developed through the study of health changes in societies that are making the transition from predominantly communicable to non-communicable disease and experiencing a rise in standards of living. It has been argued that improved living conditions act during an individual's period of physical growth to make those in the first generation who have that experience more vulnerable to diabetes, which will be most prevalent in the poorest. The social gradient in diabetes will change once 'most people in the population have several generations of economic development behind them', arguably because of environmentally driven changes in gene expression (Schooling and Leung 2010).

Health management on a population scale

Since the National Health Service began British governments have increasingly evaluated the risks, costs and benefits of new treatments and preventive health care, as well as taking account of pressures from scientists and pharmaceutical companies and lobbying from professionals, patients and the public. In the early post-war years the 'good of the community' was evident in such essential measures as food rationing and the control and prevention of tuberculosis. Improving environmental public health was also a reasonably straightforward aim. New knowledge about risks associated with some chemicals and materials, such as asbestos, and risks of injury when working with unguarded machinery led to extensive preventive regulation.

However, other new scientific knowledge has been more difficult to manage. In environmental health, for instance, risks from atmospheric pollution from coal burning were evident, but statutory control was not feasible until an alternative energy source was found and eventually the Clean Air Act was passed in 1956. Other new knowledge of potential value for environmental public health includes the addition of vitamins to cereals and bread flour and the dental protective effect of adding fluoride to the drinking water supply. But implementation of such measures now involves great ethical difficulties.

New knowledge in terms of treatments has had far-reaching effects on policy. For example, new knowledge (partly provided by the birth cohort studies) showed the benefit of birth in hospital, and policy was changed accordingly (Macfarlane and Mugford 2000). New understanding of disease processes and new pharmaceutical knowledge reduced infections and viral diseases, and many isolation hospitals were consequently closed. Comparable advances in understanding and care of mental illness reduced the risk of acute episodes, with subsequent extensive hospital closures (Department of Health 1975), but not without continuing discussion of the responsibility placed on patients and carers, and concern about preventive detention.

New knowledge about preventive care for the individual brought new problems. Public scepticism about health risks, such as excessive smoking and alcohol consumption, grew because the risk is difficult to quantify. There is also public concern about taking drugs for long-term prevention of risk development, for example in blood pressure, where symptoms are rare. The public health management dilemma is that, although on a population scale a decrease in average blood pressure equates to significant improvements in mortality (Rose 1992), the difficulty of achieving that is great because of scepticism and the financial burden for the National Health Service. Conversely, health policy innovation can be influenced by public pressure to make new knowledge available, as happened in the development of screening and new treatments for cancer of the cervix and breast. Where scientific knowledge has yet to develop effective treatments, for example for dementia, care may be very varied and in that instance has largely been left to private providers, with a government-regulated inspection system.

Methods of dealing with difficulties of whether and when to introduce new treatments include the establishment of expert groups, such as the National Institute for Clinical Excellence (established in 1999; now called the National Institute for Health and Clinical Excellence), to evaluate risk and benefit in relation to cost. The most salient professional means of establishing the safest and most effective clinical procedures is the Cochrane method of systematic reviewing; these results are published by the collaboration's database, set up in 1993.

Table 7.4 gives the dates of some important public health policy actions, enquiries and legislation that have taken place since the end of the Second World War.

Responsibility for health

The beginnings of state responsibility for health had been agreed early in the twentieth century (the National Insurance Act 1911), on humanitarian as well as pragmatic grounds, in order to maintain maximally efficient and reliable labour and defence forces, and to develop their healthy replacements in the following generation. The initial assumption that the National Health Service would diminish demand for medical care once the backlog awaiting free care had been cleared was demolished by the new powerfully effective treatments and new knowledge about the natural history of disease.

The new knowledge and the ability to measure pre-symptomatic indications of potential illness were significant for individual and public health care. Public health developed screening services to detect early signs of illness or risk, for instance in tuberculosis, some cancers and some aspects of cardiovascular disease. A public health specialist interpreted the new knowledge as showing that ill health treated by medical care was only the tip of the 'iceberg of disease' (Morris 1967: 118–25), and new screening methods would reveal the existence of the pre-symptomatic aspects beneath the surface. This kind of thinking brought the return of ideas (in the 1960s) about disease prevention that saw a role for individual responsibility, in terms, for instance, of exercise, smoking and diet (e.g. Butterfield 1968). The concept of individual responsibility prepared the way for greater state involvement in preventive health, in terms of the control of advertising and sales of tobacco and alcohol, inspection of foods and their contents, requirements for food labelling and advice about a healthy lifestyle. The responsibility for deciding is then left to the individual, who must evaluate the interpretations of science that are presented. An important aspect of this preventive strategy is that it is easier for higher socio-economic and better-educated people to evaluate and to follow. The argument about where responsibility for health should lie continues in current concerns about the state's role in controlling alcohol and recreational drug use.

Individual responsibility for health has been modified by concerns for civil and political rights of the individual. The areas where health care has to be monitored for human rights purposes have increased, for example in mental health tribunals, and there were 'concerted attempts to reduce the responsibility of the state and to emphasise people's responsibilities for their own welfare' (Feldman 2002: 72). That affected the relationship between health-care professionals and patients. On

Table 7.4 Public health policy actions

Policy action	*Date*	*Purpose*
Food rationing	1940–54	
Clean Air Act	1956	Reduced smoke from coal burning
Guillebaud Report	1956	On the cost of the National Health Service
Platt Report	1959	Concerned with the welfare of children in hospital; brought about many more visiting opportunities
Mental Health Act	1959	Introduced new emphasis on voluntary treatment and new safeguards for when compulsory treatment was to be used
Drugs (Prevention of Misuse) Act	1964	Amphetamines legally available only on prescription
Smoking advertising banned from television	1965	
Wolfenden Report and the subsequent Sexual Offences Act	1967	On prostitution and homosexual offences: decriminalised consenting homosexuality
Abortion Law Reform Act	1967	Made abortion possible on the NHS
Road Safety Act	1967	Introduced tests and limits of 80 mg alcohol in 100 ml blood in drivers
Obligatory printing of health warnings on cigarette packets	1971	
Misuse of Drugs Act	1971	Control and classification of drugs
Road Traffic Act	1972	New regulations on driving whilst under the influence of alcohol or drugs
Control of Pollution Act	1974	Concerned with management of waste, water pollution, sewage, noise
Court Report	1976	Proposed fundamental reform of child health services
Licensing Act Scotland	1976	Enabled pub opening hours to be varied by local authorities
Wilkes Report	1981	On the need for hospice care for the dying
Mental Health Act	1983	Introduced new definitions of circumstances for compulsory detention and clarified concept of consent to treatment
Human Fertilisation and Embryology Act	1990	To establish a regulatory authority
Children and Young Persons (Protection from Tobacco) Act	1991	It becomes illegal to sell tobacco to those under sixteen years of age

Policy action	*Date*	*Purpose*
Establishment of the Human Embryology Authority	1991	Regulation of fertilisation and embryology research and practice
Cochrane Collaboration established	1993	A database of systematic reviews of trials of treatments and clinical care
Disability Discrimination Act	1995	Aimed to end discrimination and open up educational, occupational and travel opportunities to the disabled
The Mental Health Act	1998	New approaches to assessment and treatment plans and more consistent safeguards for patients, having regard to the Human Rights Act 1998
National Institute for Clinical Excellence established	1999	Regulation of treatments having regard to effectiveness and cost
Disability Rights Commission established	1999	Reviewed the working of the 1995 Disability Discrimination Act
UN Declaration of Commitment on HIV/AIDS	2001	
Wanless Report	2002	'Securing our future health: taking a long-term view'
England and Wales Licensing Act	2003	Rules about opening hours for sale of alcohol made specific to premises and no longer generally applicable
Wanless Report	2004	'Improving public health and reducing health inequalities'
Scottish Licensing Act	2005	As in the English and Wales Licensing Act of 2003
Drugs Act	2005	New classification of drugs and new powers for testing those suspected of being under the influence of drugs
Mental Health Act	2007	Concerned with supervision of community care and aftercare, and definition of approved professionals to supervise care
Marmot Review	2010	Strategic review of health inequalities in England post 2010

one hand it was associated with improved communication between professionals and patients, and a greater readiness in patients to discuss what were once thought embarrassing physical or mental problems. On the other hand it is also associated with increased defensive practices by professionals, greater public scepticism about professional knowledge, lower tolerance of professional misjudgement and error and greater inclination to sue. It also brought anxieties about protection of the individual against prolongation of life once expectation of recovery has expired. Thus the nature of the relationship between patients and professional health carers gradually changed, so that now the patient is more involved in decision making about care and is asked to consent to treatment in a manner that is practically contractual.

Giving and receiving health care is, in summary, now more difficult than in the early years of the National Health Service. The complexity of contemporary decisions about treatment can be illustrated by the parental dilemma concerning vaccination of a child. Three elements have now to be considered: (1) Is the science credible and the risk understandable?, (2) Should the child be subject to the risk and the treatment?, (3) Should I have this done to help protect the whole community of children?

The complexity of government responsibility for health was emphasised by the conclusion of the Marmot Review that health and social justice are so closely related 'that the magnitude of health inequalities is a good marker of progress towards creating a fairer society' (Marmot 2010: 16).

British birth cohort and life course studies of health

The contribution from the cohort studies

The power of the birth cohort studies' contribution lies essentially in their design as prospective studies of representative populations unselected for any health characteristics. This section outlines the types of contributions that the birth cohort studies have made to understanding health.

The first study showed extensive socio-economic and geographical differences in infant health and survival and care of the mother during pregnancy and birth, two years before the National Health Service started (Joint Committee 1948; Douglas and Blomfield 1956; Wadsworth 1991). Consequently, the following two birth cohort studies in 1958 and 1970 were designed initially to show the extent of change in those outcomes. They found that the socio-economic and geographical differences were remarkably persistent, despite great improvements in survival and in care (Butler and Bonham 1963; Butler and Alberman 1969; Chamberlain *et al.* 1978). The birth cohort studies of 1991 and 2000 continued to find a concentration of early life health problems in the most disadvantaged groups (Baker and Taylor 1997; Dex and Joshi 2005).

The first two studies in particular contributed to health-care policy by showing the risks to infant and maternal health associated with home births. The studies tested hypotheses about the outcomes over time of exposure to health-damaging risks including maternal smoking in pregnancy (Butler *et al.* 1971), atmospheric pollution from coal burning (Douglas and Waller 1966) and long periods of hospital care (Douglas 1975). They showed the positive effects of health visitor care (Douglas and Blomfield 1956) and diet in infancy (Rodgers 1978), and improvement in chances of survival with cerebral palsy and confirmation that it was not associated with obstetric risk (Emond *et al.* 1989). Adverse social outcomes associated with health problems were also found, such as mild mental retardation (Maughan *et al.* 1999) and poor physical health and growth in childhood (Bartley *et al.* 1994; Walker 1982).

The scientific significance of the cohort studies of early life was shown at that time by two findings. First was the idea that perhaps disadvantaged mothers had poorer pregnancy outcomes because of their own poor early life development. Illsley and Kincaid (1963) developed this idea because short height was associated with greater perinatal risk in mothers of the 1958 cohort, who had themselves been in early life during the economic depression when the diet of disadvantaged infants was very poor. Second was the demonstration that smoking in pregnancy was related to birth outcome (Butler *et al.* 1971). Each of these findings played a significant part in the development of life course epidemiology.

Later, when adult health outcomes were measured, the significance of poor growth in early life was further developed. Many analyses of the cohorts' data showed the association, and complexity, between growth and development in early life and physical and mental health in adulthood (e.g. Wadsworth *et al.* 1985; Jones *et al.* 1994; Kuh *et al.* 1994; Power and Li 2000), including the impact of obstetric care on later cognitive function (Odd *et al.* 2009) and the relationships between early head growth and later cognitive function (Gale *et al.* 2006), maternal anxiety during pregnancy and later asthma in offspring (Cookson *et al.* 2009), early psycho-social environment and growth (Montgomery *et al.* 1997), and offspring psychological adjustment (Collishaw *et al.* 2007) and adult alcohol habits (Hope *et al.* 1988). Poor growth and physical development was related to later socio-economic and occupational disadvantage (Bartley *et al.* 1994; Montgomery *et al.* 1996), and disadvantaged growth and socio-economic circumstances were risks for later poor health life chances, raised risk of chronic illness, earlier mental and physical ageing, and premature death (Kuh and Hardy 2002; Kuh and Ben Shlomo 2004; Kuh *et al.* 2006; Power and Kuh 2006; Richards *et al.* 2004; Hertzman and Power 2006; Murray *et al.* 2007). Now the studies are examining genetic effects in relation to lifetime environmental, social and psychological risks in terms of a wide range of outcomes including cognitive function (Barnett *et al.* 2009), timing of puberty (Ong *et al.* 2009), respiratory health (Wadsworth *et al.* 2004) and type 1 diabetes (Barrett *et al.* 2009).

Future potential contributions from the cohort studies

The value of the British birth cohorts lies in their powerful design features as life course studies, and the opportunity they offer to compare life courses that occurred under different socio-economic and environmental circumstances. Each cohort carries marks or imprints of the health and health-related experiences unique to their time. The 1946 cohort were, for example, mostly conceived when food was rationed and medical care was costly and far less effective than it is today, and many of their mothers were infants during the pre-war period of economic depression and may therefore have had limited health capital to pass on to their offspring. Infants in the first cohort thus began life in hard and restricted circumstances in terms of diet and physical environment. But they then lived at least half their adult years in much more favourable conditions, and the life expectancy of their generation at middle age increased greatly compared with earlier generations (see Table 7.2). By contrast comparable health imprints of the later-born birth cohorts are progressively different. These features will be valuable for new research that will compare, at specific ages, the health and well-being capital of each cohort as a whole, in order to address questions about the effectiveness of health care and the impact of policy.

The later studies, and the new study proposed to start in pregnancy during 2012, were designed to explore further the hypotheses about effects on health and development of poor home circumstances, neglectful and inconsistent parenting and poor growth in early life. Work on the earlier cohorts is likely to continue on the interrelationship of adult health with health and experience throughout life. This work will probably follow the 1946 cohort in concentrating on indicators of rate and type of health change with age, such as decline in respiratory, memory and cardiovascular function and in strength and balance. Studies could then examine how the impact of adult life experience compares with early life development and socio-economic circumstances in their relationships with health and life expectation in later adulthood. Studies could also ask whether Brunner and Marmot's (2006) hypothesis about the relationship between long-term exposure to chronic stress and chronic physical illness may be protected against or exacerbated by early life experience, how much the relationships they observe vary across generations and whether some aspects of their findings are accounted for by epigenetic effects.

Variation in exposure to known risks during many years of life may be studied within cohorts and compared between cohorts. Inter-cohort comparisons may find that profound deprivation can produce different relationships in different cohorts and in different generations within cohorts. For example, research in the depressed Rhondda Valley in 1934 found that 'no improvement in antenatal service reduced the high maternal mortality rate until food was distributed to expectant mothers –when this was done it fell by 75 per cent.' (Burnett 1989: 271). That kind of difference was thought to affect inter-generational variation in relationships between breastfeeding and cognitive function in the 1946 cohort (Richards *et al.* 1998). Profound deprivation may affect genetic effects and gene–environment interactions differently in different generations (Kaati *et al.* 2007). No doubt the cohort studies will continue to explore how genetic influences have their effects on health and how environmental circumstances moderate genetic effects. Pooling data from several or all cohorts may be necessary.

The cohorts may be useful for new studies of lifetime effects of specific exposures. For instance, exposure to poliomyelitis during the early post-war epidemics has been associated with post-poliomyelitis syndrome in later life, and hypothesised also to increase the risk of neurological disease in later life (Martyn *et al.* 1988), and prenatal exposure to influenza has been suggested as a possible risk for later schizophrenia (Brown *et al.* 1995). Prion disease, which is thought to be associated with some meat products and has an incubation period of several decades, may be a topic for future study.

Comparisons of the health imprints of the birth cohorts will shed new light on the relative effects of childhood and early life circumstances in the development of adult health and the processes of ageing, and will show the likelihood of inter-cohort differences in health in later life. In other words it will be of predictive value for public health.

Conclusions

Since the end of the Second World War the health of the public has improved greatly in response to rising material and economic standards of living and improvements in the treatment and prevention of health problems. Demographic and epidemiological evidence makes that clear and shows the significant social impact of health changes.

Concepts of risk and causes of illness expanded greatly during the same period. As well as new knowledge from the health sciences, new ideas have been developed about how adverse socio-economic and psychological environments can precipitate mental and physical ill health. It seems likely that prolonged exposure to psychological stress triggers adverse biological reactions, and that incomplete or disrupted physical and mental development in early life can be a significant source of vulnerability to ill health at later ages throughout adulthood. The role of genetic factors in these processes is only just beginning to be studied.

Evidence of risk from prolonged exposure to stressful circumstances has so far been shown mostly in longitudinal studies that begin in middle life and in studies of countries undergoing profound social change. New research to test these ideas in the birth cohort populations would further strengthen the evidence, showing the interaction of adult stress effects with early life developmental effects.

If there is consistent evidence for these new notions of risk, then new approaches to treatment and to preventive care will be required, and changes in ways of life will need to be considered. They are likely to be as important as the changes in material and economic standards have been over the period studied.

Responsibility for health became increasingly contentious during the 1980s as individualism and 'belief in the market as the supreme arbiter of value' (Feldman 2002: 105) took hold. Responsibility is still debated and becomes more difficult as the costs of preventive health care and treatment grow and as preventive care associated with changes in lifestyle is resisted or found by many to be unattainable or too arduous to maintain. New ways of achieving preventive health care need to be developed.

References

Acheson, D., Barker, D., Chambers, J., Graham, H., Marmot, M. and Whitehead, M. (1998) *Independent inquiry into inequalities in health*, London: Her Majesty's Stationery Office.

Baker, D. and Taylor, H. (1997) 'Inequality in health and health service use for mothers of young children in South West England', *Journal of Epidemiology and Community Health*, 51: 74–9

Barker, D. J. P. (1984) *Mothers, babies, and disease in later life*, London: BMJ Publishing.

Barker, D. J. P. (1998) *Mothers and babies and health in later life*, 2nd edn, Edinburgh: Churchill Livingstone.

Barnett, J. H., Heron, J., Goldman, D., Jones, P. B. and Xu, K. (2009) 'Effects of catechol-O-methyltransferase on normal variation in the cognitive function of children', *American Journal of Psychiatry*, 166: 909–16.

Barrett, J. C., Clayton, D. G., Concannon, P., Akolkar, B., Cooper, J. D., Erlich, H. A., Julier, C., Morahan, G., Nerup, J., Nierras, C., Plagnol, V., Pociot, F., Schuilenberg, H., Smyth, D. J., Stevens, H., Todd, J. A., Walker, N. M., Rich, S. S. and the Type 1 Diabetes Genetics Consortium (2009) 'Genome-wide association study and meta-analysis find that over 40 loci affect risk of type 1 diabetes', *Nature Genetics*, 4: 703–7.

Bartley, M. J., Power, C., Blane, D., Davey Smith, D. and Shipley, M. (1994) 'Birth weight and later socioeconomic disadvantage – evidence from the 1958 British cohort study', *British Medical Journal*, 309: 1475–8.

Black, D., Morris, J., Smith, C. and Townsend, P. (1980) *Inequalities in health: report of a research working group,* London: Department of Health and Social Security.

Brayne, C., Matthews, F. E., McGee, M. and Jagger, C. (2001) 'Health and ill-health in the older population in England and Wales', *Age and Ageing*, 30: 53–62.

Breakwell, C. and Bajekal, M. (2006) 'Health expectancies in the UK and its constituent countries, 2001', *Health Statistics Quarterly*, 29: 18–25.

British Geriatric Society (n.d.) http://www.bgs.org.uk (last accessed 21 November 2010).

Brown, A. S., Susser, E. S., Lin, S. P. and Gorman, J. M. (1995) 'Affective disorder in Holland after prenatal exposure to the 1957 A2 influenza epidemic, *Biological Psychiatry*, 38: 270–3.

Brunner, E. and Marmot, M. (2006) 'Social organisation, stress and health', in M. Marmot and R. G. Wilkinson (eds) *Social determinants of health*, 2nd edn, pp. 6–30, Oxford: Oxford University Press.

Burnett, J. (1989) *Plenty and want: a social history of food in England from 1815 to the present day*, 3rd edn, London: Routledge.

Butler, N. R. and Bonham, D. G. (1963) *Perinatal mortality*, Edinburgh: Livingstone.

Butler, N. R. and Alberman, E. D. (1969) *Perinatal problems*, Edinburgh:Livingstone.

Butler, N. R., Goldstein, H. and Ross, E. M. (1971) 'Cigarette smoking in pregnancy: influence on birth and perinatal mortality', *British Medical Journal*, 1: 127–30.

Butterfield, W. J. H. (1968) *Priorities in medicine*, London: Nuffield Provincial Hospitals Trust.

Chamberlain, G. V. P., Philipp, E., Howlett, B. and Masters, K. (1978) *British births 1970*, London: Heinemann.

Collishaw, S., Maughan, B., Goodman, R. and Pickles, A. (2004) 'Time trends in adolescent mental health', *Journal of Child Psychology and Psychiatry*, 45: 1350–62.

Collishaw, S., Dunn, J., O'Connor, T. G. and Golding, J. (2007) 'Maternal childhood abuse and offspring adjustment over time', *Developmental Psychopathology*, 19: 367–83.

Colman, I., Wadsworth, M. E. J., Croudace, T. J. and Jones, P. B. (2006) 'Three decades of antidepressant, anxiolytic and hypnotic use in a national population birth cohort', *British Journal of Psychiatry*, 189: 156–60.

Cookson, H., Granell, R., Joinson, C., Ben-Shlomo, Y. and Henderson, A. J. (2009) 'Mothers' anxiety during pregnancy is associated with asthma in their children', *Journal of Allergy and Clinical Immunology*, 123: 847–53.

Department of Health (1975) *Health and personal social service statistics for England 1975*, Table 4.1, London: Her Majesty's Stationery Office.

Dex, S. and Joshi, H. (eds) (2005) *Children of the 21st century*, Bristol: Policy Press.

Dezateux, C., Foster, L., Tate, R., Walton, S., Samad, L., Bedford, H., Bartington, S., Peckham, C. and Butler, N. (2005) 'Children's health', in S. Dex and H. Joshi (eds) *Children of the 21st century*, pp. 133–58, Bristol: Policy Press.

Doll, R. (2004) 'Evolution of knowledge of the smoking picture', in P. Boyle, J. Gray, J. Henningfield, J. Seffrin and W. Zatonski (eds) *Tobacco: science, policy and public health*, pp. 1–12, Oxford: Oxford University Press.

Doll, R. and Hill, A. B. (1950) 'Smoking and lung cancer: preliminary report', *British Medical Journal*, 2: 739–48.

Doll, R. and Hill, A. B. (1956) 'Lung cancer and other causes of death in relation to smoking: a second report on the mortality of British doctors', *British Medical Journal*, 2: 1071–6.

Doll, R. and Hill, A. B. (1964) 'The mortality of doctors in relation to their smoking habits: a preliminary report', *British Medical Journal*, 1: 1451–5.

Douglas, J. W. B. (1975) 'Early hospital admissions and later disturbances of behaviour and learning', *Developmental Medicine and Child Neurology*, 17: 456–80.

Douglas, J. W. B. and Blomfield, J. M. (1956) *Children under five*, London: Allen and Unwin.

Douglas, J. W. B. and Waller, R. E. (1966) 'Air pollution and respiratory infection in children', *British Journal of Preventive and Social Medicine*, 20: 1–8.

Ebrahim, S. and Kalache. A. (eds) (1996) *Epidemiology in old age*, London: BMJ Publishing.

Emond, A., Golding, J. and Peckham, C. (1989) 'Cerebral palsy in two national cohort studies', *Archives of Disease in Childhood*, 64: 848–52.

Feldman, D. (2002) *Civil liberties and human rights in England and Wales*, 2nd edn, Oxford: Oxford University Press.

Forey, B., Hamling, J., Lee, P. and Wald, N. (2002) *International smoking statistics*, 2nd edn, Oxford: Oxford University Press.

Frankenberg, R. (1957) *Village on the border: a study of religion, politics and football in a North Wales community*, London: Cohen and West.

Gale, C. R., O'Callaghan, F. J., Bredow, M. and Martyn, C. N. (2006) 'The influence of head growth in fetal life, infancy, and childhood on intelligence at the ages of 4 and 8 years', *Pediatrics*, 118: 1486–92.

Gath, D. H., Mynors-Wallis, L. M. and Williams, J. W. (1997) 'Problem-solving treatment in general practice', in D. Clark and C. G. Fairburn (eds) *Science and practice of cognitive behaviour therapy*, pp. 415–31, Oxford: Oxford, University Press.

General Household Survey (2000) *Living in Britain*, London: Her Majesty's Stationery Office.

Grafton, P. (1981) *You, you and you: people out of step with World War II*, London: Pluto.

Grimley Evans, J. (1997) 'Geriatric medicine: a brief history', *British Medical Journal*, 315: 1075–7.

Gunnell, D. (2001) 'Early insights into height, leg length, proportionate growth and health', *International Journal of Epidemiology*, 30: 221–2.

Haworth, J. and Hart, G. (2007) *Well-being: individual, community and social perspectives*, Basingstoke: Palgrave Macmillan.

Hertzman, C. and Power, C. (2006) 'A life course approach to health and human development', in J. Heymann, C. Hertzman, M. L. Barer and R. G. Evans (eds) *Healthier societies: from analysis to action*, pp. 83–106, Oxford: Oxford University Press.

Hope, S., Power, C. and Rodgers, B. (1998) 'The relationship between parental separation in childhood and problem drinking in adulthood', *Addiction*, 93: 505–14.

House of Lords Science and Technology Committee (2006) 'Ageing: scientific aspects', House of Lords Paper 7, London: Her Majesty's Stationery Office.

Howarth, T. E. B. (1985) *Prospect and reality: Great Britain 1945–1955*, London: Collins.

Illsley, R. and Kincaid, J. C. (1963) 'Social correlates of perinatal mortality', in N. R. Butler and D. G. Bonham (eds) *Perinatal mortality*, pp. 270–86, Edinburgh: Livingstone.

Joint Committee (1948) *Maternity in Great Britain*, Oxford: Oxford University Press.

Jones, P., Rodgers, B., Murray, M. and Marmot, M. (1994) 'Child developmental risk factors for adult schizophrenia in the British 1946 birth cohort', *Lancet*, 344: 1398–402.

Jones, P., Rantakallio, P., Hartikainen, A.-L., Isohanni, M. and Sipila, P. (1998) 'Schizophrenia as a long-term outcome of pregnancy, delivery, and perinatal complications: a 28 year follow-up of the 1966 North Finnish general population birth cohort', *American Journal of Psychiatry*, 155: 355–64.

Kaati, G., Bygren, L. O., Pembrey, M. and Sjostrom, M. (2007) 'Transgenerational response to nutrition, early life circumstances and longevity', *European Journal of Human Genetics*, 15: 1–7.

Kahneman, D., Diener, E. and Schwarz, N. (1999) *Well-being: the foundations of hedonistic psychology*, New York: Russell Sage Foundation.

Kuh, D. and Hardy, R. (eds) (2002) *A life course approach to women's health*, Oxford: Oxford University Press.

Kuh, D. and Ben Shlomo, Y. (eds) (2004) *A life course approach to chronic disease epidemiology*, 2nd edn, Oxford: Oxford University Press.

Kuh, D., Wadsworth, M. E. J. and Yusuf, E. (1994) 'Burden of disability in a post-war birth cohort', *Journal of Epidemiology and Community Health*, 48: 262–9.

Kuh, D., Hardy, R., Butterworth, S., Okell, L., Wadsworth, M. E. J., Cooper, C. and Aihie Sayer, A. (2006) 'Developmental origins of adult grip strength: findings from a British birth cohort', *Journal of Gerontology (Medical Sciences)*, 61: 702–6.

Layard, R. (2005) *Happiness: lessons from a new science*, London: Allen Lane.

Li, L., Hardy, R., Kuh, D., Lo Conte, R. and Power, C. (2008) 'Child-to-adult body mass index and height trajectories: a comparison of two British birth cohort studies', *American Journal of Epidemiology*, 168: 1008–15.

Macfarlane, A. J. and Mugford, M. (2000) *Birth counts. Volumes 1 and 2*, London: Her Majesty's Stationery Office.

Marmot, M. G. (2010) *Fair society, healthy lives: the Marmot Review: strategic review of health inequalities in England post-2010*, London: Department of Health.

Marmot, M. G., Shipley, M. J. and Rose, G. (1984) 'Inequalities in death – specific explanations of a general pattern', *Lancet*, 323: 1003–6.

Martyn, C., Barker, D. J. P. and Osmond, C. (1988) 'Motoneuron disease and past poliomyelitis in England and Wales', *Lancet*, 331: 1319–22.

Marwick, A. (1982) *British society since 1945*, London: Pelican.

Maughan, B. (2002) 'Depression and psychological distress: a life course perspective', in D. Kuh and R. J. Hardy (eds) *A life course approach to women's health*, pp. 161–76, Oxford: Oxford University Press.

Maughan, B., Collishaw, S. and Pickles, A. (1999) 'Mild mental retardation: psychosocial functioning in adulthood', *Psychological Medicine*, 29: 351–66.

Middleton, N., Gunnell, D., Whitley, E., Dorling, D. and Frankel, S. (2001) 'Secular trends in antidepressant prescribing in the UK, 1975–1998', *Journal of Public Health Medicine*, 23: 262–67.

Moffitt, T. E. (2005) 'The new look of behavioural genetics in developmental psychopathology: gene–environment interplay in antisocial behaviours', *Psychological Bulletin*, 131: 533–54.

Montgomery, S. M., Bartley, M. J., Cook, D. G. and Wadsworth, M. E. J. (1996) 'Health and social precursors of unemployment in young men in Great Britain', *Journal of Epidemiology and Community Health*, 50: 415–22.

Montgomery, S. M., Bartley, M. J. and Wilkinson, R. J. (1997) 'Family conflict and slow growth', *Archives of Disease in Childhood*, 77: 326–30.

Morley, J. E. (2004) 'A brief history of geriatrics', *Journals of Gerontology. Series A*, 59: 1132–52.

Morris, J. N. (1967) *Uses of epidemiology*, Edinburgh: Livingstone.

Morris, J. N., Heady, J. A., Raffle, P. A. B., Roberts, C. G. and Parks, J. W. (1953) 'Coronary heart disease and physical activity at work', *Lancet* 265: 1111–20.

Murray, G. K., Jones, P. B., Kuh, D. and Richards, M. (2007) 'Infant developmental milestones and subsequent cognitive function', *Annals of Neurology*, 62: 128–36.

National Health Service (2009) *Prescriptions dispensed in the community; statistics for 1998 to 2008: England*, London: Health and Social Care Information Centre, NHS.

Odd, D. E., Lewis, G., Whitelaw, A. and Gunnell, D. (2009) 'Resuscitation at birth and cognition at 8 years of age: a cohort study', *Lancet*, 373:1615–22.

Office for National Statistics (1997) *Living in Britain; results from the 1995 General Household Survey*, London: Her Majesty's Stationery Office.

Office for National Statistics (2007) 'Trends in life expectancy by social class'. Available at http://www.statistics.gov.uk/downloads/theme_population/Life_Expect_Social_class_1972–05/life_expect_social_class.pdf (last accessed 30 September 2009).

Ong, K. K., Elks, C. E., Li, S., Zhao, K. H., Luan, J., Andersen, L. B., Bingham, S. A., Brage, S., Smith, G. D., Ekelund, U., Gillson, C. J., Glaser, B., Golding. J., Hardy, R., Khaw, K.-T., Kuh, D., Luben, R., Marcus, M., McGeehin, M. A., Ness, A. R., Northstone, K., Ring, S. M., Rubin, C., Sims, M. A., Song, K., Strachan, D. P., Vollenweider, P., Waeber, G., Waterworth, D. M., Wong, A., Deloukas, P., Barroso, I., Mooser, V., Loos, R. J. and Wareham, N. (2009) 'Genetic variation in *LIN28B* is associated with the timing of puberty', *Nature Genetics*, 41: 729–33.

Plant, M. and Plant, M. (2006) *Binge Britain: alcohol and the national response*, Oxford: Oxford University Press.

Power, C. and Li, L. (2000) 'Cohort study of birthweight, mortality and disability', *British Medical Journal*, 320: 840–1.

Power, C. and Kuh, D. (2006) 'Life course development of unequal health', in J. Siegrist and M. Marmot (eds) *Socioeconomic position and health: new explanations and their policy implications*, pp. 27–54, Oxford: Oxford University Press.

Prynne, C. J., Paul, A. A., Mishra, G. D., Hardy, R. J., Bolton-Smith, C. and Wadsworth, M. E. J. (2002) 'Socio-demographic inequalities in the diet of young children in the 1946 British birth cohort', *Public Health Nutrition*, 5: 733–45.

Public Accounts Committee (2009) *Reducing alcohol harm; health services in England for alcohol abuse*, London: Stationery Office.

Rachman, S. (1997) 'The evolution of cognitive behaviour therapy', in D. Clark, C. G. Fairburn and M. G. Gelder (eds) *Science and practice and cognitive behaviour therapy*, pp. 1–26, Oxford: Oxford University Press.

Reid, D. D. (1969) 'The beginnings of chronic bronchitis', *Proceedings of the Royal Society of Medicine*, 62: 311–16.

Richards, M. and Deary, I. J. (2005) 'Cognitive reserve: a model for cognitive aging and development?', *Annals of Neurology*, 58: 617–20.

Richards, M., Wadsworth, M. E. J., Rahimi-Foroushani, A., Hardy, R. J., Kuh, D. and Paul, A. A. (1998) Infant nutrition and cognitive development in the first offspring of a national UK born cohort. *Developmental Medicine and Child Neurology*, 40: 163–7.

Richards, M., Shipley, B., Fuhrer, R. and Wadsworth, M. E. J. (2004) 'Cognitive ability in childhood and cognitive decline in midlife: longitudinal birth cohort study', *British Medical Journal*, 328: 552–4.

Richards, M., Abbott, R., Collis, G., Hackett, P., Hotopf, M., Kuh, D., Jones, P., Maughan, B. and Parsonage, M. (2009) *Childhood mental health and life chances in post-war Britain: insights from three national birth cohort studies*, London: Medical Research Council Unit for Lifelong Health and Ageing.

Rodgers, B. (1978) 'Feeding in infancy and later ability and attainment', *Developmental Medicine and Child Neurology*, 20: 421–6.

Rose, G. (1992) *The strategy of preventive medicine*, Oxford: Oxford University Press.

Rutter, M. (2005) 'Environmentally mediated risks for psychopathology: research strategies and findings', *Journal of the American Academy of Child and Adolescent Psychiatry*, 44: 3–18.

Schooling, C. M. and Leung, G. M. (2010) 'A socio-biological explanation for social disparities in non-communicable diseases: the product of history?', *Journal of Epidemiology and Community Health*, 64: 941–9.

Sheridan, D. (ed.) (1990) *Wartime women: a mass observation anthology of the experiences of women at war*, London: Heinemann.

Social Trends (1970) No. 1, London: Stationery Office.

Social Trends (1980) No. 10, London: Stationery Office.

Social Trends (1990) No. 20, London: Stationery Office.

Social Trends (2009) No. 39, London: Palgrave Macmillan.

Stamatakis, E., Primatesta, P., Chinn, S., Rona, R. and Falascheti, E. (2005) 'Overweight and obesity trends from 1974 to 2003 in English children: what is the role of socioeconomic factors?', *Archives of Disease in Childhood*, 90: 999–1004.

Stark, O., Peckham, C. S. and Moynihan, C. (1989) 'Weight and age at menarche', *Archives of Disease in Childhood*, 64: 383–7.

Strachan, D. and Sheikh, A. (2004) 'A life course approach to respiratory and allergic disease', in D. Kuh and Y. Ben Shlomo (eds) *A life course approach to chronic disease epidemiology*, pp. 240–59, Oxford: Oxford University Press.

Svanborg, A. (1996) 'Conduct of long-term cohort sequential studies', in S. Ebrahim and A. Kalache (eds) *Epidemiology in old age*, pp. 57–66, London: BMJ Publishing.

Tanner, J. M., Hayashi, T., Preece, M. and Cameron, N. (1982) 'Increase in length of leg relative to trunk in Japanese children from 1957 to 1977: comparison with British and Japanese Americans', *Annals of Human Biology*, 9: 411–23.

Vyse, A. J., Gay, N. J., White, J. M., Ramsay, M. E., Brown, D. W. G., Cohen, B. J., Hesketh, L. M., Morgan-Capner, P. and Miller, E. (2002) 'Evolution of surveillance of measles, mumps, and rubella in England and Wales', *Epidemiologic Reviews*, 24: 125–36.

Wadsworth, M. E. J. (1991) *The imprint of time: childhood, history, and adult life*, Oxford: Clarendon Press.

Wadsworth, M. E. J., Cripps, H. A., Midwinter, R. and Colley, J. R. T. (1985) 'Blood pressure at age 36 years and social and familial factors, cigarette smoking and body mass in a national birth cohort', *British Medical Journal*, 291: 1534–8.

Wadsworth, M. E. J., Butterworth, S., Montgomery, S., Ehlin, A. and Bartley, M. (2003) 'Health', in E. Ferri, J. Bynner, and M. E. J. Wadsworth (eds) *Changing Britain, changing lives: three generations at the turn of the century*, pp. 207–36, London: Institute of Education Press.

Wadsworth, M. E. J., Vinall, L. E., Jones, A. L., Hardy, R. J., Whitehouse, D. B., Butterworth, S. L., Hilder, W. S., Lovegrove, J. U. and Swallow, D. M. (2004) 'Alpha1-antitrypsin as a risk for infant and adult respiratory outcomes in a national birth cohort', *American Journal of Respiratory Cell and Molecular Biology*, 31: 559–64.

Walker, A. (1982) *Unqualified and underemployed: handicapped young people and the labour market*, London: Macmillan.

Wanless Report (2006) *Securing good care for older people: taking a long-term view*, London: Kings Fund.

Warren, M. W. (1946) 'Care of the chronic aged sick', *Lancet*, i: 841–3.

Wilkinson, R. G. (2006) 'Ourselves and others – for better or worse: social vulnerability and inequality', in M. Marmot and R. G. Wilkinson (eds) *Social determinants of health*, 2nd edn, pp. 341–57, Oxford: Oxford University Press.

Wilkinson, R. and Pickett, K. (2010) *The spirit level: why equality is better for everyone*, London, Penguin.

World Health Organization (2008) *The global burden of disease*, Geneva: World Health Organization.

8 Leisure

Stability and change

Ken Roberts

Introduction

The ways in which Britons spend their free time have remained relatively stable since the 1950s. This is compared with the concurrent scale of economic restructuring (de-industrialisation) and changes in family patterns, the shape of the class structure, the age structure of the population and post-16 educational participation. Of course, there have been changes associated with, for example, the advent of multi-channel television, the expansion of information and communication technology (ICT), take-up and internet leisure use, the spread of car ownership and rising incomes enabling more people to take holidays and to spend more of them abroad, to dine out more frequently and to consume more alcohol. But against prediction, the time available for leisure has not grown dramatically. Since the 1960s leisure time has grown at around a minute per year per working age male, and hardly at all for women (Gershuny and Fisher 1999). The leisure society that was foreseen in the 1950s, 1960s and 1970s (by, for example, Glasser 1970; Jenkins and Sherman 1981) is still awaited. It is leisure spending, not time, that has grown dramatically, rising fivefold since the 1960s.

The relative stability in post-war leisure time and use contrasts in another sense with the changes in uses of leisure that preceded the 1950s. During the nineteenth century Britain was transformed from a mainly rural into a mainly urban industrial society. Routines became governed by the clock rather than by the rhythms of nature. The urban–rural contrast was one way in which sociology's founding fathers distinguished modern from traditional societies. Then, in the late nineteenth and early twentieth centuries, leisure was again transformed by:

- the one-and-a-half-day weekend;
- modern sports, for players and spectators;
- the modern holiday: a week or a fortnight spent away from home, typically at the seaside;
- mass circulation daily newspapers;
- the music hall;
- electricity, which transformed home environments.

Between the world wars there were further major lifestyle changes:

- radio broadcasting, which in Britain began in 1922 and achieved almost instant mass popularity;
- the cinema, after Hollywood began producing feature-length movies;
- recorded music, with the gramophone beginning to replace the piano as a normal source (alongside radio) of music in the home.

There were further major changes between the 1930s and 1950s. Children growing up in the digital age may become another change generation, but we will not know until they have become adults. Up until now there has been nothing comparable since the dawn of the age of television. This is despite major changes in virtually all other areas of life in Britain. With the transformation from a manufacturing to a service industry the economy has become 'post industrial' (Bell 1974). Women working full-time or part-time are now almost 50 per cent of the labour force. Manual work has become a minority occupation. The expansion of employment in professional and management occupations (now accounting for around 40 per cent of all jobs) has led to increased rates of absolute upwards job movement even though rates of relative social mobility have not changed (Goldthorpe and Mills 2008). Yet the main social class differences in uses of leisure are much as they were. The middle classes do more and have become cultural omnivores, increasingly absorbing into their leisure time traditional working class leisure pursuits such as football matches. The present-day working class simply does less of virtually everything except television viewing (Bennett *et al.* 2009; Le Roux *et al.* 2008).

Since the mid-twentieth century there has been a so-called 'gender-quake' (Wilkinson 1995). Girls now outperform boys at all levels in education. More women now hold full-time employment more or less continuously from leaving education until retirement, taking maternity leave instead of terminating employment. Since the 1970s most children have grown up in households with a working mother as a role model. The trend has been towards genderless leisure lifestyles among young adults, basically as a result of young women acting in ways that were once considered masculine, in terms for instance of alcohol consumption, smoking, drug use, playing sport and, perhaps most basically, acting independently and using public space without male 'guardians' (Sweeting and West 2003). The leisure life of partnerless teenage girls is no longer confined to a 'bedroom culture', as McRobbie and Garber (1976) described it. However, the chances of the genderless leisure of present-day young adults surviving the lifecycle squeeze – the pressure on leisure time and spending that accompanies new household and family formation – remains in doubt (Gershuny 2003).

The shape of the life course is now different from in the mid-twentieth century. The post-retirement period of life has been steadily getting longer. More people are living through their seventies and into their eighties and increasingly beyond. Men have been retiring from employment at younger ages, so for them adulthood as a period of working life has been increasingly compressed. Youth, like later life, now lasts longer, particularly for those whose education extends through further and higher education, postponing entry into adult jobs. Over the decade preceding 2008 the mean age at marriage for men increased by nearly five and a half years and for women by just over four and a half years. The provisional mean age for men marrying in 2008 was 36.5 years, and for women 33.8 years. Cohabiting before or instead of marriage has also increasingly become the norm.

The significance of these changes is hotly debated. In the pre-employment life phase, are some young adults deliberately stepping off the career ladder to enjoy a new 'emerging adulthood'? (Arnett 2005). Is leisure for them still a site where they accomplish socio-psychological developmental tasks, before moving on? (Hendry *et al.* 1993). Or are these young adults pioneering lifestyles and adopting consumption-based identities, legal or otherwise, that they may retain into adulthood? (Hollands 1995). That would mean consumer roles displacing producer roles as sources of identity, as suggested, for example, by Baudrillard (1998) and Bauman (1998). The contrary view is that a period of job experimentation and enhanced leisure time before continuous employment is simply a source of temporary identities while (usually university educated) young people progress through an extended youth life stage (Miles 2000; Côté and Bynner 2008; Hendry and Kloep 2010).

It must also be asked whether such possible reshaping of the youth phase of the life course affects the leisure lives not only of young people but also of those in later life? The cohorts born in the early post-war period are now at or approaching retirement from paid employment, and some appear to be beginning a life stage of active engagement and consumption, compared with previous generations, for whom this was a time of withdrawal from active social life (Higgs *et al.* 2009). The argument in this chapter is that the first post-Second World War cohort, the 'baby boomers', who were the first generation to be identified with a distinct 'youth' phase of the life course, are now receptive to and are pioneering a new concept of 'old age'. The traditionally low rates of leisure participation among older people, as recorded in surveys up to now, have probably been, at least in part, due to the poverty of socialisation into leisure time among children and young people born before 1945.

This argument receives support from studies that show continuity in individuals' leisure practices from youth up until late adulthood (Scott and Willits 1989). People tend to base the bulk of their leisure lives on tastes, interests and skills that were learned during childhood and youth. Adults and even seniors may take up entirely new activities, but doing so tends to be the exception rather than the rule. The football teams that we always support (or at least follow through the media) and our favourite kinds of music tend to be resilient. Some of Frank Sinatra's original fans were still packing his concerts for as long as he could perform (up to age seventy-nine).

But it may be an over-simplification to see leisure lifestyles as largely immutable. Part of the function of leisure during the teens is to define an identity that is at least temporarily distinct and independent from, if not in conflict with, that of their parents. Young people and their parents share much in common with respect to basic values associated with class and education such as political orientation, for example, but are likely to part company when it comes to attitudes to relationships, peer group activity and generally the signs and symbols of growing up (Brake 1985; Bynner and Ashford 1992). Teenage fashions and tastes in music and reading matter are taken on in response to a variety of societal forces including the blandishments of the partly commercialised wider youth culture. They may be reconstituted many times as young people grow older, finally crystallising in young adulthood into lifestyles that bear little resemblance to those when adolescence, post-puberty and increasingly pre-puberty began. While youth becomes stretched, so the scope of experimentation with lifestyle and identity extends.

The family lifecycle has been, and remains, the main driver of these changes (Rapoport and Rapoport 1975; Gershuny 2003). Family life events such as births, marriages, deaths, moving house and leaving school, and for the young family member getting a job and leaving home, are the occasions when lifestyles unfreeze and are then re-shaped. In these situations the other crucial influence for young people, the peer group, is likely to gain prominence. Individuals do not remain rigidly stuck in their ways throughout the life course, but change from the foundations laid in childhood and youth during the transitions they experience. Such changes are much more likely to be driven by age than by the pressures of historical change, although these too can play a part. The extension of global media-driven youth culture across the boundaries of the Soviet Union is seen, by some, as one of the drivers of the generational shift that led to its demise (Wallace and Kovacheva 1998). At the same time, the key features of development as expressed through, and shaped by, leisure activity (Coleman 1974; Hendry 1983) remain firmly in place (Birchwood *et al.* 2008; Roberts *et al.* 2009).

Nevertheless, a new way of using leisure may become available and sweep through the entire population, changing the leisure habits of all age cohorts. Radio and television are the main twentieth-century examples. Indeed, the commanding position of television viewing has been a stabilising anchor in everyday life throughout the last fifty years. Information technology (IT) has yet to create a comparable new wave – although since IT transformed into ICT (and the boundaries between media became increasingly blurred), especially among the younger generation, there have been signs that it will soon do so.

Deliberate attempts by governments to change how leisure time is spent have not generally met with much success in Britain. The shake-up in the management of local authority sport and leisure services through compulsory competitive tendering at the end of the 1980s had no impact whatsoever on participation rates. Nor has the subsequent spread of commercial health and fitness clubs boosted the proportion of adults taking part in keep-fit activities. Despite persistent promotion by the BBC since it was nationalised in 1927, and later on also by the Arts Council, the size and social composition of today's audience for high culture (theatre, concerts, art galleries and museums, opera and ballet) have changed little since the 1920s. When government measures were effective, as was the case with the opening of local authority indoor sport and leisure centres from the 1960s onwards (see later), this was usually because they were addressing a predisposed public. Apart from re-enforcing their attractions for each new generation of users, commercial businesses (including health and fitness clubs) know that it is futile to try to change people's basic tastes. Tour companies and beer manufacturers mainly compete for shares of their existing markets. They rarely attempt to build up entirely new markets, or to increase the total size of the existing bodies of consumers. Businesses find it much easier to hire and fire workers than to change demand for their products.

We have plenty of statistics about people's uses of their time and money. Unfortunately, the available historical data are rarely ideal for present purposes. Time use surveys have been conducted periodically in Britain since the 1960s, but not before. Since the 1970s government departments have collected data about the uses of leisure for which they are responsible (mainly the arts, sport, uses of the countryside and tourism). There are data extending much further back on cinema and football match attendances and alcohol and tobacco consumption, but rarely about the social composition of the audiences and consumers.

Nevertheless, we can compose an accurate picture of the main continuities and changes in uses of free time in Britain since the Second World War. The best way to chart these changes is on the basis of broad overlapping phases distinguished by significant shifts in behaviour and attitudes, with a degree of continuity within each of them as reflected in the experience of successive cohorts. Three such phases can be identified for present purposes, which also map on to those considered in other chapters: 'baby boomers' (1950–70), 'permissive society' (1970–90) and 'digital age' (1990 to the present day).

Austerity to affluence: the baby boomers (1950–70)

The products of the high post-war birth rates were known as 'the bulge' as they passed through Britain's schools, but the American term 'baby boomer' has stuck (Willetts 2010). The 1946 birth cohort were in the first, immediate post-war baby boom (a larger one was to follow in the late 1950s) and their early childhood was spent in what, in many ways, were wartime or pre-war social conditions.

Food rationing remained in force until 1954. This meant that children could eat only limited confectionery or meat (by subsequent standards). There were no pre-prepared meals or frozen foods. Canned foods were available but fresh vegetables were less expensive. Most mothers of primary school children were full-time housewives, and their children usually returned home for a cooked meal at mid-day. Primary age children walked to school. Bicycles were a means of transport rather than toys, and were used for road journeys when children transferred to secondary school. By this time children would be using public transport independently, to attend children's matinees at the cinema, among other things. Children's lifestyles were probably healthier than for any subsequent cohorts.

The baby boomers also benefitted from the National Health Service that began in 1948, and the antibiotics that were taming former child killers (penicillin became available from 1941). Poliomyelitis remained a threat until the Salk vaccine was introduced in 1955. All state education, including higher education, was free and those who could not otherwise afford to live away from home had access to (means-tested) maintenance grants.

The males in all cohorts born in the first thirty years of the twentieth century fought in one of the world wars, and military conscription continued until 1960. Any older brothers of the baby boomers would have done military service. The boomers grew up in its shadow, and did not know until they were teenagers that they would be the first cohort to avoid this. The implications are probably underestimated in explanations of the subsequent weakening of gender differences.

By the time the baby boomers became adults in the late 1960s, Britain was a rather different kind of society compared with that into which they had been born. It was an affluent society in which Prime Minister Harold Macmillan was able to assert that 'you never had it so good'. The baby boomers were the first post-scarcity generation whose childhoods were not marred by the kind of absolute poverty that was common up to and throughout the 1930s, or by the blight of adult unemployment (Inglehart 1977).

Recreation and leisure time

The wireless remained the main source of news and family entertainment until the early 1950s. Other forms of entertainment that had grown in popularity during the inter-war years – the cinema and watching sports, especially football matches – also enjoyed a resurgence in the late 1940s. Sales of recorded music also rose and replaced sales of sheet music as the basis for the 'hit parade'.

Alcohol consumption had been in long-term decline since the closing decades of the nineteenth century under pressure from taxation, licensing laws and temperance campaigns. In 1900 the British were consuming roughly 11 litres of alcohol per head of population aged fourteen and over. Between 1930 and 1960 the mean level of consumption fluctuated around 4 litres. In the 1940s and 1950s pubs were places for adult men. They were off-limits for most teenagers and generally for unaccompanied women. In working class neighbourhoods especially, alcohol was rarely stocked or drunk at home except at Christmas and during other celebrations. When teenagers went out, unless they stayed on the streets, those who simply wanted to socialise with each other generally went to milk bars, soon to be replaced by the more comfortable and trendy coffee bars (one example of Americanisation). These were the places where first skiffle groups, emulating American music such as blues, folk and New Orleans jazz, and later, following the sensation of Americans Bill Hayley and the Comets, the first 'pop' groups honed their skills. The Liverpool Cavern where the Beatles played in the early 1960s was dry.

Drugs were rarely encountered, if at all, by teenagers in the 1950s and those who did, because of effective propaganda, typically saw them as a 'risk too far'. Tobacco, in contrast, was everywhere. Consumption reached its historical high in the 1950s with 80 per cent of males smoking and most households containing at least one adult cigarette smoker. There were warnings from epidemiological research and from doctors that smoking caused lung cancer (Doll and Hill 1956). Smokers were aware of this, but young smokers especially preferred to continue smoking, confident that medicine would have found a cure before they became vulnerable. The associations of smoking with masculinity, maturity and an adult lifestyle, and the need to keep up with the group, reinforced by advertising – as in the 'Marlboro Man' – ensured continuing recruitment to the habit (Bynner 1969).

As the baby boom generation became adults, leisure time became more plentiful in post-war industrial Britain. The two-day weekend became the norm. Standard working hours (often supplemented by overtime) were reduced to forty per week; white-collar grades worked less. Two weeks annual holiday on top of statutory holidays had been made a statutory right in 1939. In post-war Britain the holiday away from home – usually in Britain – became common in all social strata. The 1950s was the era of Pontins and Butlins. Blackpool, Margate, Skegness or a caravan on the North Wales coast were highlights in families' annual leisure calendars.

Impact of television

The 1950s was the start of the age of television. Broadcasting by the BBC had commenced in 1936, was suspended during wartime, and then resumed, and sales of TV sets began to soar. By the end of the 1950s over 90 per cent of households had a (monochrome) receiver. Television was an instant success. As soon as receivers were installed they were switched on throughout broadcasting hours (just teatime and evenings at that time) whenever anyone was at home. By the mid-1950s the television audience had grown to a size capable of supporting a free-to-air, advertising-funded channel, and the Independent Television (ITV) network began broadcasting in 1955. ITV changed the broadcasting culture. It gave viewers more choice: a different kind of soap opera to those previously offered by the BBC, game shows and interviewers who did not address government ministers as 'Sir'.

There was widespread interest at the time in how children were being affected by television, which replaced horror comics as the main perceived threat to their moral welfare. Research at the time found that hours devoted to homework, sport and clubs were unaffected (Himmelweit *et al.* 1958). The main casualties from the time absorbed by television were the radio and cinema. In the early 1950s the UK population was visiting the cinema on average once per fortnight. By 1963, as Table 8.1 shows, the cinema had lost over 70 per cent of its audience of a decade previously. The cinema's decline continued until the 1980s when it had dropped, on average, to just one visit a year. Since then cinema attendances have recovered, but only to the level of the 1970s.

Sports participation by young people was largely unaffected by the coming of television, but was extremely low by all subsequent standards. Few girls did any sport regularly. Among boys football was the only sport that involved substantial numbers, and most of them ceased playing organised football soon after they left school (Emmett 1971).

By the 1950s adults were deserting the cinema (they had television at home) and so teenagers (who had no homes of their own) became the core cinema audience.

Table 8.1 Cinema admissions in the UK in millions

1953	1285.0
1958	755.0
1963	357.0
1968	237.0
1973	134.0
1978	126.0
1983	63.0
1988	75.0
1993	99.0
1998	135.2
2000	142.5
2004	171.3
2008	164.0

Sources: *Annual Abstract of Statistics* (2006); *Social Trends* (2004, 2008, 2010).

Films that incorporated teenage characters, especially if they also included teenagers' music, attracted mass teenage audiences. *Blackboard Jungle*, first shown in 1955, which featured Bill Haley's band playing 'Rock Around the Clock', was in many respects a turning point in tastes and behaviour, leading to dancing in the aisles, wrecked seating and the first cinema bans. Affluent teenagers were purchasing their own transistor radios and portable record players and became the main purchasers of recorded music whose tastes dictated the hit parade. They were a cohort that had grown up in the age of radio and recorded music. For them, the recorded sound was the 'real thing', on which you could hear the top recording stars and which live performers often found difficult to replicate for live audiences, hence the advent of lip synching.

Membership of youth clubs and the uniformed youth organisations slumped in the post-war years. The inter-war years had been the heyday of these organisations. Television was not responsible. A government enquiry (Albermarle Report 1960) concluded that draughty church halls were simply unable to compete with the glitzy dance palais for affluent older teenagers' time and money. The lifestyles associated with the dance hall, including easily available cigarettes and alcohol, added to their appeal.

The affluent teenager

In the 1950s the affluent young worker appeared, and the teenage consumer became an important market segment for clothing, transport, films and music (Abrams 1961). Full employment enabled teenagers to leave school at fifteen and then advance rapidly towards adult earnings. Consumer goods and services followed teenagers' tastes. The baby boomers were the first cohort to grow up in a society in which credit was readily available to 'take the waiting out of wanting'. Hire purchase was used to acquire expensive consumer durables such as television sets and washing machines. By the time that the 1946 birth cohort was aged twenty, car ownership was spreading rapidly. In 1951 just 14 per cent of households had motor cars, rising to 52 per cent in 1971 and 78 per cent in 2008, when 34 per cent of households had two or more cars (Table 8.2).

Home ownership as an aspiration was also on the way to becoming the norm. All these trends depended on the availability of credit. Those who could not afford their own homes, or who preferred not to incur debt in order to acquire them, tended to rent privately or, until the acceleration of privatisation much later in the 1980s, to live in local authority (council) housing. The baby boomer house owner occupiers became indebted in young adulthood and many remained so throughout their adult lives. As house prices rose, mortgages could be increased (using the property as collateral) to finance the purchase of cars, holidays and home improvements. It remains to be seen how the baby boomers will behave in later life, post-retirement (Higgs *et al.* 2009). Will they re-mortgage their now privately owned homes, if necessary, to sustain levels of consumer spending?

Protest and delinquency

The youth cultures of the 1950s were linked, in media discourse, to rising levels of juvenile delinquency (Radzinowicz and King 1979). They were seen later by some academic analysts as the means by which especially male working class identity could be established as a form of resistance to the essentially middle class norms and values associated with schooling (Hall and Jefferson 1976; Willis 1977). Leaving school at the minimum age of fifteen to enter a manual job and earn money offered the opportunity to achieve status in leisure life outside, some of which tipped over into delinquency of various kinds. Delinquency levels were to be far surpassed later in the twentieth century, but in the 1950s recorded crime

Table 8.2 Per cent of households in Great Britain with and without regular use of a car

	No car	*One car*	*Two or more cars*
1951	86	13	1
1961	69	29	2
1971	48	44	8
1981	40	45	15
1991	32	45	23
1997	30	45	25
2008	22	44	34

Sources: *Social Trends* (1999, 2010).

was rising at as rapid a rate as recorded in any subsequent decade. The crime rate roughly doubled in the 1950s, then again in the 1960s, again in the 1970s and yet again in the 1980s, before stabilising in the 1990s (Table 8.3).

Teenage promiscuity was another headline issue and the cause of a moral panic in the 1950s. Pre-marital sex was on the increase. The proportion of births to unmarried mothers had reached what was regarded as a disturbing level (around 5 per cent of all births). Shotgun weddings had become common. The typical age of first marriages fell. Most girls were marrying in their late teens or early twenties. However, very early pregnancy was not evenly spread; much of it could be seen as prompted by the unstimulating experience of factory work with the highest prevalence among working class young women (Griffin 1985). Nevertheless, by today's standards for most young people, 'youth' at that time was a relatively brief flowering.

Not everyone was enthusiastic about the quality of life in post-war Britain. By the end of the 1950s a new generation of 'angry young men' (and some young women) – novelists and screen and stage writers – were expressing 'angst' and protesting against the vacuity of life in the affluent society. John Osborne (*Look Back in Anger*), John Braine (*Room at the Top*), Alan Sillitoe (*Saturday Night and Sunday Morning*) and Shelagh Delaney (*A Taste of Honey*) appeared to speak for large sections of the baby boomer generation.

In 1959 the Campaign for Nuclear Disarmament (CND) organised the Aldermaston march. This was the first of the new social movements. The baby boomers grew up in an era of de-colonisation. The politically aware grew up treating equality between nations as normal. They urged politicians to 'make love not war'. During the 1960s opposition to the Vietnam War became a *cause célèbre*. The baby boomers who became university students (less than 10 per cent of them – 9 per cent in the 1946 cohort but only 5 per cent of women) experienced the birth of second-wave feminism and the turmoil that erupted on campuses throughout the Western world in the late 1960s. The products of these movements are now our rulers, but are probably not as out of touch with today's youth as were Winston Churchill, Anthony Eden, Harold Macmillan and Alec Douglas-Home in the 1950s and 1960s. Only a minority of students (Blackstone *et al.* 1970), and a much smaller proportion of all young people, were part of the politicised counter-cultures of the 1960s, but others became silent social revolutionaries.

Table 8.3 Recorded crimes per 1,000 population

1951	12.0
1961	17.5
1971	33.5
1981	59.7
1991	104.0
2001	98.1

Source: Walker *et al.* (2009).

Around 90 per cent of the baby boomers were still living with their two natural parents when they reached age sixteen. Clearly, many were unimpressed by stable family lives, as in US folk singer Joni Mitchell's living in 'little boxes made of ticky-tacky'. Their parents' marital and sexual fidelity was also no longer accepted as model behaviour set against the 'permissiveness' that the advent of the contraceptive pill in 1961 heralded, and this defined the next historical phase.

Permissive society? (1970–90)

Cohorts born at this time have no popular name. Attempts have been made to characterise them as Generation X or Y, or Thatcher's children, because Britain was changing. As we have seen in the first section of this chapter, by the end of the period the economy was post industrial, almost 50 per cent of the workforce was women and the male breadwinner family was a thing of the past. Conjugal relationships were less stable. Leisure also changed, but here the changes were incremental and gradual; there was no clear rupture with the lifestyles of the baby boomers.

The 'swinging sixties' is remembered as the decade when Britain became a permissive society. This reputation was founded on a number of liberalising developments including legislation. The effects of these changes unfolded over the next 30 years:

- pre-marital sex with a series of partners became common and socially acceptable;
- typical ages of first marriages and births to women rose to the late twenties;
- cohabitation was normalised as a prelude or alternative to marriage;
- divorce and separation rates rose, and by the end of the 1990s over one-third of first marriages were ending in divorce or separation;
- more mothers were lone parents and more children were experiencing family and household reconstitution;
- the birth rate sank beneath the replacement level in the 1970s and remained sub-replacement until the twenty-first century;
- the proportion of all births in which the mother was unmarried rose, reaching 44 per cent in 2006.

Children born in 1958 became teenagers when gays were already 'out'. The following decades witnessed gay pride marches, the creation of gay villages and the rise of the 'pink pound' market, and paved the way for civil partnerships ('gay marriages'), which finally became legally sanctioned in 2005.

Competing demands of work

The 1970 Equal Pay Act and the 1975 Equal Opportunities Act reflected the fact that women were spending more of their adult lives in the labour market and expected equal treatment. By the end of the twentieth century it had become common for mothers-to-be to take maternity leave instead of terminating their employment, and to return to work well before their children reached primary school age.

In total, households containing adults of working age were doing more paid work. Overall, between 1961 and 2001 there was a substantial decline in the average amount of time per day that men spent working. The decline was due mainly to later entry into the workforce because of extended education, and earlier retirements. Women, overall, were doing more paid work in 2001 than in 1961 (although still far less than men, on average), due mainly to the higher rate of labour market participation by women. Women were spending slightly less time on housework and childcare, whereas men were doing more housework in 2001 than in 1961 (although still far less than women). Total time devoted to housework and childcare increased. Women's leisure time hardly changed but as Table 8.4 shows men had gained an average of around fifty minutes extra leisure time per day by the end of the 1990s.

For people in paid employment, the earlier long-term decline in weekly hours of work bottomed out in the 1970s, and by then a historical reversal was under way: the working time of managers and professionals was pulling ahead of the hours worked by manual employees. From the 1970s and over the next three decades, leisure spending ('recreation and culture' in Table 8.5) in Britain increased eightfold. Spending abroad (basically on holidays) increased eightfold, and spending on communications (basically telephone and more recently the internet) increased tenfold. Meanwhile, for the working population leisure time hardly changed except that holiday entitlement grew from two to four, five or six weeks plus public holidays. Thus, complaints spread about 'time crunch', alongside demands for a better work–life balance. Schoolchildren no longer had mothers at home to cook a midday meal and more children were returning from school to empty houses or flats. The motor car, in fact often more than one per household, became taken for granted as the means to enable families to cope with daily routines, which often included ferrying children to and from school and to and from out-of-home leisure activities.

Mobility

By 1960 Britain was already on the verge of the age of mass motoring. In 1959 the M1 opened and the first mini-car rolled from the assembly line. In the 1940s, as before the war, the private motor car was a luxury. By the 1970s to be a carless

Table 8.4 Average (mean) minutes per day spent on paid work, unpaid work and leisure time, all UK adults aged 20–60 years

	Paid work 1961	*Paid work 2001*	*Unpaid work 1961*	*Unpaid work 2001*	*Non-work 1961*	*Non-work 2001*
Men	434	323	83	146	923	971
Women	183	203	303	277	954	959

Source: Gershuny (2005).

Table 8.5 Growth in UK household expenditure in real terms, 1971–2007 (1971=100)

Housing, water and fuel	161
Transport	273
Recreation and culture	841
Restaurants and hotels	214
Food and non-alcohol drinks	158
Household goods and services	305
Clothing and footwear	516
Alcohol and tobacco	91
Communication	1,031
Health	220
Education	233
Miscellaneous	311
Spending abroad	807
All household expenditure	267

Source: *Social Trends* (2009).

household was a serious disadvantage because, as car ownership spread, public transport declined. Car ownership has had many consequences. Mass motoring released waves of day trippers heading for coastal resorts, inland places of natural beauty and heritage sites, and theme parks became commercially viable. The motor car liberated the journey to work from public transport. It widened employers' catchment areas and the places where workers could seek employment without moving house. Cars also changed neighbourhoods. From the 1950s television was keeping people in while the car enabled them to go out in private to shop and to seek recreation beyond walking distance from their homes. Streets became unsafe for children to play out in let alone to make bicycle journeys. Thus, the bicycle became another toy. It became normal for children to be driven to school, and for leisure. However, by the end of the 1970s around 40 per cent of all households were still carless (Table 8.2), and since 1990 this proportion had changed very little until recently.

Holidays

Since the 1970s tourism has been Britain's fastest growing leisure industry as it has in many other countries. By the end of the century, on some criteria (turnover rather than numbers employed), tourism was the world's largest single industry. The main development in the UK was the diversion of holidaymakers from domestic to overseas resorts. The first overseas air package holidays from the UK were marketed (by Horizon) in 1950, but it was not until the 1970s that the overseas package became the standard holiday. Since then children have grown up with an expectation of foreign travel, and an English seaside resort like Blackpool was no longer seen as a proper holiday. UK destinations became places for weekend breaks and day trips and business conferences. Later cohorts may feel differently, but those who grew up in the 1970s and 1980s expected to be able to drive and fly.

However, we should note that, since 1970, when annual monitoring of holiday-making began, each year 40 per cent of the UK population has not taken a holiday (at least three nights away from home, not with relatives) (Table 8.6). This proportion has not declined, while the other 60 per cent have been increasingly taking more holidays (two or three rather than just one per year), and they have been travelling further, although the Mediterranean is still the most popular destination.

As it matured the holiday market segmented. The standard package of sun, sea and sand has remained the leader, but specialist segments now offer cultural, city and farm holidays and also 'eco-tourism'. Senior citizens became a distinct market segment, and so did young singles. Ibiza was the first, offering an all-night party experience (often heightened with drugs). Such 'ravers' transplanted the experience into Britain, then in the early 1990s the scene moved indoors and became 'clubbing' (Critcher 2000), a standard youth *rite de passage* since then.

Youth organisations

During the 1960s and 1970s the older youth organisations revived by targeting children. Cubs, brownies, Morris dancing and other dance, drama and sports classes flourished as out-of-school activities by providing places outside the home for children to play and socialise safely. By then older teenagers had different amusements. The remaining youth clubs and uniformed organisations were places for the under sixteens (typically very much under sixteen). As was shown later, the sixteen-year-olds who belonged to local authority youth clubs were usually less educationally successful working class young people, and their attendance was associated with marginally increased risks of social exclusion at age thirty, whereas participation in the typically more middle class and more regimented sports and community clubs, and involvement in the arts and in church-based groups, reduced the risks (Feinstein *et al.* 2006; Robson 2003). Government policy followed in the 2005 Green Paper, *Youth Matters* (DfES 2005), to introduce a more structured youth club experience – 'somewhere to go, something

Table 8.6 Per cent of residents of Great Britain aged sixteen and over taking holidays (foreign and domestic) of four nights or more

	One holiday	*Two or more*	*None*
1971	44	15	41
1978	42	20	38
1988	37	24	39
1998	34	25	41

Source: *Annual Abstract of Statistics* (2000).

to do, someone to talk to' – in place of the 'hanging around' that was seen as reinforcing disaffection.

In the 1960s, aided later by the loosening of licensing policies, the long-term decline in alcohol consumption was reversed, a recovery that has been gradual, but dramatic in scale over the last fifty years (Table 8.7). There has not been a sudden twenty-first-century upsurge in 'binge drinking', an ever-present phenomenon. No-one would suspect from twenty-first-century newspaper headlines that the steepest recent decline has actually been in alcohol consumption by sixteen to twenty-four-year-olds (Table 8.8). During the 1960s and 1970s alcohol became available in most restaurants, supermarkets and grocery stores rather than in only a limited number of 'off-licences'. The trade was successful in marketing its products to a wider section of the public. By the end of the 1950s pubs were welcoming female customers with refurbished lounges and drinks such as lager and lime, Pony and Cherry B, the precursors of 'alcopops'. Alcohol then became an integral part of Britain's youth cultures and spread across university campuses in the 1960s, and 'fun pubs' targeted the youth market. By the 1980s most older teenagers were drinking regularly. By the twenty-first-century regular intoxication had become normal teenage fun (Griffin *et al.* 2009). By the 1980s alcohol was stocked in most homes and was part of virtually all leisure occasions – an evening out at the theatre, a sports event or a family gathering.

Drug use also spread steadily among young people from the 1960s onwards. As with alcohol, students were in the vanguard. By the 1990s the 'sensible' use of recreational drugs had been normalised among all socio-demographic groups of young people (Parker *et al.* 2002). Tobacco, in contrast, was by then in long-term decline.

Television

As we saw in the previous section, television gained its commanding position in leisure time in the 1950s. For children who grew up subsequently there was simply more of it. BBC2 began broadcasting in 1964, colour television was available from 1967 and Channel 4 from 1982. Satellite broadcasting commenced only

Table 8.7 Estimated UK consumption of absolute alcohol; litres per person aged fourteen years and over per annum

	Beer	*Spirits*	*Wine*	*Cider*	*Total*
1957	3.88	0.82	0.31	0.11	5.12
1967	4.57	1.08	0.63	0.12	6.40
1977	5.59	1.82	1.12	0.21	8.75
1987	4.97	2.13	1.75	0.29	9.13
1997	5.26	1.77	2.23	0.57	9.83
2007	4.48	2.40	3.52	0.81	11.20

Source: *Alcohol consumption in the UK*, IAS Factsheet, 22 October 2010.

Table 8.8 Average mean alcohol consumption (units per week)

Men	*1992*	*1994*	*1996*	*1998*	*1998*[a]	*2000*[a]	*2001*[a]	*2002*[a]	*2005*
16–24	19.1	17.4	20.3	23.6	25.5	25.9	24.8	21.5	18.2
25–44	18.2	17.5	17.6	16.5	17.1	17.7	18.4	18.7	16.2
45–64	15.6	15.5	15.6	17.3	17.4	16.8	16.1	17.5	17.7
65 and over	9.7	10.0	11.0	10.7	10.6	11.0	10.8	10.7	10.4
Total	15.9	15.4	16.0	16.4	17.1	17.4	17.2	17.2	15.8
Women	*1992*	*1994*	*1996*	*1998*	*1998*[a]	*2000*[a]	*2001*[a]	*2002*[a]	*2005*
16–24	7.3	7.7	9.5	10.6	11.0	12.6	14.1	14.1	10.9
25–44	6.3	6.2	7.2	7.1	7.1	8.1	8.3	8.4	7.1
45–64	5.3	5.3	5.9	6.4	6.4	6.2	6.8	6.7	6.3
65 and over	2.7	3.2	3.5	3.3	3.2	3.5	3.6	3.8	3.5
Total	5.4	5.4	6.3	6.4	6.5	7.1	7.5	7.6	6.5

Source: Goddard (2006).

Note
a Weighted to adjust for seasonality.

in 1988, and Channel 5 was not launched until 1997. Before the 1980s, the most important development was probably the extension of broadcasting into daytime. Weekend television and daytime programmes during school holidays became popular with children. In 1983 breakfast time television was launched, first by the BBC and two weeks later by ITV's TV-am. This commercial competitor signed up the 'famous five', very well-known news presenters. The station floundered financially until 'the five' were replaced by the more child friendly 'Roland Rat'.

Broadcasters knew that any child in the room was likely to control the channel selector. It is not surprising therefore that children were increasingly becoming an attractive section of the consumer market and were targeted by commerce and its advertisers. Confectionery and toys were advertised during children's programmes, or at least when children were a significant section of the audience, thus, 'pester power' was strengthened. What were previously youth fashions and music were marketed to pre-teen 'tweenies'. There were warnings that children were being 'sexualised'. Youth was being extended upwards as young people remained in education and on training schemes (or unemployed) for longer, and was simultaneously extending downwards.

Children were allegedly becoming 'couch potatoes', watching television rather than doing anything active. They were probably eating more and taking less exercise, but not because they were doing less organised sport. Participation in organised sport was rising from the 1960s onwards. Schools were broadening the sports curriculum, indoor sports halls were being constructed and equipped, and waterlogged playing fields were being partly replaced by all-weather outdoor surfaces. Simultaneously, from the late 1960s local authorities were opening indoor sport and leisure centres, part funded by the Sports Council. National surveys throughout the 1990s and subsequently found that boys and girls in successive cohorts were doing more and more sport during term times and during school holidays as well (Sport England 2003). Overall, children at leisure were less active than senior citizens, but not through avoiding sport but because so many were taken to school and to leisure facilities, including sport, by car (Fisher 2002).

From the 1960s young males became a major section of the crowds at certain sports events, especially football matches. Adults were withdrawing in favour of television and shopping. Meanwhile, football grounds became an alternative to city centres for groups of young males. This was the background to the emergence of 'soccer hooliganism', which remained a headline issue until the post-1991 Premier League 'all-seater' stadiums and higher ticket prices changed the demography of crowds again. Soccer hooliganism was one part of rising crime in this age group, which, coupled with high levels of youth unemployment until the late 1980s, did not stabilise until the 1990s, when 'fear of crime' had become an issue in its own right.

Race relations

After the Second World War immigration from the colonies and new Commonwealth began to transform Britain into a multi-cultural society. The first Immigration Act restricting the entry of citizens of the colonies and Commonwealth was passed in 1962. Up to then black and Asian immigrants were new, and racial discrimination was widespread, blatant and legal. Job and accommodation adverts often said 'no coloureds'. This was the Britain into which the baby boomers were born and in which they were reared. The first Race Relations Act, outlawing overt discrimination, was passed in 1965 and the 'no coloureds' adverts disappeared immediately. In 1968 the act was strengthened and a Community Relations Commission was established to foster harmonious race relations. In 1976 a further act outlawed indirect discrimination and replaced the Community Relations Commission with a Commission for Racial Equality, which had powers to prosecute cases of discrimination. In 2007 this Commission was absorbed into the newly created Equality and Human Rights Commission. By then the size of Britain's minority communities, and their composition, had changed. At the beginning of the twenty-first century they amounted to 8 per cent of adults and around 12 per cent of children in schools in England and Wales. Most members of Britain's ethnic minorities were then British born and bred. Thus, since the 1960s, depending on where they lived, children grew up in a multi-cultural Britain where discrimination was officially wrong and unlawful and where racism became widely regarded as offensive.

One effect of immigration has probably been to accelerate secularisation – the decline in church attendance and belief in God. It is not that Britain's ethnic minorities tend to be irreligious: Afro-Caribbeans tend to be assiduous religious observers – Hindu and Islamic minorities similarly. The situation is rather that if all religions are equal, can any be right?

Divided Britain

By the 1980s children and young people were being reared in a much more unequal and divided society than the Britain in which the baby boomers had grown up. These divisions had arisen in an age when general respect for authority was in decline. It is difficult to pinpoint the precise causes of this trend. The mass media and the popular cultures that they nurtured, and a decline in religious belief, were likely to have contributed. On the other hand willingness to question and, if necessary, to defy can have very different consequences depending on the context. It may produce more enquiring young minds – those that have been progressing into higher education in greater numbers. It may also produce young people who are simply truculent and defiant.

During the 1980s, and ever since, economic inequalities and associated inequalities such as health have been widening (Wilkinson and Pickett 2009). As the recession of the 1980s passed, there were more good jobs, but also more lousy jobs (Goos and Manning 2003) and much higher levels of unemployment. More disaffected teenagers were truanting from school. Lower-grade GCSE passes and lower-level vocational qualifications were of dubious labour market value (McIntosh 2002). Young people seem to have grasped the implications of this. After the age of sixteen those with no qualifications or with poor qualifications were at risk of becoming NEET (not in education, employment or training). They were likely to encounter trouble with the police and courts (SEU 1999). As explained earlier, rates of teenage delinquency rose steadily from the 1950s to the 1990s. Among the cohort born in 1958, there was little if any disadvantage to leaving school with no qualifications whatsoever, whereas among the 1970 birth cohort who left school in the 1980s it was a serious handicap (Bynner and Parsons 2002).

These widening educational and labour market divisions corresponded and interacted with other ways in which Britain became more divided. It is claimed that there has been no overall decline in social capital (trusted social relationships) (Harper 2001); however, certain types of social capital have become more strongly class related. Membership of voluntary associations became more concentrated within the middle class. The male working class lost its former levels of membership of trade unions and working men's clubs (Table 8.9). Nowadays working class social capital is built mainly through informal relationships (Li *et al.* 2002, 2003, 2005).

Alongside these trends in social relationships and social capital, differences and divisions in 'cultural capital' – that is, the 'know-how' that offers entry into middle class structures of opportunity and privilege (Bourdieu and Passeron 1977) – have also changed. The main division in cultural consumption is no longer between highbrow and lowbrow/popular culture, but between voracious and omnivorous cultural consumers and a mainstream whose cultural consumption is uniformly popular and almost wholly through television and other media (Bennett *et al.* 2009; Le Roux *et al.* 2008; Sullivan and Katz-Gerro 2007).

Digital age (1990 to the present)

Perhaps the most profound of the leisure transformations considered so far is only at the beginning of its realisation. The development of digital technology, and especially the internet, is less than twenty years old. It is necessary to have been born since 1990 to have grown up to find, already available, what is still the current range of digital technologies.

Computer games

These have been marketed since the 1970s. By the 1990s they could be played on a household TV set, a dedicated console, a general purpose PC or a handheld device. They could be uploaded from a DVD or over the internet. It is very unlikely that anyone born and reared in Britain since 1990 has not been a player. The industry is huge, global and still growing.

Digital television

The launch of British Sky Broadcasting in 1988 instantly multiplied the number of TV channels that subscribers could access. Then from 1998 Sky Digital further

Table 8.9 Membership of voluntary associations in Great Britain, 1972–99

	Men 1972 (%)	*Men 1999 (%)*	*Women 1992 (%)*	*Women 1999 (%)*
Sports/hobby clubs	25	26	11	14
Trade unions	40	22	16	16
Professional associations	11	14	–	8
Social/working men's clubs	28	18	8	7
Tenants'/residents' groups	4	7	8	9
Political parties	7	2	3	2
Environmental groups	–	4	4	3
Voluntary services groups	–	3	5	5
Parents'/school associations	5	2	7	7
Religious/church groups	10	7	12	11
Other community/civic groups	–	2	3	2
Women's institutes/groups	–	–	4	4
Scouts/guides organisations	–	1	–	2
Pensioners' groups	–	1	–	–
Other organisations	15	8	9	7
At least one membership	77	59	53	51

Source: Li *et al.* (2002).

multiplied the available channels. By then, in some parts of the country, cable was a multi-channel alternative to satellite. Freeview and FreeSat subsequently became additional options. Analogue switch-off will see all households with digital and therefore multi-channel TV by 2012.

Since 1988 children and adults in homes with satellite dishes have been able to watch any kind of programme at any hour of the day or night. Nearly all the new channels carry advertising. In the 1970s over 80 per cent of TV broadcasting in Europe was public service; today over 80 per cent is commercial (Hesmondhalgh 2007). Adults have not lengthened their hours of viewing since the 1970s, but they are now paying much more per hour. Top sport is now played for a (sometimes global) TV audience. Children have become supporters of teams that they watch only on TV. Most Manchester United supporters have now never been to Old Trafford; many of them live in China. For these new fans, the TV spectacle is the 'real thing'.

Mobile phones

In 1991 Nokia marketed the first mobile phone that was to achieve global mass sales, albeit mainly to business users. This phone was a heavy, cumbersome device by subsequent standards. It was only from the mid-1990s, when mobiles had become lighter and smaller, that take-up by private citizens took off. Parents began to decide that their children needed mobiles before they could be allowed to go out independently. Children soon found that they needed mobiles to keep in touch with friends (Green and Singleton 2009). Twenty-first-century models offer more than voice communication – recorded music, texting, images and sometimes internet access.

The internet

Yahoo was launched in 1994. It had the first user-friendly search engine. This was the trigger that by the end of the century had virtually every business, every school and many voluntary societies and clubs creating their own websites. By then private households were also going online and by 2000 most young people were online regularly (Russell and Drew 2001). Young people downloading through the internet sent tremors through the recorded music industry. A cohort of listeners has been formed for whom recorded music has always been free, for whom chat rooms and socialising sites have always been everyday milieu, who blog regularly and for whom it has always been possible to lead a 'second life' in virtual reality.

Gambling

The start of the UK's National Lottery in 1994 changed the gambling culture. For the very first time in the modern age gambling was state promoted as a harmless flutter. Also for the very first time, gambling could be advertised. Other types of gambling demanded, and were given, a more-or-less level playing field. The industry boomed. Instead of steel mills, cities bid for casinos as a means of reviving their economies. Coincidentally, gambling became available through digital TV and over the internet, effectively beyond the control of national governments.

Lifestyle impact

Contrary views have been expressed on the likely long-term social impact of digital technologies. Some say that basically nothing will change; people will just do familiar things in different or additional ways, such as sending emails instead of letters, shopping online instead of by mail order, and keeping in touch with friends, family and work colleagues through mobiles and the internet as well as meeting face to face. Others argue that virtually everything will change; that we are on the threshold of a global network society in which global communities will be formed and new social movements will be mobilised, and where anything (including work and study) can be done at any place and at any time. The truth is that we cannot be sure yet; at least, not until the first cohorts who were born in the digital age have become adults.

How can we know how current, let alone future technologies, will be used thirty years from now? Electricity was brightening homes by the end of the nineteenth century, but no-one then envisaged all the domestic gadgets that would be electrically powered by the 1930s. Wireless communication and moving pictures had been demonstrated by 1900, but no-one then realised that by 1930 most households would have purchased domestic radio receivers, mainly to listen to light entertainment, or that cinemas would be open and under construction throughout all modern societies to satisfy the public's appetite for feature movies. Then again, set these uses against views of those such as H. G. Wells and Lord Reith, who saw broadcasting as transforming society through the huge educational and cultural opportunities it offered. The Open University founded in 1968 is perhaps the closest to realising their aspirations.

The rest of leisure

Alongside the above developments, alcohol consumption and drug use have first stabilised and then begun to decline, as have crime rates, while tobacco use has continued its long-term decline – a trend that will surely continue following the 'smoking ban' in public places which was implemented in 2007. Children and young people are now doing even more sport than in the 1990s, but many continue to lapse in young adulthood, just as they did in the 1950s.

All of the above developments have been in the context of continuities in how the British spend their leisure time (Table 8.10). Television became a staple time filler in the 1950s and has remained so ever since. Listening to the radio has remained almost as common, and the listening audience has actually recovered to pre-TV levels thanks to the introduction of FM band and digital technologies, an expanded number of stations and the radio becoming a standard car fitting. Visiting friends and relatives has remained near universal, unaffected by additional ways of keeping in touch. The majorities who listen to recorded music and read books are now slightly larger majorities than in the 1970s. Dressmaking, needlework and sewing have become less popular, whereas more people are gardening and undertaking DIY home improvements (no doubt related to the spread of home ownership). However, these are still minority uses of free time.

Politics

The digital generation is far less political than the baby boomers and their immediate successors. This applies however 'political' is measured: expressed interest in politics, frequency of political discussions and activity, trust in politicians and voting in elections. These trends have also occurred among adults who nowadays are less likely to be firmly attached to any political party than were voters from the 1940s up to the 1970s. A consequence is that most young people no longer inherit any party loyalties from their families, and tend to be even less political than their parents. These trends are not UK specific: they have occurred throughout Europe (see Benedicto and Blasco 2008).

Table 8.10 Percentages participating in selected leisure activities (four weeks preceding interviews) by age group, 2002

	16–19 years	*20–24 years*	*25–29 years*	*30–44 years*	*45–59 years*	*60–69 years*	*70 years and over*
Watching TV	100	99	99	99	99	99	99
Listening to radio	92	93	93	92	89	82	76
Listening to records/tapes	98	97	95	91	83	71	57
Reading books	63	67	66	65	67	64	64
Singing/playing an instrument	21	15	12	12	10	7	7
Dancing	21	23	14	11	8	9	5
Painting	24	13	11	11	7	8	5
Writing stories/poetry	12	5	4	4	3	2	2
Running arts events	4	2	2	2	3	4	2
Performing in a play	8	3	3	2	2	1	0

Source: Fox and Rickards (2004).

Another trend is for young people's political activity (such as occurs) to be outwith the main political parties. They are more likely to associate with, and to participate in events organised by 'new social movements' concerned with, for example, the environment, peace, feminism, race equality. Any groups in which young people participate now are likely to be virtual (internet) groups. If young people are mobilised, this is most likely to be via email, text or mobile phone. However, the numbers involved in any action are a minority of their age group, although it is true that much larger numbers will sign a petition or take part in a consumer boycott.

As with many other trends it is difficult to pinpoint *the* cause. The media and politicians all have their favourite explanations (see Kimberlee 2002). It is a paradox of our time that there is more information, more easily accessible, and it is easier to be involved, yet young people avoid involvement. Almost certainly this is at least partly because politics has ceased to offer exciting and challenging alternatives, such as capitalism versus socialism. This is the context in which the main response by young people has been to concentrate on building the best possible lives for themselves in the world as they find it and exercise their political inclination and actions on single issues such as the environment and race relations.

It is still too early to tell whether the latest cohorts of young adults will be more willing than their predecessors to accept limits on their motoring and air travel. The baby boomers grew up in the era of the Cold War and in the shadow of 'the bomb'. The digital cohort have grown up in a society which realises that fossil fuels will eventually be exhausted, and in which climate change is a serious threat confronting humankind. They may accept that lifestyles need to change. They may also say, just like their predecessors, preferably not yet and not here.

The leisure life course in successive cohorts

The introduction and subsequent sections of this chapter have highlighted the major changes that have transformed Britain since 1945. The economy has become post industrial. Risks of unemployment and the challenges associated with occupational redundancies have risen. The types of jobs that are available have changed. Rates of divorce, separation, and family and household reconstitution have risen. More and more women are now spending their entire adulthood in the labour market except for short interruptions. Young people are remaining longer in education. Routes through childhood, youth and into adulthood have been individualised. It has become rarer for groups of children from the same neighbourhoods to attend the same local schools, then progress into the same workplaces and settle and spend their adulthoods in the same neighbourhoods and in the same company. It is possible to imagine that individuals have been cut adrift from social moorings, 'bowling alone', to use the social capital writer Putnam's (2000) expression.

This overlooks the fact that average tenure in a job has actually lengthened (Taylor 2002), and that the careers of most adults who were already established in their occupations survived the economic restructuring of the late twentieth century (Buchholz *et al.* 2009). Individuals retain the same biological parents, siblings and children throughout their lifetimes. Social networks can simply evolve rather than weaken if and when circumstances change. Leisure has been another great stabilising force. Television (sometimes the same series) has been a huge constant since the 1950s. People tend to retain tastes and interests acquired when young. Changes in how individuals spend their leisure time are more likely to be driven by life course than historical changes. Cohorts have different formative experiences, but the changes from cohort to cohort as regards uses of leisure since the 1950s have been minor compared with those that occurred during the previous century. Since 1945 there have been no wars that have mobilised the entire population and transformed people's lifestyles.

Other chapters in this book explain fully the senses in which the baby boomers can be regarded as the lucky generation (technically a cohort). They grew up when Britain was becoming what was christened a welfare state, which promised security from cradle to grave. They benefitted from the National Health Service that began in 1948. The baby boomers benefitted from free secondary education for all (conferred by the 1944 Education Act). Those who were offered places received higher education free, and means-tested maintenance grants were available. Local authorities were building council houses to ensure that all citizens had satisfactory accommodation. The cash benefits offered by the welfare state were never sufficient to lift the recipients well clear of poverty, but the baby boomers were unlikely to need these benefits before they retired, by when over a half could supplement their state pensions with occupational pensions, often indexed to final salaries.

The British cohort studies provide the means of monitoring the outcomes of the changes historically and predicting their continuity or demise. Of major interest here is the area in which future transformations are likely to be most dramatic of all – digital technology. As earlier on with radio, television and the telephone, it begins to become unthinkable that a family can be without the latest technological advance. Yet for economic or personal reasons such as physical difficulties, old age and an inability or unwillingness to learn, a substantial minority of the present adult generation is likely to remain unengaged for some time. Such a 'digital divide' thus isolates people further from services and facilities that are important to the quality of their lives. For example, banks are scheduled over the next few years to phase out cheques in favour of electronic money transfer, hard-copy paid-for newspaper sales are declining, and shopping, advertising and communications more generally are increasingly done online. Cohort study research will supply the vital means of monitoring both the take-up of new technology and the exclusion processes and their outcomes for those who do not have it.

Leisure activity more generally can be both a source of identity and cultural expression and a life course outcome in its own right. The football supporter has 'tribal loyalty' to his or her favoured team and to other supporters. But at the same time the additional leisure time that retirement and/or redundancy offers gives opportunities for the passion to be pursued further. The cohort study again enables these life course effects and their longer-term outcomes across different cohorts to be kept continually under review, and signals the lack of, or inadequacy of, the facilities to sustain them.

Future research based on the cohort studies can add to the evidence base on these matters in a number of ways. The origins of 'leisure tastes' and their reinforcement or reconstitution over time illuminates the functions that leisure performs at different ages and at different times in helping to build and re-enforce identity in various ways. The idea of the 'leisure career' captures these different components of leisure life with stable and more fluid features as reflected in changes in them with age and across time. This includes the way tastes and interests are expressed and shaped in response to societal and commercial pressures while retaining a higher degree of constancy than in other life course areas.

The variety of leisure orientations and their dynamic relation with other life course features such as education, work and family life also merits more investigation – along the lines of the work on out-of school leisure contexts. Particularly, the long-term outcomes of connections between later leisure and experience in the late teens and twenties are yet to be studied. The extension of single status over a much longer period than in the past and the impact of the ICT revolution offer much scope for cohort study enquiry. Are much the same processes and functions occurring under the guise of new lifestyles and identities? Or is the post-industrial 'digital generation' significantly different in these respects from the generations that preceded it? How can policy best intervene to modify, if not change, the leisure tastes of each generation to move them away from their more damaging contemporary forms of expression, such as binge drinking, drugs and crime?

In a world that is changing so dramatically we need to understand how the past was experienced in order to gain the necessary insights into how the future is to be managed. In this sense the cohort studies supply the crucial underpinning for the well-being that remains the universal goal.

References

Abrams, M. (1961) *The teenage consumer*, London: London Press Exchange.

Albermarle Report (1960) *The youth service in England and Wales*, London: HMSO.

Annual Abstract of Statistics (2000) No. 136, London: Stationery Office.

Annual Abstract of Statistics (2006) No. 142, London: Palgrave Macmillan.

Arnett, J. J. (2005) *Emerging adulthood: the winding road from late teens through the twenties*, Oxford: Oxford University Press.

Baudrillard, J. (1998) *The consumer society: myths and structures*, London: Sage.

Bauman, Z. (1998) *Work, consumerism and the new poor*, Buckingham: Open University Press.

Bell, D. (1974) *The coming of post-industrial society*, New York: Harper Colophon Books.

Benedicto, J. and Blasco, A. L. (eds) (2008) 'Young people and political participation: European research', *Young People's Studies Magazine*, 81, Observatory of Youth in Madrid.

Bennett, T., Savage, M., Silva, E., Warde, A., Gayo-Cal, M. and Wright, D. (2009) *Culture, class, distinction*, London: Routledge.

Birchwood, D., Roberts, K. and Pollock, G. (2008) 'Explaining differences in sport participation rates among young adults: evidence from the South Caucasus', *European Physical Education Review*, 14: 283–300.

Blackstone, T., Gales, K., Hadley, R. and Lewis, W. (1970) *Students in conflict: LSE in 1967*, London: Weidenfeld and Nicolson.

Bourdieu, P. and Passeron, J.-C. (1977) *Reproduction in education, society and culture*, London: Sage.

Brake, M. (1985) *Comparative youth culture*, London: Routledge.

Buchholz, S., Hofacker, D., Mills, M., Blossfeld, H.-P., Kurz, K. and Hofmeister, H. (2009) 'Life courses in the globalization process: the development of social inequalities in modern societies', *European Sociological Review*, 25: 53–71.

Bynner, J. (1969) *The young smoker*, London: HMSO.

Bynner, J. and Ashford, S. (1992) 'Teenage careers and leisure lives', *Leisure and Society*, 15: 499–519.

Bynner, J. and Parsons, S. (2002) 'Social exclusion and the transition from school to work: the case of young people not in education, employment or training NEET', *Journal of Vocational Behaviour*, 60: 289–309.

Coleman, J. (1974) *The nature of adolescence*, London: Routledge and Kegan Paul.

Côté, J. and Bynner, J. (2008) 'Changes in the transition to adulthood in the UK and Canada: the role of structure and agency in emerging adulthood', *Journal of Youth Studies*, 11: 251–68.

Critcher, C. (2000) 'Still raving: social reaction to ecstasy', *Leisure Studies*, 19: 145–62.

DfES (Department for Education and Skills) (2005) *Youth matters*, London: Stationery Office.

Doll, R. and Hill, A. B. (1956) 'Lung cancer and other causes of death in relation to smoking: a second report on the mortality of British doctors, *British Medical Journal*, 233: 1071–6.

Emmett, I. (1971) *Youth and leisure in an urban sprawl*, Manchester: Manchester University Press.

Feinstein, L., Bynner, J. and Duckworth, K. (2006) 'Young people's leisure contexts and their relation to adult outcomes', *Journal of Youth Studies*, 9: 305–28.

Fisher, K. (2002) 'Chewing the fat: the story time diaries tell about physical activity in the United Kingdom', Working Paper 2002–13, Colchester: Institute for Social and Economic Research, University of Essex.

Fox, K. and Rickards, L. (2004) *Sport and leisure: results from the sport and leisure module of the 2002 General Household Survey*, London: Stationery Office.

Gershuny, J. (2003) 'Time, through the life course, in the family', Working Paper 2003–3, Colchester: Institute for Social and Economic Research, University of Essex.

Gershuny, J. (2005) 'Busyness as the badge of honour for the new superordinate working class', *Social Research*, 72, 287–315.

Gershuny, J. and Fisher, K. (1999) 'Leisure in the UK across the 20th century', Working Paper 99–3, Colchester: Institute for Social and Economic Research, University of Essex.

Glasser, R. (1970) *Leisure: penalty or prize?*, London: Macmillan.

Goddard (2006) 'Smoking and drinking among adults, 2005', Table 2.18, p. 74, London: Office for National Statistics.

Goldthorpe, J. H. and Mills, C. (2008) 'Trends in intergenerational class mobility in modern Britain: evidence from national surveys, 1972–2005', *National Institute Economic Review*, 205: 83–100.

Goos, M. and Manning, A. (2003) 'Lousy jobs and lovely jobs: the rising polarization of work in Britain', Working Paper, London: Centre for Economic Performance, London School of Economics.

Green, E. and Singleton, C. (2009) 'Mobile connections: an exploration of the place of mobile phones in friendship relations', *Sociological Review*, 57: 125–44.

Griffin, C. (1985) *Typical girls*, London: Routledge.

Griffin, C., Bengry-Howell, A., Hackley, C., Mistral, W. and Szmigin, I. (2009), 'Every time I do it I absolutely annihilate myself: loss of (self-) consciousness and loss of memory in young people's drinking narratives', *Sociology*, 43, 457–76.

Hall, J. and Jefferson, T. (eds) (1976) *Resistance through rituals: youth subcultures in post-war Britain*, London: Hutchinson University Library.

Harper, R. (2001) *Social capital: a review of the literature*, London: Office for National Statistics.

Hendry, L. B. (1983) *Growing up and going out*, Aberdeen: Aberdeen University Press.

Hendry, L. B. and Kloep, M. (2010) 'How universal is emerging adulthood? An empirical example', *Journal of Youth Studies*, 13: 169–79.

Hendry, L. B., Shucksmith, J., Love, J. G. and Glendinning, A. (1993) *Young people's leisure and lifestyles*, London: Routledge.

Hesmondhalgh, D. (2007) *The cultural industries*, 2nd edn. London: Sage.

Higgs, P. F., Hyde, M., Gilleard, C. J., Victor, C. R., Wiggins, R. D. and Jones, I. R. (2009) 'From passive to active consumers? Later life consumption in the UK from 1968–2005', *Sociological Review*, 57: 102–24.

Himmelweit, H., Oppenheim, A. N. and Vince, P. (1958) *Television and the child*, Oxford: Oxford University Press.

Hollands, R. G. (1995) *Friday night, Saturday night*, Newcastle: Department of Social Policy, University of Newcastle.

Inglehart, R. (1977) *The silent revolution*, Princeton: Princeton University Press.

Jenkins, C. and Sherman, B. (1981) *The leisure shock*, Methuen: London.

Kimberlee, R. H. (2002) 'Why don't British young people vote at general elections?', *Journal of Youth Studies*, 5: 85–98.

Le Roux, B., Rouanet, H., Savage, M. and Warde, A. (2008) 'Class and cultural division in the UK', *Sociology*, 42: 1049–71.

Li, Y., Savage, M. and Tampubolon, G. (2002) 'Dynamics of social capital: trends and turnover in associational membership in England and Wales, 1972–1999', *Sociological Research Online*, 7: 3.

Li, Y., Savage, M. and Pickles, A. (2003) 'Social capital and social exclusion in England and Wales (1972–1999), *British Journal of Sociology*, 54: 497–526.

Li, Y., Pickles, A. and Savage, M. (2005) 'Social capital and social trust in Britain', *European Sociological Review*, 21: 109–23.

McIntosh, S. (2002) 'Further analysis of returns to academic and vocational qualifications', Research Report 370, Nottingham: Department for Education and Skills.

McRobbie, A. and Garber, J. (1976) 'Girls and subcultures: an exploration', in J. Hall and T. Jefferson (eds) *Resistance through rituals: youth subcultures in post-war Britain*, pp. 209–22, London: Hutchinson University Library.

Miles, S. (2000) *Youth lifestyles in a changing world*, Buckingham: Open University Press.

Parker, H., Williams, L. and Aldridge, J. (2002) 'The normalization of "sensible" recreational drug use: further evidence from the north-west England longitudinal study', *Sociology*, 36: 941–64.

Putnam, R. D. (2000) *Bowling alone: the collapse and revival of American community*, New York: Simon and Schuster.

Radzinowicz, L. and King, J. (1979) *The growth of crime*, London: Penguin Books.

Rapoport, R. and Rapoport, R. N. (1975) *Leisure and the family life-cycle*, London: Routledge.

Roberts, K., Pollock, G., Tholen, J. and Tarkhnishvili, L. (2009) 'Youth leisure careers during post-communist transition in the South Caucasus', *Leisure Studies*, 28: 261–77.

Robson, K. (2003) 'Teenage time use as investment in cultural capital', Working Paper 2003–12, Colchester: Institute for Social and Economic Research, University of Essex.

Russell, N. and Drew, N. (2001) 'ICT access and use: report on the benchmark survey', Research Report 252, Sheffield: Department for Education and Employment.

Scott, D. and Willits, F. K. (1989) 'Adolescent and adult leisure patterns: a 37-year follow-up study', *Leisure Sciences*, 11: 323–35.

SEU (Social Exclusion Unit) (1999) *Bridging the gap*, London: Social Exclusion Unit.

Social Trends (1999) No. 29, London: Stationery Office.

Social Trends (2004) No. 34, London: Stationery Office.

Social Trends (2008) No. 38, London: Palgrave Macmillan.

Social Trends (2009) No. 39, London: Palgrave Macmillan.

Social Trends (2010) No. 40, London: Palgrave Macmillan.

Sport England (2003) *Young people and sport in England: trends in participation 1994–2002*, London: Sport England.

Sullivan, O. and Katz-Gerro, T. (2007) 'The omnivore thesis revisited: voracious cultural consumers', *European Sociological Review*, 23: 123–37.

Sweeting, H. and West, P. (2003) 'Young people's leisure and risk-taking behaviours: change in gender patterning in the West of Scotland during the 1990s', *Journal of Youth Studies*, 6: 391–412.

Taylor, R. (2002) *Britain's world of work – myths and realities*, Swindon: Economic and Social Research Council.

Walker, A., Flatley, J., Kershaw, C. and Moon, D. (2009) *Crime in England and Wales 2008/9*, Home Office Statistical Bulletin 11/09, Volume 1, London: Home Office.

Wallace, C. and Kovacheva, S. (1998) *Youth and society: the construction and deconstruction of youth in Europe*, London: St. Martin's Press.

Wilkinson, H. (1995) *No turning back: generations and the gender quake*, London: Demos.

Wilkinson, R. and Pickett, K. (2009) *The spirit level: why more equal societies almost always do better*, London: Allen Lane.

Willetts, D. (2010) *The pinch: how the baby boomers took their children's future – and why they should give it back*, London: Atlantic Books.

Willis, P. (1977) *Learning to labour*, Farnborough: Saxon House.

9 Generation and change in perspective

John Bynner and Michael Wadsworth

The transformation of Britain in the sixty-five years since the end of the Second World War has fundamentally changed the British way of life and the nature of the life course. The preceding chapters provided an overview of historical change in each of eight areas that comprised the context of cohort members' development: politics, citizenship, family, education, the economy, labour market and skills, health and health care, and leisure. Changes in each of these areas have been examined with respect to the statistical profile compiled from large-scale cross-sectional surveys, and the policies and the legislation that made up the distinctive sets of circumstances characterising each of the post-war generations' lives. Experience of change was brought into the picture by way of the cohort studies, which map the life histories, starting from birth, of large representative sections of the population over the period. Further questions about them arose that can uniquely be addressed through new research using the data from these cohort studies.

This chapter identifies a number of cross-cutting themes emerging from the previous chapters' historical overviews and develops more fully the ideas presented for next research steps within the life course framework (Elder and Giele 2009; Heinz *et al.* 2009). These steps include both the ways in which cohort study data accumulated since the war can be used to address critical questions about the changing British life course, and also some of the challenges such research presents. The chapter concludes with an optimistic view about problems and prospects that underpin the case for continual investment in these unique research resources.

Generation and change

Although each of our domains raises questions about continuities and breaks in experience and circumstance across the period, broadly four periods can be identified in which the period of birth made a difference to the shaping of the life course and the adult identities constructed through it:

- 1946–60: adversity to affluence;
- 1960–75: permissive society;

- 1975–90: individualised society;
- 1990 to present day: digital world.

The first period (1946–60) is identified with a well-recognised generation, the famously US-named 'baby boomers'. This is because of the far-reaching influence this group exercised in shaping the lives of the generations following, which David Willetts argues in *The Pinch* was on balance to the latter's detriment (Willetts 2010). Following the period of immediate post-war austerity, expansion of opportunities in education, employment and housing in the 'never had it so good' late 1950s (from a speech by Prime Minister Harold Macmillan to a Tory Party rally on 20 July 1957) were later tempered by a steady shift of the costs of opportunity from the state to the individual and his or family.

These generational distinctions are however only a rough guide to differences related to periods because clearly there is overlap between them. Austerity affected some baby boomers more than others and did not cease overnight in 1961. There are also significant differences in the staging of development from one domain to the next. Health, for example, showed continuities in a generally upwards direction as reflected in longevity across the whole period from the establishment of the NHS in 1948 (Chapter 7). This compares with the consequences of a 'boom and bust' economy resulting in a cyclical experience of unemployment and step changes brought about by new technology and globalisation (Chapters 5 and 6).

Periods reflect slices of historical time whereas cohorts, subject only to human mortality, extend across all of them. The concept of generation, with its emphasis on common features and influences on development linked to a period of birth, provides a useful lead into the consideration of cross-cutting themes and issues that can be identified across the domains. The term 'baby boomers' expresses this kind of communality and its far-reaching effects. We then recast the themes in the more operational terms of the life course perspective as a precursor to identifying examples of key questions for further research. The approach rests on the principle that the different components of experience in different areas of life come together in the development of the life course as a whole.

Shifting boundaries

The high hopes of a more equitable and less deferential post-war society, in which the five evils that Beveridge identified were eliminated, were moderated by continuing post-war austerity. Relative affluence and economic self-confidence followed, but soon began to give way over time to the reality that Britain was as much subject to worldwide economic phenomena and globalisation pressures as any other nation. Whatever the political complexions of different governments across the period, and the economic pressures to which they were responding, one of the most striking features of the period was the gradual diminution of, first, the British Empire, and then the Commonwealth, as the main trade arena (Chapter 2).

In place of the pre-war colonial arrangements initially the countries of early post-war Europe filled the gap, by establishing the Common Market. Subsequently the countries of Asia, including post-colonial countries such as India, Malaysia and Indonesia, as well as most recently China, increased their dominance as trading partners (Chapter 5). Their more efficient means of production and competitive low-paid labour force contributed to the demise of large sectors of British manufacturing (Chapter 6). Coupled with the break-up of the Soviet Union at the end of the 1980s, following the fall of the Berlin Wall in 1989, a further set of new markets and partners in the European Union emerged, together with a basis for military and strategic realignment in which long-standing military alliances such as NATO looked less tenable. There were also new markets and new trading arrangements with ex-Communist countries, some of which subsequently joined the European Union. Such *globalisation* of trade (Albrow and King 1990) changed the nature of production and distribution, so that governments had also to attract inward investment through lowered labour costs, a strong skills base and such incentives as favourable tax. The aim was to persuade industries to move production to countries that offered the best deals.

Collective versus individual interest

The nascent welfare state established after the war through the National Health Service, the new benefits system to accompany it and the 1944 Education Act were strongly affected by shifts in the political landscape in Britain (Chapter 2). The euphoria of victory under the leadership of Winston Churchill gave way to the commitment to abolish forever the material and aspirational impoverishment of many for the benefit of the affluent few that had prevailed in recession-plagued pre-war Britain. Following the landside victory of the 1945 Labour government under Clement Attlee there was commitment to massive reconstruction including the nationalisation of private industries such as coal and steel and transport.

The tight wartime control of government expenditure continued to the point that the expansionist 1951 Conservative government and the 1964 Labour government that followed were able to preside over a period of economic growth. However, by the 1970s the strains were beginning to show, for example in the form of the miners' strike and in 1972 (to conserve energy) the imposition by the Conservatives under Edward Heath of the 'three-day week'. In the grip of, on the one hand, antiquated industrial capital and lack of investment and, on the other, industrial militancy through strong trade unions, resisting the drive for change, culminating in the 'winter of discontent', it is not surprising that Britain attracted the label of 'sick man of Europe'.

The Conservative government elected in 1979 under Margaret Thatcher was committed to monetarism and market mechanisms for solving economic problems and to the philosophy of heightened individualism summed up in the words 'there is no such thing as society, only men and women and their families' (Women's Own 1987). This was further reflected not only in the challenges to the power of traditional collectivist working class institutions, such as trade unions, but also in the collective strength of the professions such as medicine and the law, which were seen as vested interests. A bonfire of restrictive practices and legislation controlling the labour market was the consequence, together with proposals for a taxation system that ultimately reached the height of individualism, through the idea of the 'poll tax' piloted in Scotland. The ensuing riots destroyed the legislation but in the process changed the political landscape. There was a boost to Scottish nationalism paving the way to devolution.

The more general reaction was a disillusion with individualism in such a 'raw form' in favour of a more liberalised and welfarist approach in which individual freedoms gave way to statutory rights to equal treatment under the law. The Blair government, elected in 1997, continued the agenda of privatising state enterprises such as London Transport and 'reforming', through market testing, public services, while also promoting the attack on poverty and its consequences for children, as epitomised in the legislation on *Every Child Matters* and the SureStart programme (Chapter 3). It also initiated for the first time, through the Social Exclusion Unit, a coherent youth policy directed at meeting the needs of young people (e.g. SEU 1999; Bynner *et al.* 2004). The government gained the advantage of the digital revolution, which through the 1980s, with consolidation in the 1990s, transformed the nature of employment and many other facets of individual and community life (Ashworth 1987).

White heat of science and technology

Each government had its own approach to managing the economy (Chapters 2, 5 and 6). The early post-war commitment to nationalisation of often failing industries faced growing hostility because of their perceived inefficiency, and gave way under Harold Wilson to harnessing the 'white heat' of the science and technology revolution to the nation's interest. But compared with other European countries, such as Germany, Britain was only partially successful in improving industrial output, because of under-investment. Will Hutton's book *The State We're In* gives a good summary of the kind of financial and shareholder culture which worked against the reconstruction of industrial processes that was needed (Hutton 1995). Nevertheless the investment in education and science expanded educational opportunity during the period, being seen as one of the key components of economic growth. There was a commitment to expansion in the form of new universities and the postponement of school leaving (Chapters 4 and 6). Initiatives between universities and the new technological and science-based industries resulted in the development of 'science parks', which helped to bridge the gap (and shorten the time lapse) between new contributions to scientific knowledge and their practical applications. That was especially valuable in computing technology, software development and pharmacological and biotechnical industries. This new source of highly specialist expertise and knowledge helped attract inward investment from the globalised industries.

The generational effects of the digital revolution have yet to be fully documented and understood (Chapters 6 and 8), but one major feature is growing reliance on digital means of communication and collecting information on an unprecedented scale. Automation and weak competitiveness had shifted employment increasingly away from manufacturing towards a service economy. This included the 'hollowing out' of the middle area of the labour market comprising intermediate-skilled non-manual jobs. The 'hourglass' society was said to be taking over (Hutton 1995), with a high-skilled university-educated set of professionals at the top end, a disappearing intermediate workforce and a marginalised unskilled population at the bottom end who had not benefited from the massive educational expansion through which the upper tier had been constructed (Chapter 6).

Disadvantage, social mobility and inequality

As the chapters demonstrate, the intertwining of these different themes – economy, technological change and political philosophy – provided the context in which the different generations grew up. At the same time some, if not all, of the major evils identified by Beveridge remained remarkably resistant to the attempts to eradicate them in the way that especially the first post-war Labour government had believed possible. The key challenges were the long-term effects of poverty and disadvantage in the circumstances in which babies were born and children grew up (see Chapters 3 and 7). Poverty was ameliorated to a certain extent by the progressive tax and benefits system, but its long reach extended through the life course of children and their families in what Conservative minister Sir Keith Joseph described as 'cycles of deprivation' (Welshman 2007). Much thought, academic endeavour and time and energy in legislative and policy development were given throughout the sixty-five post-war years to schemes designed to break that cycle.

The other sources of economic disadvantage were identified with demographic characteristics such as social class, gender, ethnicity and disability – the markers of inequality. All governments in different ways attempted to meet these challenges, with the education system seen as a particularly valuable instrument for improving social mobility, but not just in the limited sense of people moving up the socio-economic scale to be replaced by others moving down. The aim was to establish, within the limits set by individual aptitude, higher sets of standards for all, not only economically but also socially and in health and education. The key policy goal, following in the footsteps of the Scandinavian welfare states, was a more *equal* society (Chapters 2–7). A. H. Halsey's overview of the findings from the 1960s Educational Priority Area programme summed up the aspiration unambiguously:

> In other words, the goal should not be the liberal one of equality of access but equality of outcomes for the median member of each non-educationally defined group, i.e. the average woman or negro or proletarian or rural dweller should have the same level of educational attainment as the average male, white, white-collar suburbanite.
>
> (Halsey 1972: 8)

Continuing adjustments to the schooling system, ranging from the move to comprehensives early on in the period, to more independent institutions such as the more recently established academies – with accountability not to local authorities but to local interest groups and parents – contributed to whittling away the state at local level. However, local authorities re-established their role, particularly during Labour's periods of office, through partnership agendas such as in the initiation of the SureStart programme directed at combating pre-school educational disadvantage.

Successes in combating disadvantage were most obviously seen in connection with gender (Chapter 3). The concept of clearly differentiated roles of men and women still prominent in the 1940s and 1950s increasingly gave way to one in which occupational careers were seen as the right of both. Coupled with the expansion of maternity leave and provision for paternity leave, universal nursery care was made available in the late 1990s to ensure that parents, especially mothers, could exercise a choice whether to continue to work full time, focus on bringing up children, or combine the two. The changes are reflected in the earnings gap between men and women, with a much wider distribution of incomes of the male kind increasingly appearing for women, and the gender difference in mean earnings steadily reducing. However, the kind of 'glass ceiling' at the top levels of business to which women had only limited access is still reflected in the persisting 20 per cent male–female earnings gap among thirty-year-olds reported in *Changing Britain, Changing Lives* (Dearden *et al.* 2003). There was also the price to be paid of widening inequality among women.

Individualisation and risk

The theme of *individualism* has been mentioned earlier, but needs to be linked with another major theme, developing particularly through the latter part of the period, that of *individualisation* coupled with risk (see Chapters 2–4, 6 and 7). Through the early part of the post-war period, family and work were the cornerstones of socialisation into adult roles and responsibilities. Education was seen as the means of mediating, and therefore potentially moderating, the effects of family background on subsequent achievement and the career pursued. Selection into further and higher education provided the main route to the professions, and early school leaving to the unskilled and semi-skilled sectors of the labour market.

Ulrich Beck's important book, *Risk Society*, written in 1986 followed by others co-authored with such social analysts as Anthony Giddens and Scott Lash (1994), suggested that children growing up in the complex world of the 1980s and beyond were obliged to depend much more than their predecessors on their own personal resources. This was in place of their families, workplaces and communities, which had been the basis of socialisation into adult roles and identities in the past. The pathways through life were beset with challenging choices and continual risks, many unpredictable, about the consequences of the choices made in a society in which marketable skills were increasingly at a premium. Commitment to long-term partnerships and parenthood was challenged by the need to extend the educational career and the consequent prolonging of single status. At the same time a minority of women, typically with poor educational records and poor employment prospects, were continuing to leave school at the earliest age to start families. Polarising pressures of this kind are a distinctive feature of the latter part of the period.

Downsizing and redundancy in response to technological transformation and recession were continually replacing existing means of production and employment with consequent large-scale unemployment (see Chapters 5 and 6). Occupational profiles needed to offer more than one skills set for a particular kind of job. Prospective employees needed to have flexibility, creativity, the ability to work in teams, and work experience itself in order to be employable. Detachment from the traditional socialisation experiences of home, school and workplace placed increasing reliance on individual agency in growing up. A good side of this could be the positive career route of achievement and affluence, but the negative route risked *social exclusion* for the individual, and for society the disintegration of traditional social capital and societal cohesion (Atkinson 1998).

There were two unforeseen concomitants of such developments. First was the significant rise in mental illness, particularly experienced by young people, including psychological distress and depression, and even suicide (Maughan *et al.* 2008). The other was rising disaffection among sections of the younger population, as reflected in rising crime rates and general alienation from the adult world at an unprecedented level. Anti-social behaviour was not a new phenomenon but had rarely before been seen on such a large scale, nor to the point at which it needed to be certified in the form of an 'ASBO' (anti-social behaviour order) in the attempt to control young people's public activity.

However, the pressure towards taking individual responsibility for actions was associated also with greater concern for and new delineation of the rights of individuals, exemplified in the Children's Act of 1989 and subsequent legislation concerning children and the family (Chapter 3), in the statutory rights of those with mental ill health (Chapter 7) and in the Human Rights Act of 1989. But although respecting the rights of the individual these changes helped to bring, for example in health, demands for greater individual responsibility in aspects of lifestyle (e.g. smoking) known to have adverse effects on health. Existing and proposed new legislation to control the health-related habits of individuals for the greater benefit of society continues to be a source of division and controversy.

Cultural and recreational continuity and lifestyle change

Despite the general tendencies in all of these areas towards instability and change, in one area the picture is of relative calm and continuity (Chapter 8). Leisure lives of individuals follow patterns across the life course that, it can be argued, have not changed significantly across the generations. Thus cultural tastes ranging from opera to pop music are renewed afresh through each generation, retaining their function in supplying certain kinds of recreational and cultural fulfilment, and also a means, particularly for young people, of shaping identity through a critical period of their lives.

Some leisure behaviours such as drinking alcohol, smoking and, increasingly, using recreational drugs were continually under attack from governments and the media. This was justified on the grounds of, on the one hand, damage to health (Chapter 7) and, on the other, the fuelling of anti-social behaviour and crime (Chapter 8). In other recreational areas the same kinds of orientation often influenced by the family and the local community continued to maintain their appeal. Active participation in sport or as spectators attracted a fierce loyalty from young people and adults alike, creating some intergenerational continuity and solidarity alongside hostility in response to such behaviour as soccer hooliganism.

The electronic media such as television and radio differentiate in their own ways changes in tastes through time and between groups defined by social class, religion and ethnic identity. Social capital, said to be disappearing in some contexts, thrived in others. The internet supplies a means of 'bridging' between groups and between ages. The traditional English pursuits persist – reading books remains popular, especially for the older generation. Electronic media increasingly play a part, both in personal leisure pursuits and particularly collectively through networking websites, linking young people across the world (Howard 1998).

Such havens of stability underpin the essential continuities of individual and social life in Britain, and too much may be made of the effects on identity of all the other more dramatic and traumatic changes to which each generation's lives have been subjected. Risky behaviour is perhaps always inevitable but so is resilience – the human facility to transcend obstacles to fulfilment, whatever their source (Schoon 2006).

The life course and cohort study

Cohort studies are first and foremost about the human life course. The great value of the historical overviews that this book provides is the illumination of a key component of the life course, which is often unacknowledged in research using cohort study data. Understanding the context of people's lives is of central importance to interpreting many of the research findings about them. In line with Phelps *et al.*'s (2002) *Looking at Lives*, an edited collection of autobiographical accounts by leaders of US longitudinal studies, the British birth cohort studies may be viewed as an aggregation of the life histories obtained from a large, representative sample of individuals sharing a common period of birth. With data about cohort members collected in comparable form at regular intervals, the studies enable us to obtain a statistical picture of the life courses of a whole society. That is, we can expose to scrutiny the British life course and variations within it identified with different demographically or experientially defined sections of the population – the young, the old, the married, the divorced, the sick, the healthy.

The longitudinal and repeated measures aspects of cohort study data sets also enable us to go further towards explaining how outcomes in people's lives, such as ill health or occupational achievement and failure, may arise from conditions and experience encountered earlier (Wadsworth 1991). We cannot prove causality for what are passive observations without any manipulation of data through allocation of 'subjects' to 'treatments' as in the 'true experiment'. But nevertheless we can gain a powerful purchase on the likely direction of causation in the identification of shaping influences in the lives of the cohort members involved, because of our knowledge of their sequencing in time. The cohort study can therefore be seen as offering important insights into, for example, the effect of a new policy intervention, by comparing those who have experienced the intervention with those who have not, within a given cohort or between successive cohorts. This is while recognising that the randomisation of individuals to treatments demanded by the 'true experiment' as a basis for causal inference can be approached in the longitudinal survey only by statistical modelling of the cause and effect processes involved, that is, by statistically controlling the effects of confounding variables from which 'selection biases' are derived. In other words the cohort study offers a quasi-experimental approach to understanding cause and effect, including that arising from social and health interventions (Shadish *et al.* 2001).

What is described as the 'life course perspective' focuses particularly on four features of development: 'trajectories', 'transitions' and 'turning points', and, a fourth factor critical in establishing and shaping them, 'intergenerational transfer' (Robins and Rutter 1990; Elder 1998; Kuh and Ben Shlomo 2004; Mortimer and Shanahan 2006)

Trajectory reflects the fact that development in the different domains of life from childhood through adolescence to adulthood is to a certain extent predictable. Outcomes at any given stage in life in the family, education, employment, health, politics and leisure domains will be a product of the individual's attributes and environment. They also originate in the circumstances (social and physical), exposures and experiences through which development and growth begin from conception onwards and then continue in through the individual adjusting to and in some circumstances (later) actively changing them. In health the individual's initial position on the distribution at the start of the trajectory is of great importance, and is strongly influenced by the socio-economic circumstances of the parents, as well as by genetic aspects of inheritance. Prenatal growth and growth during the early postnatal years take place in a window of opportunity uniquely available at that stage in life (Barker 1998). Because of this one-off opportunity, the interaction of growth and physical development with the environment of early life genetic influences has been said to establish the individual's biological capital (Barker 1998). Life course health research into biological capital is concerned to establish how far its influence may be detected at later ages throughout life, and whether through interaction with intrinsic and extrinsic influences of all kinds throughout life the effects of poor biological capital may be escaped. The process of transmission of adverse early biological influences throughout life has been characterised as one of 'accumulation' (e.g. of risk experience) (Blane 2006) and as a chain of predisposing influences (Rutter 2005).

The trajectory links *transitions* – some statutory such as leaving school, some by choice such as moving house, and some biological such as puberty and the menopause – and *turning points* – in which the predicted direction of a trajectory is not borne out. The fluidity of some aspects of development is evident in the shift from downwards (negative) to upwards (positive) directions, and life course studies enable the key components of such 'escapes from disadvantage' to be identified (e.g. Douglas *et al.* 1968; Pilling 1990; Werner 1989; Barker 1998; Kuh and Ben Shlomo 2004).

Intergenerational transfer in its most direct form is through genetic inheritance, and through what passes from parents to child in the form of the prenatal environment, which influences many aspects of opportunities for good health throughout life. Of equal significance is the transfer of cognitive, social and psychological resources in the acquisition of behavioural and emotional styles and attitudes, as well as material, cultural and economic resources from one generation to the next (Côté and Levine 2002). Teenage pregnancy, for example, is increasingly uncommon in contemporary society, and is more likely to be experienced by girls whose own mothers similarly had their first child as teenagers (Hardy *et al.* 1998). Such phenomena gave rise to the idea of 'cycles of deprivation' (and achievement) whereby the processes of marginalisation on the one hand and continued upwards mobility on the other tend to be replicated within families (Rutter and Madge 1976; Welshman 2007; Blanden and Machin 2010).

Trajectories, transitions, turning points and intergenerational transfers make the point that experience in any one domain of life, for example the labour market, is integrally connected with experience in others, for example the family, the workplace, the community and health. The interactions between trajectories in different domains in aggregate constitute the construction of the life course as a whole. Life course research identifies four key sets of influence in the developmental processes involved. *Location in historical time and space* embraces the culture, institutions and social structure that frame the social world in which the individual is located. *Linked lives* emphasises the role of social relations and social integration in life course construction, in the family, the school, the workplace and the community. *Human agency* refers to the marshalling of the developing individual's resources (cognitive, social and psychological) in deciding and pursuing courses of action. *Timing (of events and transitions)* encompasses the intersection of the birth cohort of which the individual is a member (*cohort effect*), the period when data are collected (*period effect*) and chronological *age* reflecting the stage of life reached (*age effect*). The distinctive feature of this framework is the emphasis it places on the role of the physical and social environment in the shaping of the life course not only in their immediate 'proximal' (relational) and 'distal' (cultural structural) effects (Bronfenbrenner 1979) but also historically. At the same time the exercise of agency, founded on the personal attributes and identity we possess, supplies the means of changing the context of development for the future.

Strengths and challenges

Mapping out in detail the key constructs and components of the life course in the terms set out above points to the multi-disciplinary strengths of the British birth cohort studies as a resource for research. It also points to the challenges in using them, some of which are unique to the British studies and others common to all longitudinal enquiries (Magnusson and Bergman 1990; Lynn 2009). The scientific power of the British studies lies in the fact that in some form, although by no means entirely consistently, we have since the Second World War five studies through which the life course can be examined and changes in it identified, in response to an external changing context. Each study in isolation is subject to the problem that any two of the three external timing effects – age, cohort – are confounded with the third (period), which means that one has to be assumed constant if the effects of the other two are to be separated (Hobcraft *et al.* 1982; Bynner 2005). For example, the period effect may be assumed to be relatively unimportant in the aetiology of a given disease so a single cohort's data are sufficient for research on it. As data are collected at much the same ages in the five British studies, carrying out cross-cohort analysis for cohort members of the same age is another way of achieving this objective, for example comparing the three earliest cohorts in their early thirties as in *Changing Britain, Changing Lives* (Ferri *et al.* 2003).

As we saw in Chapter 1 there are basic design differences between the studies. For example, in the approach to sampling in the 1946 study, largely for cost and information technology reasons, it was decided to follow up a sub-sample (stratified by class – see Appendix 1) of the original cohort's births occurring over one week, compared with follow-up of all births in one week in the 1958 and 1970 studies. The more recent studies differ again from the earlier ones in taking a whole year's births rather than just one week's. Other variations in the more recent studies include over-sampling some sections of the population as opposed to giving all individuals equal probability of being sampled. In the 1991–2 birth cohort study the sample is based in one area of the country. The 2000 study includes all babies born in one year in 400 electoral wards, this time weighted towards disadvantage and ethnic minority status and with additional sample boosts in Scotland, Wales and Northern Ireland (the last followed up in a UK cohort study for the first time). These inconsistencies can present problems for interpretation, but none is insurmountable.

Data adjustments can be used to deal with sampling issues and mixed or incomplete measurement can be to an extent approximated through multiple imputation. Other more difficult issues reside in the ecology of development. The early studies were all based on individuals growing up in relative isolation from each other. The theme of 'linked lives' raises the question of data collection from other family members, peer groups and the community. We have to acknowledge that these kinds of effects on development cannot be pursued in all studies to the same extent. The Millennium Cohort Study (2000–1) study, for example, targeted fathers especially (alongside mothers) for data collection. The household panel studies such as the British Household Panel Study fill this gap more fully by surveying annually all household members over the age of sixteen. In its newly established form, 'Understanding Society', the study collects data on this basis from 40,000 households annually. Future birth cohort studies are likely to collect data on all family members but not necessarily at the same depth for all of them.

Measurement across time has to be assumed rather than fully established, namely that the validity and meaning of measurement using different instrumentation for a given scientific purpose are consistent across cohorts and, in the case of international comparative studies, across nations and cultures. Thus, the measurement of cognitive development, let alone the attitudes and values associated with it, is not impervious to the effects of secular change. We seek the most stable measurement of the kind that factual demographic or health indicators supply, but in either case changes over time also occur in concepts and methods of operationalisation. For attitudinal and behavioural data such methods as latent variable modelling are often used to improve measurement stability across time.

Potential next steps in research

Despite the challenges in implementing fully the life course perspective using cohort study data the research strategies it offers supply probably the best framework for deciding where investment in further cohort research is likely to be most effective and for realising to the full the studies' potential in addressing key questions about human development. The first strategy, now largely accepted by science and government funding sources, is to continue the studies throughout the whole of cohort members' lives. The value of such data multiplies as each study progresses. This is because each new item of information in the longitudinal record links to the ever-expanding bank of data already collected – all of which can be capitalised on to the full. The second strategy is to make good where necessary the gaps in individual records, by means of administrative data – if necessary going back to hospitals, general practitioners and schools where data about cohort members were collected and may still be available. The third strategy is to ensure that, with the help of expert users, coverage of each new follow-up maintains continuity with past surveys, while at the same time meeting the full range of contemporary scientific and policy demands.

Given the extensive database we can begin to sec how data collected in the cohort studies, and the new data that might be collected in subsequent sweeps, make it possible to address the research questions highlighted in the preceding chapters and classified broadly as follows: changing life course, politics, family, education, economy and skills, health and leisure.

Changing life course

The themes of trajectories, transitions and turning points arise strongly through the chapters, especially in relation to critical stages in the life course where policy interventions for particular purposes are likely to have most impact. A valuable research initiative will be to chart the ways in which trajectories and transition outcomes have shifted across the cohorts in each of these domains from the earliest in 1946 to the most recent in the 2000 study. What are the transition outcomes at each age and life course stage and what produced turning points in them in each new era?

Intergenerational transfers arise in relation to the question of whether social mobility within cohorts and between cohorts has been changing. Because so much of this research depends on standard socio-economic classifications based on occupation, which is available in all cohort studies, we have a ready-made means of measuring this key feature of individual lives, both in the children's and the parents' generations within families. However, the work needs to be extended to include other classifiers such as income and health and other features of mobility besides that arising from the parents' position relative to that of their grown-up offspring. For example, to what extent are income and health equality increasing or declining between the generations, taking all relevant confounding factors such as material circumstances at birth into account?

An important research development in each of these areas would be to extend comparison cross-nationally. The establishment of comparable cohort studies in other countries offers the opportunity not only of pooling data, but also of testing the effects of different transition systems on variations in the timing and duration of life course stages and their outcomes in each country.

Politics

Each cohort has been exposed in different ways to the changing political context and the different political philosophies to which successive governments were attached. There are two main questions to address: (1) What are the impacts of such contextual shifts on political trajectories comprising voting participation and interest and their outcomes for different cohorts at different ages? (2) What are the origins of political attitudes, values and behaviours that make up political agency, and how do they develop with age?

For example, in relation to (1) we need to explain the relationship in the 1980s and 1990s between the widening of educational opportunity and the shift to the political right. In relation to (2) we need to know what characterises – in social class, education and family terms – the politically active, including the up to 70 per cent who are likely to vote in a general election. These contrast with the 30 per cent who are politically disaffected, cynical or apathetic. Why has the latter group expanded over the last twenty years? Is there evidence to support the theory of class de-alignment, suggesting a steady haemorrhaging of support away from traditional class-based party politics?

The hypothesis of steady decline in social capital, and its counterparts – increasing individualisation coupled with risk and lack of social cohesion – raises wider questions about the robustness of the foundations of contemporary civil society. What forms the foundations of 'civic lives' and social capital in a community setting and what is the basis of their demise? Does the internet offer forms of political communication and routes to social participation that will ultimately replace traditional modes of political expression and action, or is it merely a means of enhancing them? Answering these questions will require mapping the political context on to experience, undertaking data analysis at a number of levels, from society as a whole, through the community and the family, down to the individual.

Family

Changes in family structure and role are one of the most striking features of the post-war period, pointing to the need for cohort study research in a number of areas. To what extent are family careers and experiences, such as teenage motherhood, repeated in the following generation, and is this less true for later cohorts of young women when teenage motherhood is less common? Other themes to pursue include the negative consequences of long-term family adversity and the avoidance of, or escape from, its negative consequences; the effects of children's agency interacting with that of their parents and other family members and the role of community social capital in child outcomes; and the impact of the changing life course of women and men on the timing of parenthood, child development, family structure and functioning.

Further questions extend the picture about the origins and consequences of changing family life for all family members. To what extent do the trajectories that bear out the known long-term effects of childhood circumstances and experience vary between cohorts? For example, members of the 1970 and later cohorts were much more likely to experience family breakdown in childhood than previous cohorts, and this can be followed through to examine later life developments in psycho-social health, physical health and health-related behaviour, as well as the trajectories of educational and occupational development.

Family policy, which was only weakly formulated, if at all, in the early part of the post-war period, has become increasingly significant in its effects on family life and the domestic roles of men and women, especially in relation to matters of equality. We need to understand the interactions of family policy with policy in other areas such as housing and the tax and benefits system in shaping family outcomes. What impact do they have on differentiated household roles and gender equality?

Education

Each of the cohorts experienced radical educational interventions, both at the level of the system as a whole, for example the move to comprehensive schools and more recently the conversion of some of them into academies, and at the level of the school and the classroom with respect to curriculum and assessment. Cross-cohort comparisons will aid understanding of the way these policy regimes have impacted on educational outcomes, both in terms of exam success and qualifications, and in the broader areas of educational aspiration, personal and social development and health and lifestyle. The growth of disaffection and anti-social behaviour is countered by intervention to build pro-social values through bridging social capital to the local community and raising civic awareness. The successes and failures of such interventions with different groups of pupils is an important target for research.

The period of post-16 education is becoming ever more important in contemporary society in which skills and qualifications count increasingly as key signifiers of employability and subsequent occupational achievement. There has been a transformation of the means by which young people progress towards adulthood through the development of further education, and apprenticeship, while entry into higher education has steadily risen. At the same time up to one-sixth of the 1970 cohort drifted into non-engagement with education, employment or training (NEET). More research is needed on the aptitudes and characteristics of individuals (and the origins of those aspects of motivation) that drive experience during this period from age thirteen years onwards, and how that experience has influenced the future pathways that these young people take. Among all the different and effectively competing routes to adulthood that characterise the English 'system', what are the wider social, personal and community benefits and economic returns to be gained from choosing or being selected to enter each of them?

Economy, labour market, employment and skills

Each of the five birth cohort samples had a quite different economic experience, from their family of origin to their own adult economic circumstances and now, in the oldest cohort, to their retirement. They were also subjected to a series of changing economic scenarios and different political agendas in response to them – for example nationalisation versus privatisation, Keynesianism versus monetarism, low-tech versus high-tech industry, supply-side versus demand-side management – against the backcloth of cycles of 'boom and bust'. Such political 'climates' affected each cohort differentially. Cross-cohort comparisons can usefully point to the way that different groups were affected, both in the short term and in the long term, as reflected in variations in educational attainment, in employment and unemployment, in earnings and savings, in occupational progression and in material circumstances including home ownership.

Changes in the preparation for the transition from school to work reflect the accompanying transformations of the labour market. The predictable trajectory of leaving school early without qualifications to enter an unskilled job has declined with much emphasis instead (since the end of the 1970s) on the need for skills and qualifications to match the rising expectations of employers. Such changes raise questions of occupational identity. How does each new generation see their relationship with the labour market? What are the main influences shaping occupational career, including active labour market policies and training provision? What are the roles of family, peers and schooling in the shaping of occupational aspirations and to what extent are they transferred across the generations? What are the labour market returns to skills (including the basic skills of literacy and numeracy) and the different post-16 routes to acquiring them? Is digital competence acquiring the status of a basic skill and is lack of such competence the precursor of another long-term route to social exclusion?

Health

The health sciences will continue to be very concerned with trajectories, for example of physical development and growth, cognitive development and adult functional change, for instance in blood pressure and memory, and their relationship with earlier life from the earliest time onwards. Transitions and turning points will continue to be studied in terms, for instance, of the search for what drives the beginnings and end times of fertility, and the beginnings of age-related decline in physical and mental function, and the onset of chronic disease. Intergenerational transfer in health studies is increasingly concerned with the role of genetics, the impact of environment on genetic effects and external and internal influences during childhood and adolescence on health-related habits such as nutrition, smoking and exercise.

Comparisons between the British birth cohorts are also likely to be concerned with differences in impacts of improvements in health care. It would be helpful, for example, to ask what benefit or otherwise to life course health the later cohorts gained from their protection from the childhood experience of infectious and viral disease. Similarly, there is likely to be concern with the long-term and whole-cohort impact of new kinds of care, for example anti-depressant medication and medication to control aspects of risk for cardiovascular health. Is there, for instance, a price to pay, in health terms, for the long-term use of these kinds of pharmaceutical preventive treatments? As prolonged stress is now clearly identified as likely to trigger biological pathways to ill health, the hypothesised increase in stress of various kinds can be tested by cross-cohort comparisons. The cohorts will be valuable for identifying the factors that increase the risk of prolonged stress and the factors that protect against it, and for studying health effects of variations in the length of prolonged exposure to stress and in the ages at which prolonged exposure occurred. Conversely, identification of well-being and its association with physical and mental health will continue to be an important element in the work of each birth cohort.

Public health interest in the cohorts will be likely to include the study of why socio-economic variation in many aspects of health persists. Studies may also want (as already described in Chapter 7) to identify in the earlier cohorts the risks for premature decline in adult health and the onset of disability and debilitating mental and physical ageing processes so that they can assess the likely upcoming burden of ageing in later-born cohorts.

As well as cross-cohort comparisons it may be valuable for genetic studies to pool cohort data in order to increase sample sizes for studies of specific pathways to risk and in cases in which the incidence of a particular illness is low.

Leisure

Unlike the story of change accompanying each new cohort's lives in other areas, leisure is an area where, except superficially, tastes and preferences have been more stable. Young people use the symbols of adulthood, such as drinking and smoking, in their quest for adult identity, but at the same time have their own ways of resisting the responsibility that adulthood implies. The role of these development processes within and between cohorts in young people's identity development needs investigating as does the narrowing generational gap through early adulthood.

To what extent are demographic changes such as the extension of singlehood and longevity post retirement impacting on lifestyles, leisure interests and needs? How are their effects differentiated by gender, socio-economic status, education and ethnicity?

In studies of the impact of change perhaps the key questions to address are about the ever-accelerating trends towards digitalised experience in place of that of social relations of a direct kind in the peer group and in the community. Do the new forms of social networking represent new forms of social capital or do they remain distinctly different from what that term fundamentally describes – trust-based social relationships? Are new kinds of identity and personality being shaped through internet exposure or is so much of the hyperbole about this new development no more than that – an exaggeration of the significance of technological enhancement, which, as earlier, will continually be overcome by direct social experience? Are there in all these areas differences identifiable with gender, class, ethnicity and social class? Does it matter where you live and who you are as to the way in which digital experience affects your life? Is the generation gap in digital competence another barrier to continuing social participation and inclusion – especially for the elderly?

Conclusion

The book has focused on a rather neglected aspect of research using the British birth cohorts' data, namely the differences in historical contexts experienced by the respondents in each of them. Deeper understanding of the life course requires attention to the political, educational and socio-economic context of lives through the periods in which they were lived. Each successive cohort is subject to a continuing and new set of influences while at the same time contributes itself to shaping the life course of the cohorts following, directly through family relationships and indirectly through the wider socio-economic environment. The historical context of the period supplies the basis of the cycles of interacting influences involved. Disentangling these will be one of the next major steps in multi-disciplinary longitudinal and life course research. The study of birth cohorts conducted in the British context as suggested here offers an example of the kind of research that is needed.

Each of the five large-scale birth cohort studies still collects data, and the time span that each data set covers is therefore considerable. The earliest of the five studies, which began in 1946, is currently (2009–10) collecting data from its sample at ages sixty-three to sixty-four years. Its archive includes data from parents who were born between 1882 and 1931. The most recent study's children have yet to reach ten years of age and none of their parents was born before 1970. This unique historical span points to the studies' power existing in the mass of information collected on human development across the life course at different times. Despite the formidable challenges in analysing the data linked across them, the scientific potential of the life course data that the birth cohort studies comprise is uniquely valuable. The full exploitation of the scientific resources they represent will constitute a major contribution to the knowledge and understanding of the foundations of well-being.

References

Albrow, M. and King, E. (1990) *Globalization, knowledge, and society*, London: Sage.

Ashworth, J. M. (1987) *IT futures . . . IT can work*, London: National Economic Development Office.

Atkinson, A. B. (1998) 'Exclusion, employment and opportunity', Case Paper 4, London: Centre for the Analysis of Social Exclusion, London School of Economics.

Barker, D. J. P. (1998) *Mothers and babies and health in later life*, 2nd edn, Edinburgh: Churchill Livingstone.

Beck, U. (1986) *Risk society*, London: Sage.

Beck, U., Giddens, A. and Lash, S. (1994) *Reflexive modernization, politics, tradition and aesthetics*, Cambridge: Polity Press.

Blanden, J. and Machin, S. (2010) 'Intergenerational inequality in early years assessments', in K. Hansen, H. Joshi and S. Dex (eds) *Children of the 21st century: the first five years*, pp. 153–68, Bristol: Policy Press.

Blane, D. (2006) 'The life course, the social gradient, and health', in M. Marmot and R. G. Wilkinson (eds) *Social determinants of health* 2nd edn, pp. 54–77, Oxford: Oxford University Press.

Bronfenbrenner, U. (1979) *The ecology of human development*, Cambridge, MA: Harvard University Press.

Bynner, J. (2005) 'Longitudinal cohort designs', in K. Kempf-Leonard (ed.) *Encyclopedia of social measurement, vol 2*, pp. 591–9, San Diego: Elsevier.

Bynner, J., Londra, M. and Jones, G. (2004) *The impact of government policy on social exclusion among young people*, London: Social Exclusion Unit, Office of the Deputy Prime Minister.

Côté, J. E. and Levine, C. G. (2002) *Identity formation, agency, and culture*, London: Lawrence Erlbaum.

Dearden, L., Goodman, A. and Saunders, P. (2003) 'Income and living standards', in E. Ferri, J. Bynner and M. Wadsworth (eds) *Changing Britain changing lives*, pp. 148–93, London: Institute of Education Press.

Douglas, J. W. B., Ross, J. M. and Simpson, H. R. (1968) *All our future*, London: Peter Davies.

Elder, G. H. (1998) 'The life course and human development', in R. M. Lerner (ed.) *Handbook of child psychology, volume 1: theoretical models of human development*, pp. 939–91, New York: Wiley.

Elder, G. H. and Giele, J. Z. (eds) (2009) *The craft of life course research*, New York: Guilford Press.

Ferri, E., Bynner, J. and Wadsworth, M. (2003) *Changing Britain, changing lives: three generations at the turn of the century*. London: Institute of Education Press.

Halsey, A. H. (1972) *Educational priority: problems and policies*, London: Her Majesty's Stationery Office.

Hardy, J. B., Astone, N. M., Brooks-Gunn, J., Shapiro, S. and Miller, T. L. (1998) 'Like mother, like child: intergenerational patterns of age at first birth and associations with childhood and adolescent characteristics and adult outcomes in the second generation', *Developmental Psychology*, 34: 1220–32.

Heinz, W. R., Huinink, J. and Weymann, A. (eds) (2009) *The life course reader: individuals and societies across time*, Frankfurt: Campus Verlag.

Hobcraft, J., Menken, J. and Preston, S. (1982) 'Age-period and cohort effect in demography: a review', *Population Index*, 48: 4–43.

Howard, S. (1998) *Wired up: young people and the electronic media*, London: UCL Press.

Hutton, W. (1995) *The state we're in*, London: Hutton Cape.

Kuh, D. and Ben Shlomo, Y. (2004) *A life course approach to chronic disease epidemiology*, 2nd edn, Oxford: Oxford University Press.

Lynn, P. (2009) *Methodology of longitudinal surveys*, Chichester: John Wiley.

Magnusson, D. and Bergman, L. R. (1990) *Data quality in longitudinal research*, Cambridge: Cambridge University Press.

Maughan, B., Collishaw, S., Meltzer, H. and Goodman, R. (2008) 'Recent trends in UK child and adolescent mental health', *Social Psychiatry and Psychiatric Epidemiology*, 43: 305–10.

Mortimer, J. T. and Shanahan, M. J. (2006) *Handbook of the life course*, New York: Springer.

Phelps, E., Furstenberg, F. F. and Colby, A. (eds) (2002) *Looking at lives: American longitudinal studies of the 20th century*, New York: Russell Sage Foundation.

Pilling, D. (1990) *Escape from disadvantage*, London: Falmer Press.

Robins, L. and Rutter, M. (1990) *Straight and deviant pathways from childhood to adulthood*, Cambridge: Cambridge University Press.

Rutter, M. and Madge, N. (1976) *Cycles of disadvantage*, London: Heinemann.

Rutter, M. (2005) 'Environmentally mediated risks for psychopathology: research strategies and findings', *Journal of the American Academy of Child and Adolescent Psychiatry*, 44: 3–18.

Schoon, I. (2006) *Risk and resilience: adaptations in changing times*, Cambridge: Cambridge University Press.

SEU (Social Exclusion Unit) (1999) *Bridging the gap: new opportunities for 16–18 year-olds not in education employment or training*, London: Stationery Office.

Shadish, W. R., Cook, T. D. and Campbell, D. (2001) *Experiments and quasi-experiments for generalised causal inference*, Boston: Houghton-Mifflin.

Wadsworth, M. E. J. (1991) *The imprint of time*, Oxford: Clarendon Press.

Welshman, J. (2007) *From transmitted deprivation to social exclusion*, Bristol: Policy Press.

Werner, E. E. (1989) 'Vulnerability and resiliency: a longitudinal perspective', in M. Brambring, F. Lösel and H. Skowronek (eds) *Children at risk: assessment, longitudinal research and intervention*, pp. 158–72, Berlin: Walter de Gruyter.

Willetts, D. (2010) *The pinch: how baby-boomers took their children's future – and why they should give it back*, London: Atlantic Books.

Women's Own (1987) Interview, 31 October.

Appendix 1 Key elements of the five large-scale British birth cohort studies

This appendix provides basic information about the five large-scale British birth cohort studies. As each has collected an enormous amount of data readers should visit the websites (details are given below) and see the references given in the first chapter, and for an overview see also Bynner and Joshi's (2007) 'Building the evidence base from longitudinal data: the aims, content and achievements of the British birth cohort studies' (*Innovation: the European Journal of Social Science Research*, 20: 159–79). In addition, summary papers have been published on the 1946 cohort [Wadsworth, M. E. J., Kuh, D., Richards, R. and Hardy, R. (2006) 'Cohort profile: the 1946 national birth cohort', *International Journal of Epidemiology*, 35: 49–54], the 1958 cohort [Power, C. and Elliott, J. (2006) 'Cohort profile: the 1958 British birth cohort', *International Journal of Epidemiology*, 35: 34–41], the 1970 cohort [Elliott, J. and Shepherd, P. (2006) 'Cohort profile: the 1970 British birth cohort', *International Journal of Epidemiology*, 35: 836–43] and the 1991–2 or ALSPAC study [Golding, J., Pembrey, M., Jones, R. and the ALSPAC study team (2001) 'APLSPAC – the Avon Longitudinal Study of Parents and Children: 1. Study methodology', *Paediatric and Perinatal Epidemiology*, 15: 74–87]. The Millennium Cohort Study is summarised in Dex, S. and Joshi, H. (2005) *Children of the 21st Century*, Bristol: Policy Press.

Table A1.1 Sampling and contact details of the 1946 birth cohort, the Medical Research Council (MRC) National Survey of Health and Development (NSHD)

Start date	*1946*
Website	http://www.nshd.mrc.ac.uk
Sampling frame	All births during seven consecutive days in March in England, Wales and Scotland
Sample size for first data collection	16,695
Sampling frame for follow-up	All singleton births to married women during 7 consecutive days in March in England, Wales and Scotland were sampled to include all those whose fathers were in non-manual or agricultural employment and one in four of those whose fathers were in manual employment
Sample size at outset of follow-up	5,362
Responding sample members at the most recently completed data collection	4,432 (at age 53 years)
Number of data collections	Thirteen data collections between birth and age 20 years; twelve data collections after age 20 years and up to current age of 64 years

Table A1.2 Sampling and contact details of the 1958 birth cohort, the National Child Development Study (NCDS)

Start date	*1958*
Website	http://www.cls.ioe.ac.uk
Sampling frame	All births during 7 consecutive days in March in England, Wales and Scotland; all those born on the selected days during school-age follow-ups, whether or not they had been born in England, Wales or Scotland
Sample size at outset	17,634
Responding sample members at the most recently completed data collection	15,451 (at age 42 years)
Number of data collections	Five data collections between birth and age 20 years; four data collections after age 20 years and up to current age of 52 years

Table A1.3 Sampling and contact details of the 1970 birth cohort (BCS70)

Start date	*1970*
Website	http://www.cls.ioe.ac.uk
Sampling frame	All births during 7 consecutive days in April in England, Wales, Scotland and Northern Ireland; all those born on the selected days during school-age follow-ups, whether or not they had been born in England, Wales or Scotland
Sample size at outset	17,287
Responding sample members at the most recently completed data collection	15,503 (at age 30 years)
Number of data collections	Four data collections between birth and age 20 years; two data collections after age 20 years and up to current age of 40 years

Table A1.4 Sampling and contact details of the 1991–2 Avon Longitudinal Study of Parents and Children (ALSPAC)

Start date	*1991–2*
Website	http://www.bristol.ac.uk/alspac
Sampling frame	All eligible pregnancies in the English county of Avon between April 1991 and 31 December 1992
Sample size at outset	14,541
Responding sample members at the most recently completed data collection	7,942
Number of data collections	Twenty data collections between birth and current age of 18–19 years

Table A1.5 Sampling and contact details of the 2000–1 Millennium Cohort Study

Start date	*2000–1*
Website	www.cls.ioe.ac.uk
Sampling frame	All live births for 12 months in England and Wales beginning 1 September 2000, and in Scotland and Northern Ireland beginning 1 December 2000
Sample size at outset	18,818
Responding sample members at the most recently completed data collection	15,246
Number of data collections	Four data collections between birth and current age of 9–10 years

Appendix 2 Timeline of salient events, Acts of Parliament and enquiries, 1942–2010

Figures in brackets identify the chapter which refers to that item, and the marginal colour line indicates the political persuasion of the government in power.

1942	Publication of the Beveridge Report *Social Insurance and Allied Services* (1, 2, 7)
1944	The Bretton Woods Agreement establishes the International Monetary Fund and a system of fixed exchange rates and parameters for international trade (5, 6)
1944	Education Act (2, 4, 6, 8)
1944	Publication of White Paper on employment policy, which recommends government to maintain high employment
1945	Education (Scotland) Act (4)
1945	*Election of Labour government with Clement Atlee as Prime Minister to replace wartime coalition*
1945	Family Allowance Act (3)
1945	The Percy Report on higher technological education published (4)
1946	The Barlow Report on scientific manpower published (4)
1946	National Insurance Act (3)
1947	The Advisory Council on Scientific Policy established
1947	Foundation of the British Geriatric Society (7)
1948	National Health Service begins (2, 7, 8)
1948	British Nationality Act (5)
1948	Children Act establishes children's departments in local authorities and employed childcare officers (3)
1951	*Election of Conservative government with Winston Churchill as Prime Minister*
1951	Introduction of the General Certificate of Education (GCE) Ordinary and Advanced levels replacing School Certificate and Higher School Certificate (4)
1954	Food rationing ends (7, 8)
1955	Churchill resigns and Anthony Eden becomes Prime Minister
1955	ITV begins broadcasting (8)

1956 Report of the Royal Commission on Marriage and Divorce (commissioned in 1951) (3)
1956 Report of the Guillebaud Committee on the cost of the NHS (commissioned in 1953) (5, 7)
1956 White Paper on technical education published (4)
1956 Clean Air Act regulates pollution from coal burning (7)
1957 Eden resigns and Harold Macmillan becomes Prime Minister
1957 Publication of Wolfenden Report on homosexual offences and prostitution, originally commissioned in 1954 (7)
1958 Campaign for Nuclear Disarmament inaugurated (8)
1959 Mental Health Act sets up the Mental Health Tribunals (7)
1959 The Crowther Report *15 to 18* published (commissioned in 1956); includes recommendation to raise the school leaving age to sixteen years, which is implemented in 1972/3 (4)
1959 The first motorway (M1) opens (8)
1959 Obscene Publications Act makes exceptions for work shown to be in the interests of science, literature, the arts or learning
1960 The Albermarle Report on services for youth published (commissioned in 1958) (8)
1960 Compulsory military conscription (National Service) ends (8)
1960 Betting and Gaming Act legalising off-course betting and bookmakers (8)
1961 The oral contraceptive licensed for use (3, 7, 8)
1962 Commonwealth Immigrants Act (8)
1963 Macmillan resigns and Alec Douglas Home becomes Prime Minister
1963 The Newsom Report *Half our Future* on secondary education published (commissioned in 1961) (4)
1963 Report of the Committee on Higher Education (the Robbins Report) published (commissioned in 1961), recommending expansion of the university system (4)
1964 Industrial Training Act established the Industry Training Boards (6)
1964 Election of a Labour government with Harold Wilson as Prime Minister
1964 Child Poverty Action Group founded (3)
1964 Married Women's Property Act increases entitlement
1964 Obscene Publications Act includes prosecution of those publishing obscene material for gain
1965 The Race Relations Act (8)
1965 The Government's National Plan sets targets for industry
1965 Circular 10/65 recommends comprehensive schooling to local authorities (4)
1965 The Sports Council established (7, 8)
1966 First credit cards introduced (5)
1967 The Family Planning Act permits local health authorities to provide contraceptive advice regardless of marital status (3)

1967 Publication of the Plowden Report *Children and their Primary Schools* (commissioned in 1963) (4)
1967 The Abortion Law Reform Act (7)
1967 Sexual Offences Act legalises homosexual acts between consenting adults (3, 7)
1967 North Sea gas production begins (6)
1968 Race Relations Act amendments and establishment of the Community Relations Commission (8)
1968 The Open University is founded (4, 8)
1968 Theatres Act ends theatre censorship
1969 Divorce Reform Act (operative in 1972) added 'no fault' to existing grounds for divorce (3, 8)
1969 Publication of the 'Black Papers' in opposition to education reforms (4)
1969 Government publishes *In Place of Strife* with proposals for reducing strike action (5, 6)
1970 Election of a Conservative government with Edward Heath as Prime Minister
1970 Equal Pay Act (3, 8)
1970 Local Authority Social Services Act sets up unified social services departments to help families through casework (3)
1971 Introduction of compulsory health warning on tobacco products packaging (7, 8)
1972 Miners' strike (5, 6, 8)
1972 Publication of the White Paper *Education: A Framework for Expansion* (4)
1973 Britain joins the European Economic Community (2, 5)
1973 Organization of the Petroleum Exporting Countries (OPEC) quadruples oil prices (5)
1973 Employment and Training Act establishes the Manpower Services Commission (4, 6)
1973 Education Act raises the school leaving age to sixteen years (4)
1973 Matrimonial Causes Act provides framework for divorce on grounds of irretrievable breakdown of marriage (3)
1974 Imposition of the three-day working week to conserve energy (6)
1974 Election of a Labour government with Harold Wilson as Prime Minister
1974 Publication of the Finer Committee Report on one-parent families (commissioned in 1969) (3)
1975 North Sea Oil production begins (2, 5, 6)
1975 Sex Discrimination Act makes it illegal to discriminate on grounds of sex or marital status (3)
1975 Equal Opportunities Act (8)
1976 Resignation of Prime Minister Harold Wilson and James Callaghan becomes Prime Minister
1976 Race Relations Act amendment and Commission for Racial Equality established to replace the Community Relations Commission (8)

1977 Publication of the Green Paper *Education in Schools* (4)
1978 The Warnock Report *Special Educational Needs* published (commissioned 1974 under the Conservative government) (4)
1979 Election of a Conservative government with Margaret Thatcher as Prime Minister
1979 Employment Protection Act (3)
1979 A further OPEC increase in oil prices (5, 6)
1980 Housing Act permits sale of local authority-owned housing to tenants (3)
1980 End of provision of free school milk (7)
1980 Publication of the Black Report *Inequalities in Health* (commissioned by the Department of Health in 1977) (7)
1980 Education (Scotland) Act (4)
1981 Youth Opportunities Training Programme established (6)
1981 Social Democratic Party formed (2)
1983 Mental Health Act redefines types of detention and work of the Mental Health Tribunals (7)
1983 Youth Training Scheme introduced (6)
1984 Matrimonial and Family Proceeding Act (3)
1984 Miners' strike (5, 8)
1985 The Swann Report *Education for All* on education for children in ethnic minority groups published (commissioned in 1979) (4)
1986 De-regulation of financial markets – the 'big bang' (5, 6)
1986 National Vocational Qualifications established (6)
1986 Social Security Act signals a move away from universal benefits to means testing (3)
1986 General Certificate of Secondary Education (GCSE) introduced (4)
1986 Sex Discrimination Act removes restrictions on women's employment and brings Britain into line with EU sex discrimination legislation
1988 Education Reform Act introduces the National Curriculum and the Universities Funding Council (4)
1988 Social Democratic Party merges with the Liberal Party (2)
1988 Satellite television broadcasting begins (8)
1989 Children's Act establishes the centrality of children's interests and parental responsibility rather than parental rights (3)
1989 Introduction in Scotland of the community charge or 'poll tax' to replace domestic rates (8)
1990 Poll tax riots opposing their introduction in England (8)
1990 Election of a Conservative government with John Major as Prime Minister
1990 Taxation Act establishes independent taxation of husbands and wives (3)
1990 Human Fertilisation and Embryology Bill sets up monitoring of fertility treatment and research using human embryos (7)
1991 Child Support Act sets up the Child Support Agency to ensure payments from absent parents (3)
1991 White Paper *Education and Training for the 21st Century* published (4)

1991 Strengthening of content of printed warnings on tobacco products packaging (7)
1991 The first mobile phone marketed (8)
1992 Incorporation of polytechnics into the university system (4)
1992 Office for Standards in Education (OFSTED) established (4, 6)
1992 White Paper *Choice and Diversity: A New Framework for Schools* published (4)
1992 Further and Higher Education Act grants university status to polytechnics (4)
1992 The Maastricht Treaty signed establishing the European Union in 1993 with UK as a member (5)
1993 Education Act with increased emphasis on parental choice and autonomy for schools (4)
1994 Yahoo, the first user-friendly search engine, launched (8)
1994 UK National Lottery inaugurated (8)
1994 Criminal Justice and Public Order Act makes it illegal to transmit obscene images electronically
1995 Disability Discrimination Act (7)
1996 Family Law Act intended to reduce costs of 'quickie' divorce and easier settlement of responsibilities more easily (3)
1996 Food labelling regulations come into force (7)
1997 *Election of a new Labour government with Tony Blair as Prime Minister*
1997 Qualifications and Curriculum Authority established (4)
1997 The Dearing Report *The National Committee of Inquiry into Higher Education* published (commissioned 1996) (4)
1997 The White Paper *Excellence in Schools* published (4)
1997 Quality Assurance Agency established (6)
1997 The National Literacy Strategy introduced (4)
1998 Human Rights Act (7, 8)
1998 Further education colleges incorporated into the university system (6)
1998 Publication by the Home Office of *Supporting Families*, the first overt family policy document (3)
1998 Department of Social Security review of child support policy (3)
1998 Publication of the Acheson Report *Independent Inquiry into Inequalities in Health* (commissioned in 1997) (7)
1998 The SureStart pre-school programme begins with the aim of improving childcare, early education, health and family support (3, 4, 9)
1998 The Scotland Act paves the way for the Scottish Assembly (2)
1998 Government of Wales Act creates the National Assembly for Wales (2)
1999 National minimum wage first established (6)
1999 Report of the Royal Commission on Long-term Care for the Elderly published (commissioned 1997) (3, 7)
1999 Government pledge to halve child poverty by 2010 and to eradicate it by 2020 (3)

1999 Moser Report *A Fresh Start* published – concerned with basic skills (commissioned in 1998) (6)
1999 National Institute for Clinical Excellence (NICE) established (7)
1999 SEU publishes *Bridging the Gap* – government report on advising young people on educational and occupational choice (6)
2000 SEU publishes *Disadvantaged Youth* (6)
2000 Skills for Life initiative (6)
2000 Standards in Scotland's Schools Act introduces a legal basis for children's rights (4)
2002 The Adoption and Children Act permits adoption by single persons or same-sex couples (3)
2002 Publication of the independent Wanless Report, *Securing our Future Health: Taking a Long-Term View* (commissioned 2001) (7)
2002 Introduction of City Academies (4)
2003 Government publishes *Every Child Matters*, an integrated programme for the well-being of children (3, 4, 8)
2003 Further strengthening of content of printed warnings on tobacco products packaging (7)
2004 Children Act emphasises the need for preventive strategies to ensure positive outcomes (e.g. good health) for all children, and unifies children's services under directors of children's services with multi-disciplinary teams and databases. (3)
2004 (Effective 2005) Civil Partnership Act (3)
2004 Publication of the Tomlinson Report on post-16 qualifications reform (4)
2004 Educational Maintenance Allowance launched (2005 in Scotland) (6)
2005 Disability Discrimination Act (amendments to the 1995 Act) (7)
2005 Mental Capacity Act introduces new safeguards in relation to deprivation of liberty (7)
2005 Publication of Green Paper *Youth Matters* on provision for young people (4, 8)
2005 Ban on advertising tobacco products (7, 8)
2006 Report of the independent Leitch Review of Skills published (commissioned in 2004) (4, 6)
2006 The Wanless Report *Securing Good Care for Older People: Taking a Long-Term View* published (7)
2006 House of Lords Science and Technology Committee's report *Ageing: Scientific Aspects* published (also a follow-up report in the same year) (7)
2007 Resignation of Prime Minister Tony Blair and Gordon Brown becomes Prime Minister
2007 Mental Health Act introduces community treatment orders and new codes of practice (7)
2007 Tobacco smoking banned in public places (7, 8)
2007 Food labelling (declaration of allergens) regulations come into force (7)
2007 National Learning and Skills Council established (6)
2007 Equality and Human Rights Commission established (8)

2007 Ban on smoking in public enclosed spaces, and legal age for purchase of tobacco in any form raised from sixteen to eighteen years (7, 8)

2008 Education and Skills Act extends participation in education to age eighteen years as from 2015 (4)

2008 Bank crisis and recession begins (5, 6)

2008 The Human Fertilisation and Embryology Act required the 'need for supporting parenting' (rather than necessarily a father) and allows naming of both same-sex partners on a birth certificate (3, 7)

2008 The Child Maintenance and Enforcement Commission replaces the Child Support Agency (3)

2010 Election of a coalition Conservative/Liberal Democrat government with David Cameron as Prime Minister

2010 White Paper on proposals for a National Care Service (3)

2010 Marmot Review, *Fair Society, Healthy Lives: A Strategic Review of Health Inequalities in England Post-2010*, published (7)

Index